T0336904

Assistive and Augmentive Communication for the Disabled:

Intelligent Technologies for Communication, Learning and Teaching

Lau Bee Theng
Swinburne University of Technology, Malaysia

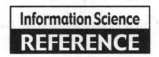

Information Science
REFERENCE

Senior Editorial Director:	Kristin Klinger
Director of Book Publications:	Julia Mosemann
Editorial Director:	Lindsay Johnston
Acquisitions Editor:	Erika Carter
Development Editor:	Joel Gamon
Production Editor:	Sean Woznicki
Typesetters:	Jennifer Romanchak, Deanna Zombro & Michael Brehm
Print Coordinator:	Jamie Snavely
Cover Design:	Nick Newcomer

Published in the United States of America by
    Information Science Reference (an imprint of IGI Global)
    701 E. Chocolate Avenue
    Hershey PA 17033
    Tel: 717-533-8845
    Fax: 717-533-8661
    E-mail: cust@igi-global.com
    Web site: http://www.igi-global.com/reference

Copyright © 2011 by IGI Global. All rights reserved. No part of this publication may be reproduced, stored or distributed in any form or by any means, electronic or mechanical, including photocopying, without written permission from the publisher.
Product or company names used in this set are for identification purposes only. Inclusion of the names of the products or companies does not indicate a claim of ownership by IGI Global of the trademark or registered trademark.

Library of Congress Cataloging-in-Publication Data

Assistive and augmentive communication for the disabled : intelligent technologies for communication, learning and teaching / Lau Bee Theng, editor.
   p. cm.
 Includes bibliographical references and index.
 Summary: "This book provides benefits to professionals and researchers working in various disciplines in the field, such as special education, healthcare, computational intelligence and information technology offering insights and support to individuals who are concerned with the development of children and adults with disabilities"--Provided by publisher.
  ISBN 978-1-60960-541-4 (hbk.) -- ISBN 978-1-60960-542-1 (ebook) 1. People with disabilities--Means of communication. 2. Communication devices for people with disabilities. 3. Assistive computer technology. I. Theng, Lau Bee, 1974-
 HV1568.4.A83 2011
 681'.761--dc22
                  2010054436

British Cataloguing in Publication Data
A Cataloguing in Publication record for this book is available from the British Library.

All work contributed to this book is new, previously-unpublished material. The views expressed in this book are those of the authors, but not necessarily of the publisher.

Editorial Advisory Board

Bong Chin Wei, *Universiti Sains Malaysia, Malaysia*
Justo A. Diaz, *University of Auckland, New Zealand*
Lee Bee Wah, *Cambodia Methodist International School, Cambodia*
Lee Seldon, *Multimedia University, Malaysia*
Marlene Valerie Lu, *Swinburne University of Technology, Malaysia*
Nia Valeria, *Swinburne University of Technology, Malaysia*
Ong Chin Ann, *Swinburne University of Technology, Malaysia*
Wang Yin Chai, *Universiti Malaysia Sarawak, Malaysia*

Table of Contents

Chapter 10
The Outdoor Wireless Healthcare Monitoring System for Hospital Patients
Xiaoxin Xu, Zhejiang University, China
Mingguang Wu, Zhejiang University, China
Bin Sun, China JiLiang University, China
Jianwei Zhang, China JiLiang University, China
Cheng Ding, HangZhou Meacon Automatic Technology Co., Ltd, China

Detailed Table of Contents

Chapter 1

Vivi Mandasari, Swinburne University of Technology, Malaysia
Marlene Valerie Lu, Swinburne University of Technology, Malaysia
Lau Bee Theng, Swinburne University of Technology, Malaysia

Asperger Syndrome is a developmental disorder under the umbrella term of Autism Spectrum Disorders, and it is a milder variant of autism. It is characterized by a significant difficulty in communication, prominently in social interaction and non-verbal communication. Since a decade ago, there have been a variety of tools for teaching and assisting children with AS in the acquisition of social skills, ranging from the simple picture exchange system to the high-end virtual reality system. This chapter discusses on the effectiveness of integrating Social Story, 2D animations and video instruction for teaching social skills to children diagnosed with Asperger Syndrome in an interactive manner. The prototype has been developed, implemented, and evaluated in an experimental way. This chapter will discuss on the evaluation process, results, findings, and areas for further exploration.

Chapter 2

Georgios Dafoulas, Middlesex University, London, UK
Noha Saleeb, Middlesex University, London, UK

The significance of newly emergent 3D virtual worlds to different genres of users is currently a controversial subject in deliberation. Users range from education pursuers, business contenders, and social seekers to technology enhancers and many more who comprise both users with normal abilities in physical life and those with different disabilities. This study aims to derive and critically analyze, using grounded theory, advantageous and disadvantageous themes, and their sub concepts of providing e-learning through 3D Virtual Learning Environments (VLEs), like Second Life, to disabled users. Hence providing evidence that 3DVLEs not only support traditional physical learning, but also offer e-learning opportunities unavailable through 2D VLEs (like Moodle, Blackboard), and offer learning opportunities unavailable through traditional physical education. Furthermore, to achieve full potential from the above-mentioned derived concepts, architectural and accessibility design requirements of 3D educational facilities proposed by different categories of disabled students to accommodate for their needs, are demonstrated.

Chapter 3

Ong Chin Ann, Swinburne University of Technology, Malaysia
Marlene Valerie Lu, Swinburne University of Technology, Malaysia
Lau Bee Theng, Swinburne University of Technology, Malaysia

The main purpose of this research is to enhance the communication of the disabled community. The authors of this chapter propose an enhanced interpersonal-human interaction for people with special needs, especially those with physical and communication disabilities. The proposed model comprises of automated real time behaviour monitoring, designed and implemented with the ubiquitous and affordable concept in mind to suit the underprivileged. In this chapter, the authors present the prototype which encapsulates an automated facial expression recognition system for monitoring the disabled, equipped with a feature to send Short Messaging System (SMS) for notification purposes. The authors adapted the Viola-Jones face detection algorithm at the face detection stage and implemented template matching technique for the expression classification and recognition stage. They tested their model with a few users and achieved satisfactory results. The enhanced real time behaviour monitoring system is an assistive tool to improve the quality of life for the disabled by assisting them anytime and anywhere when needed. They can do their own tasks more independently without constantly being monitored physically or accompanied by their care takers, teachers, or even parents. The rest of this chapter is organized as follows. The background of the facial expression recognition system is reviewed in Section 2. Section 3 is the description and explanations of the conceptual model of facial expression recognition. Evaluation of the proposed system is in Section

4. Results and findings on the testing are laid out in Section 5, and the final section concludes the chapter.

Chapter 4

Tee Zhi Heng, The University of Nottingham Malaysia Campus,
*   Malaysia*
Ang Li Minn, The University of Nottingham Malaysia Campus,
*   Malaysia*
Seng Kah Phooi, The University of Nottingham Malaysia Campus,
*   Malaysia*

This chapter presents a novel application for wireless technology to assist visually impaired people. As an alternative to the medical model of rehabilitation, the information explosion era provides the foundation for a technological solution to lead the visually impaired to more independent lives in the community by minimizing the obstacles of living. A "SmartGuide" caregiver monitoring system is built as a standalone portable handheld device linked. The objective of this system is to assist blind and low vision people to walk around independently especially in dynamic changing environments. Navigation assistance is accomplished by providing speech guidance on how to move to a particular location. The system delivers dynamic environmental information to lead the visually impaired to more independent lives in the community by minimizing the obstacles of living. Information of changing environments such as road blockage, road closure, and intelligent navigation aids is provided to the user in order to guide the user safely to his or her destination. This system also includes a camera sensor network to enhance monitoring capabilities for an extra level of security and reliability.

Chapter 5

Nia Valeria, Swinburne University of Technology, Malaysia
Marlene Valerie Lu, Swinburne University of Technology, Malaysia
Lau Bee Theng, Swinburne University of Technology, Malaysia

Communication through speech is a vital skill, an innate ability in most human beings intended to convey thoughts, needs, and it is the very foundation of literacy. However, some people find it as one of the challenges in their lives, particularly children with Cerebral Palsy. Children with such disability suffer from brain injuries before, during, and after birth that evidently affect their motor, cognitive, and linguistic skills. Some of the additional complexities may also cause hearing, visual, and speech impairments that further decrease their learning abilities. Their development milestones in learning is slower than a typical child, thus they require intensive personal drilling. It is believed that the cognitive skills in these children can be improved to enable them to lead a more productive life. That was an antecedent that strongly motivated us to develop the proposed Virtual Collaborative Learning Tool. It aims to assist the learning ability of the targeted children through a responsive avatar of their parents, teachers, or caretakers. A preliminary study was conducted on voluntary participants to evaluate the effectiveness of the proposed learning model. The results showed 80% of the participants were able to answer questions provided within the program.

Chapter 6

Technology can be used to assist people with disabilities in their daily activities. Especially when the users have communication deficiencies, suitable technology and tools can solve such needs. We envision that context awareness is a potential method suitable to provide services and solutions in the area of Assistive and Augmentative Communication (AAC). In this chapter, the authors give an introduction to context awareness and the state of the art. This is followed with the elaboration on how context awareness can be used in AAC. The Context Aware Remote Monitoring Assistant (CARMA) is presented as an application designed for a care assistant and his patient. A demonstration of a context aware component implemented in the CARMA application is shown in this chapter. An experiment that investigates movement recognition using an accelerometer in a smartphone and the obtained results are presented. This chapter ends with a discussion on challenges, future work and the conclusion.

Chapter 7

A computational model of non-visual spatial learning through virtual learning environment (VLE) is presented in this chapter. The inspiration has come from Landmark-Route-Survey (LRS) theory, the most accepted theory of spatial learning. An attempt has been made to combine the findings and methods from several disciplines including cognitive psychology, behavioral science and computer science (specifically virtual reality (VR) technology). The study of influencing factors on spatial learning and the potential of using cognitive maps in the modeling of spatial learning are described. Motivation to use VLE and its characteristics are also described briefly. Different types of locomotion interface to VLE with their constraints and benefits are discussed briefly. The authors believe that by incorporating perspectives from cognitive and experimental psychology to computer science, this chapter will appeal to a wide range of audience - particularly computer engineers concerned with assistive technologies, professionals interested in virtual environments, including computer engineers, architect, city-planner, cartographer, high-tech artists, and mobility trainers, and psychologists involved in the study of spatial cognition, cognitive behaviour, and human-computer interfaces.

Chapter 8

The aim of this chapter is to identify those face areas containing high facial expression information, which may be useful for facial expression analysis, face and facial expression recognition and synthesis. In the study of facial expression analysis, landmarks are usually placed on well-defined craniofacial features. In this experiment, the authors have selected a set of landmarks based on craniofacial anthropometry and associate each of the landmarks with facial muscles and the Facial Action Coding System (FACS) framework, which means to locate landmarks on less palpable areas that contain high facial expression mobility. The selected landmarks are statistically analysed in terms of facial muscles motion based on FACS. Given that human faces provide information to channel verbal and non-verbal communication: speech, facial expression of emotions, gestures, and other human communicative actions; hence, these cues may be significant in the identification of expressions such as pain, agony, anger, happiness, et cetera. Here, the authors describe the potential of computer-based models of three-dimensional (3D) facial expression analysis and the non-verbal communication recognition to assist in biometric recognition and clinical diagnosis.

E-learning systems generally rely on good visual and cognitive abilities, making them suitable for individuals with good levels of intelligence in these areas. A group of such individuals are those with Non-Systemising Impairments (NSIs), such as people with autism spectrum conditions (ASCs). These individuals could benefit greatly from technology that allows them to use their abilities to overcome their impairments in social functioning and emotion recognition in order to develop pro-social behaviours. Existing systems such as PARLE and MindReading are discussed, and a new one, the Visual Ontological Imitation System (VOIS), is proposed and discussed. This chapter details an investigation into the acceptability of these systems by those working in social work and advocacy. The study found that VOIS would be well received, although dependency on assistive technology and its impact on how others view individuals with NSIs still need to be addressed by society and its institutions.

Advances in embedded computing systems have resulted in the emergence of Wireless Sensor Networks (WSNs), which provide unique opportunities for sensing physical environments. ZigBee-compliant WSN platforms have been proposed for healthcare monitoring, smart home, industrial monitoring and sensor, and other applications. In this chapter, the authors, using TI CC2430 and CC2431 chipsets with Z-Stack, designed an outdoor patients' healthcare monitoring system for tracking patients and helping doctors and nurses to keep tabs on patients' health remotely. Furthermore, several important techniques are elaborated, including reliable communication, localization algorithm, and backup power, which can enhance the system performance. Finally, some suggestions for future development are presented.

Preface

Assistive and augmentive communication (AAC) is an emerging area that receives much support from the disabled community. It enables communication for those with impairments or restrictions on the production or comprehension of spoken or written language. There are unaided and aided AAC systems. Unaided systems do not require any external device for their use, but include facial expression, vocalizations, gestures, and signed languages. On the other hand, an aided AAC uses either an electronic or non-electronic device to transmit messages such as communication books or voice output devices using symbols. Since the skills, areas of difficulty, and communication requirements of AAC users vary greatly, an equally diverse range of communication aids and devices exists to meet these demands. For the low-tech aided AAC, communication is done through letters, words, phrases, pictures, and/or symbols on a board or in a book for access. As for high-tech aided AAC, electronic devices with storage and retrieval of messages allow the user to communicate with others using recorded speech output. There are high-tech aided AAC which use dedicated devices developed solely for communication, and non-dedicated devices, such as computers, adapted for use as communication with some external devices and software packages.

AAC has been a great assistance to people with cerebral palsy, autism, brainstem stroke, traumatic brain injury, and other disabilities. It helps them to learn, communicate, and gain social abilities. For young children, it develops their vocabulary from scratch and helps them learn the speech proficiency to go to school, improve their literacy, and gain employability in the market. Foremost, it improves the quality of their life.

There are many AAC tools being developed by various industry giants being distributed to fit into the general public needs. In fact, there are various niche researches going on in the research institutions, universities, and non-profit organizations that have not been publicized or commercialized widely. Hence, we gathered the recently completed and ongoing research in AAC and shared them with other researchers. All the chapters were peer-reviewed by members of our editorial board before they were accepted.

We anticipate this book will benefit professionals and researchers working in the field of assistive and augmentative technology in various disciplines, such as special education, healthcare, computational intelligence, and Information Technology. Moreover, the book also provides insights and support to individuals who are concerned with the development of children and adult with disabilities.

Lau Bee Theng
Swinburne University of Technology, Malaysia

Chapter 1
2D Animated Social Story for Assisting Social Skills Learning of Children with Autism Spectrum Disorder

Vivi Mandasari
Swinburne University of Technology, Malaysia

Marlene Valerie Lu
Swinburne University of Technology, Malaysia

Lau Bee Theng
Swinburne University of Technology, Malaysia

ABSTRACT

Asperger Syndrome is a developmental disorder under the umbrella term of Autism Spectrum Disorders, and it is a milder variant of autism. It is characterized by a significant difficulty in communication, prominently in social interaction and non-verbal communication. Since a decade ago, there have been a variety of tools for teaching and assisting children with AS in the acquisition of social skills, ranging from the simple picture exchange system to the high-end virtual reality system. This chapter discusses on the effectiveness of integrating Social Story, 2D animations and video instruction for teaching social skills to children diagnosed with Asperger Syndrome in an interactive manner. The prototype has been developed, implemented, and evaluated in an experimental way. This chapter will discuss on the evaluation process, results, findings, and areas for further exploration.

DOI: 10.4018/978-1-60960-541-4.ch001

Copyright ©2011, IGI Global. Copying or distributing in print or electronic forms without written permission of IGI Global is prohibited.

INTRODUCTION

Asperger Syndrome (AS) is a type of Autism Spectrum Disorder (ASD) with symptoms of impairment in social communication, interaction and coordination skills.

Hagiwara and Myles (1999) were the first to conduct a study to use multimedia approach combining Social Stories, visual symbols and computer-based instruction. Social story is a strategy designed to teach autistic children social skills and behavior management skills by addressing specific social situations and how to cope with them. Since then, there are many studies and research to find the effectiveness of Social Story by combining it with other intervention mode; Roger and Myles (2001) who combined Social Story with Comic Strip Conversations, Thiemann and Goldstein (2001) combined Social Story with multi-component intervention which includes Social Stories, cue cards, role-play and video feedback. Schneider and Goldstein (2009) had compiled the studies of Social Story for Children with ASD from the year of 1995 to 2006. He concluded that the effectiveness of Social Story alone is hard to be measured as it is combined with other modes of interventions (Crozier & Tincani, 2005). Thus, it is inconclusive to denote that the positive behavior changes are resulted from the Social Story intervention itself or a combination of Social Story with other interventions (Schneider & Goldstein, 2009).

Despite the unclearness of the effectiveness of Social Story itself, Schneider and Goldstein (2009) also reported that additional components such as visual schedules may be useful for optimizing the children's performance rather than by using Social Story individually. Same result was reported by Mancil, Haydon, and Whitby (2009) who found that Social Stories in Power Point format produces slightly better outcome than the Social Stories in the paper format. Students also indicated that they liked the computer-assisted format (Mancil et al., 2009; Heimann, Nelson, Tjus, & Gillberg, 1995). The uses of computer based teaching aids have also been demonstrated to decrease inappropriate behaviors and improve vocabulary acquisition among children with ASD, as well as increase their social skills (Sansosti & Powell-Smith, 2008).

Based on the research and studies conducted which were briefly cited and discussed above, we concluded that social story is more effective when incorporated with some visual stimuli to enhance learning and understanding by providing an attractive and enjoyable learning environment. It is agreed that learning is most effectual when motivated. With that we propose the combination of social story, 2D animation and video instruction as an interactive pedagogical tool for ASD children. This chapter will present our attempts in assisting children with AS in social and communication skills building by using the proposed prototype. It is anticipated to be more effective in assisting them to attain social skills and real-life adaptive skills.

Copyright © 2011, IGI Global. Copying or distributing in print or electronic forms without written permission of IGI Global is prohibited.

AUTISM SPECTRUM DISORDER AND ASPERGER SYNDROME

Autism Spectrum Disorder defines any developmental disabilities that have been caused by brain abnormality with the results of impaired social interaction, difficulties in verbal and non-verbal communications, and unusual, repetitive, or severely limited activities and interest (Johnson, 2008).

ASD generally characterized by a triad of impairments in social communication (verbal and non-verbal) (e.g. not understanding common gestures, facial expressions or affective responses), reciprocal social interaction (impaired relationship) (e.g. they may appear indifferent to other people) and repetitive behaviors and interests (rigidity of thought). This triad of impairments includes difficulty in understanding non-literal communication and articulating thoughts and ideas, expressing and reading emotions, participating in interpersonal imaginative play (Tartaro & Cassell, 2008; Tartaro, 2007; Cheng, Moore, McGrath, & Fan, 2005).

Social behavior and social ethics are the core deficit in ASD with a range of problems, which includes failure to develop peer relationships appropriate to their developmental level, abnormality in voice and speech intonation, impairment in the use of multiple non-verbal behaviors (such as eye to eye gaze, facial expression, gestures) and failure to enjoy, share interest or achievement with other people spontaneously (Weiss, LaRue, & Newcomer, 2009).

Due to the inability to conform to social standards, ASD children tend to isolate themselves by spending their time interacting with objects, and as the result of this, the visual portion of their brain becomes highly developed (Kalb, 2009; National Autistic Society, 2008). Children with ASD are a better visual learner than auditory learner. They understand better from reading or through graphical illustration than through spoken instructions. Thus, visual strategies are widely employed to help them in communication learning.

Study by Capps, Kehres, and Sigman (1998) compares the behavior of 15 children with ASD and 15 children with developmental delays by comparing their language ability within the context of a semi-structured conversation. The finding revealed that ASD children failed in most occasions to respond to questions and comments, unable to contribute new relevant ideas in discussion and have a tendency of making tangential remarks. It is observed that they have difficulty in relating their personal experience to others. The result also showed that both groups of children did not show any difference in their gesture; however several children with ASD enhanced their communication through dramatization and pointing.

As to date, there is still not a single known cause for ASD. However, it is generally accepted that ASD is caused by the abnormalities in the brain structure or function (e.g. Sparks et al., 2002). Brain scans showed the differences in the shape

Copyright © 2011, IGI Global. Copying or distributing in print or electronic forms without written permission of IGI Global is prohibited.

and structure of the brain in children with ASD versus neuro-typical children (Autism Society, 2008).

Research on the causes and treatment of ASD is expanding rapidly, with the aim to understand the underlying brain abnormalities and causes of ASD in order to improve prevention, early detection, diagnosis and treatment (Fombonne, 2003). Improvement in diagnostic techniques will allow ASD children to be appropriately identified and treated (Loomis, 2008). Many had agreed that the syndrome can be cured if the interventions are carried out at the earliest possible time (Evans, nd; Dawson et al, 2009). With early treatment, children with ASD can gain improved communication and social skills (Holmes, 2009; Dawson et al, 2009). This suggestion has been supported by an experiment at the Mind Institute of the University of California (Holmes, 2009; Dawson et al, 2009).

There are five spectrums of autism that are different from each other. The three main types of ASD that are most studied are Asperger's Syndrome, Pervasive Developmental Disorders – Not Otherwise Specified (PDD-NOS) and Autistic Disorder, and two rare, severe autistic-like conditions, which are Rett's Syndrome and Childhood Disintegrative Disorder (Hirsch, 2009; American Psychiatric Association, 2009; Matson & Neal, 2009; Bregman, 2005; Dixon, Garcia, Granpeesheh, & Tarbox, 2009). In this chapter, the discussion will focus on Asperger Syndrome.

The etymology of autism was introduced by a psychiatrist, Paul Bleuler in 1912. The term was derived from the Greek word to describe a condition of "self state" where individuals are engrossed in their own world. The first autistic condition known as "Asperger Syndrome" was discovered by an Austrian pediatrician, Hans Asperger to describe a less severe form of autism in people with higher intelligence quotient but have difficulty time fitting in socially. The factor that distinguishes between autism and Asperger Syndrome is the severity of disorder in terms of social interaction, communication skills and peculiar mannerism. Asperger Syndrome is the mildest form of autism, also called as "high-functioning autism". However, there were some debates between researchers that defined Asperger Syndrome as an extension of high-functioning autism. The debate has reached a convergent point with mutual agreement that autism is not a categorical diagnosis but rather a cluster of symptoms falling along a spectrum. While the debate still continues, majority of researchers considers AS distinct from high-functioning autism (Dixon et al., 2009).

Social maturity and social reasoning in children with AS were delayed and some aspects of their social abilities were typical throughout their development stage. They have the desire to socialize and be accepted by their peers but they are crippled by their inability to establish a reciprocal communication in any social interaction and unable to project appropriate non-verbal communication behavior. The children's use of language was pedantic, they are deeply absorbed in highly specific topics of

Copyright © 2011, IGI Global. Copying or distributing in print or electronic forms without written permission of IGI Global is prohibited.

their interest on which they are extremely knowledgeable, they dominate the interaction, had clumsy motor skill and they are lack of empathy (Matson & Neal, 2009; Attwood, 2006). The do not possess social intuition or understand social cues, such as not knowing when and how to terminate a conversation appropriately (Sigafoos, Schlosser, O'Reilly, & Lancioni, 2009), and some children had an unusual prosody that affected the tone, pitch and rhythm of speech. Their grammar and vocabulary may have been relatively advanced but, at the end of the conversation, they projected an impression that evidently reveals their inability to have a typical conversation.

People with AS perceive and view the world differently than typical people (Attwood, 2006). Children with AS have verbal abilities, but they also have difficulties in pragmatics, or in using language to convey meaning in a communicative context. These pragmatic abilities are important for initiating and sustaining reciprocal social interaction (Tartaro & Cassell, 2008).

Several studies suggested that children with high-functioning autism performed well on the recognition of simple emotions (happiness, sadness, anger, fear). However, they exhibit difficulties in explaining the causes of simple and complex emotions (e.g. surprise). They also experience incomplete understanding of socially complex emotions, which are compounded with social understanding of cultural norms, conventions, and rules of behaviors. Another social cognition problem affiliated with social detachment is the insensitivity of ASD children in responding to social stimuli (responding to name calling, participating in a play group). Instead, they have a circumscribed and obsessive interest in the physical aspect of the social situation rather than being engaged in the social experiences. For instance, in a setting where two or more children are playing with some toys, ASD children will not be drawn to join in but rather they will have a fixation on other physical elements such as the toys or other objects.

Children with AS can manage by themselves with their deficits, however, personal relationship and social situations are challenging for them (Evans, nd). In order to lead an independent life, Bauminger (2002) suggested that children with high functioning autism need help in understanding social norms and rules and in processing social information. Intervention should thus focus on facilitating the child's social understanding, should teach the ability to read social cues in different social situations; enhance the capacity for making accurate social interpretation, and expand the child's repertoire of behavioral alternatives for different social tasks.

One successful example of people with Asperger Syndrome is Temple Grandin – an American academic and researcher of various books about ASD. Like her, many people with AS or HFA managed to achieve high level of academic achievement and have independent lives (Parsons et al, 2000).

Copyright © 2011, IGI Global. Copying or distributing in print or electronic forms without written permission of IGI Global is prohibited.

SOCIAL STORY FOR CHILDREN WITH ASD

There have been many intervention approaches in assisting children with ASD to acquire social skills. From the various kinds of teaching and learning methods and strategies adapted for ASD children, this chapter will focus solely on Social Story.

Social Story is a promising intervention for children with ASD (Heward, 2006). Social Story was developed by Carol Gray in 1991 as an intervention strategy that teaches children with ASD self awareness, self-calming and self management skills. Based on Scurlock (2008), a social story is a brief, written narrative that depicts events or situations in a person's life focusing on social cues and re-enforcing pro-social behavior. Social Story provides concrete information to help children with ASD to improve their reaction and responses in social situations and to tolerate change. Social story is a great tool for teaching a skill through direct instructions in a controlled environment. It aims at improving Theory of Mind deficits in ASD children by cultivating a better understanding of the beliefs, thoughts and feelings of others. This will help strengthen their intuitive skills and instill in them a sense of ethics (Gabbert, 2010). Social stories are commonly used to explain social situation and concepts and educate them on the typical rules and conventions of our social and cultural milieu. It inculcates the expected social behaviors from the characters involved in a social situation, explains simple steps for achieving certain goals or outcomes, teaches new routines and anticipates actions in a format that is easily understood. However, the purpose of social stories is to describe the situation, not direct the child's behavior. A social story uses specific types of sentences to teach social skills, however, is a short, straightforward description of social situations which provide details of what a person might expect from a situation, and describes what may be expected of the person. Carol Gray suggested the usage of specific types of sentences to relate the stories effectively. This includes descriptive, perspective and directive sentences. Descriptive sentence is used to describe a situation and social setting while perspective is used to relay people's thoughts and feelings. Directive sentence is used to indicate the expected responses to a particular situation.

Providing social stories before an event or activity can decrease a child's anxiety, improve his behavior, and help him understand the event from the perspective of others (Heward, 2006).

Children with ASD are often visual learners, so the story could includes drawings, picture, and even real objects to be attached to each page (Heffner, 2002; Heward, 2006; Gabbert, 2010). The goal of the social story is to increase the child's understanding of social situation and to make him more comfortable in, and possibly suggest some appropriate responses for the situation in question (Wallin, nd).

Copyright © 2011, IGI Global. Copying or distributing in print or electronic forms without written permission of IGI Global is prohibited.

Existing researches and studies had been using the traditional paper-based Social Story and the combination of Social Stories with other intervention, such as in Power Point presentation. However, the current available Social Story formats have been not really interesting and interactive. Some social stories are depicted with picture cues to make it more appealing but the effectiveness of this approach is uncertain as static pictures failed to portray the non-literal components in communication such as body language, facial expression and gesture. It requires a more interactive and dynamic approach. To deviate from the typical social stories presentation format, some researchers had adapted the presentation format of Social Story into computerized presentation format. They found that that the presentation of computer format is as effective as the traditional paper presentation (Mancil et al., 2009; Sansosti & Powell-Smith, 2008; Hagiwara & Myles, 1999). There were a few results being published on how stories changed the behavior of ASD children.

Despite receiving positive responds and outcomes, there are factors affecting the adaptation of traditional social stories into classroom lessons in a consistent manner. Crozier and Tinccani (2007) deduced that it is time consuming for teachers to read each social story before an activity especially when handling a large group of ASD children. The inconsistent deployment of social stories will decrease its effectiveness as a tool in remediating unruly behavior.

Scattone (2007) did a study that integrated social story with video modeling as an approach to improve conversation skills of children with Asperger Syndrome. Scattone believe this method has a profound impact in teaching conversational skill to autistic children. It was a successful intervention with different level of improvement for each skill but the effectiveness of video modeling as part of the enhancement to a traditional social story intervention is uncertain. Moreover, the processes involved in video production require extensive planning; it is time-consuming and is resource intensive.

The embodiment of 2D animation around social stories hopes to address certain issues stipulated above. It is intended to break the monotony of typical social stories format and to capture and engage children's attention using visual effects and vibrant colors. This prototype incorporated a video avatar of an instructor reading the social stories, assuming the role of the teacher. This technique is used to gear the children towards self-learning with minor supervision and to shift from a "teacher-centered approach" where students became passive learners by listening and reciting what have been taught to "learning through direct experience" where they can relate what they see to the real object within their environment. This hopes to alleviate the usability and efficacy of social stories techniques through the application of currently available technology as a means to enhance and enrich the learning process, thus breaking the typical norm of social stories represented in text form.

Copyright © 2011, IGI Global. Copying or distributing in print or electronic forms without written permission of IGI Global is prohibited.

Figure 1. 2D animated social story interface

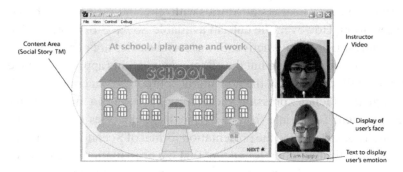

PROTOTYPING

Our prototype contains interactive 2D animation to enhance the content of the Social Story. This is a novel way of presenting Social Story as to date. The prototype is designed to display in full screen mode to avoid any distractions from the desktop background display. It starts off with a simple animation for 8 seconds before the program displays a list of three Social Stories to choose from. Once the selection has been made, the respective animation and video of instruction of the social story content will be displayed.

Quizzes will appear at the end of each story. The participant is then required to answer one question related to the story by selecting only one of the choices given. He will be given unlimited attempts to answer the question and a correct answer will be indicated with a hand clapping animation. The prototype realizes two main features (see Figure 1) that is social story designed with 2D animations and avatar for Instructor.

The social stories were adopted accordingly from previously published papers. They were depicted in a 2D animated form and were used to benchmark the effectiveness of the prototype. The 2D animated social stories were created using Adobe Flash. Figure 2 illustrated four screenshots of the prototype. In a clockwise manner, the upper left interface showed a list of stories for the participant to select, the upper right showed an example of the question asked, the lower right is a screenshot to indicate a correct answer and the lower left screenshot indicated a wrong answer.

There is an avatar of the instructor's face in the form of video. The avatar is embedded into the system with the purpose of manifesting the presence of the instructor to extend a personalized attention and verbal prompts while the participant is using the system. The avatar is created in a series of prerecorded videos for different social interaction scenarios during the learning.

Copyright © 2011, IGI Global. Copying or distributing in print or electronic forms without written permission of IGI Global is prohibited.

Figure 2. Few interfaces of 2D animated social story

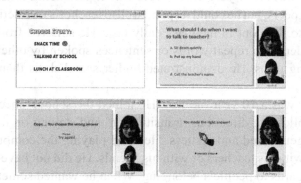

EVALUATION

After the prototyping, we conducted a series of field testing to evaluate the appropriateness and efficacy of the model. This section discusses the evaluation setup for the proposed prototype in the aspects of participants, materials, environment, observation procedures, target behaviors and social stories used.

Participants

There are a few criteria to consider when selecting the participants.

1. She\He has been diagnosed with Autism.
2. She\He has demonstrated off-task problem behaviors and has impaired verbal and/or social communication (currently or in the past) for the targeted off-task problem behaviors.
3. She\He should be able to operate computer by using a mouse or touchpad.
4. She\He should be functioning intellectually at the trainable mentally impaired range or above and have basic language skill (Del Valle, McEachern, & Chambers, 2001) for the social story to work out best.

Participant 1 was a 10 year old boy. He joined the school since 2006. He had a very good drawing and coloring skills. He was the advanced student among his classmates. He was good in mathematics and had shown some creativity in building Lego blocks. However, he had difficulties in expressing his emotions while communicating with his teachers or friends. He could not initiate conversation and interact with his peers. However, he showed the ability in following directions, taking turns and staying on the task.

Copyright © 2011, IGI Global. Copying or distributing in print or electronic forms without written permission of IGI Global is prohibited.

Participant 2 was an 11 year old boy. He was experiencing difficulties in communicating with peers, but he could respond well to teacher's instruction. His teacher often asks him to help out in the class daily task. He suffered from echolalia, an involuntary tendency to repeat words or sentences spoken by others. He had difficulties in taking turns. He demonstrated higher social skills than the other two participants.

Participant 3 was a 10 year old boy. He joined the school since 2010. He had difficulties in following directions, transitioning, and staying on the task. During class, he often gets bored and restless. He liked playing the computer. He hardly communicated with his teachers or with his friends. He did not have a sense of proprietary with regards to people's belonging. When he wanted something he would just get it without asking for permission.

Materials

Materials used in this study included a notebook with integrated camera, 2D Animated Social Story prototype, and the notebook's touchpad for navigation. Observation notes were used to record the significant behavior of the participants.

Consent was obtained from the participant's parents, principal and teacher for all the three phases (baseline, intervention and maintenance) and to be conducted in the participants' classroom between their study break with the presence of other students, teachers and class helpers.

Environment

Our research was conducted in a special school for mentally retarded children. Each class has one teacher and one helper with a maximum cap of 17 children. The students come from various intellectually disabled groups: downs syndrome, autistic and various types of brain damage with additional problem such as physical handicap, hearing or speech impairment and behavioral problems.

The field test took place in the respective participant's classroom. All the phases (Baseline, Intervention and Maintenance) were conducted at the same time and place each day. All of the three participants were in the classroom with about 10 to 15 students, depending on the class's daily attendance. There was a teacher and a class helper in each class, together with the researcher as the observer.

Observation Procedures

The observations were conducted at the baseline stage for one week. It was carried out to investigate the behaviour of our targeted participants and to detect any behav-

Copyright © 2011, IGI Global. Copying or distributing in print or electronic forms without written permission of IGI Global is prohibited.

ioral anomalies. It provides a basis to compare the participants' behavior after the intervention was executed. After the baseline phase, we compiled a list of students' profiles with their impairments and targeted behavior. Then, we proceeded to the intervention phase where the participants went through the 2D animated stories. The intervention sessions were held for one week. Each day, participants went through the 2D animated social stories with the researcher for about 2 to 3 sessions. Each session took about 10-15 minutes.

The maintenance phase was conducted after the intervention phase by observing the participant's behavior in their classroom. The maintenance sessions were held for two weeks. The maintenance sessions took place immediately after the intervention session. The participants were observed in their classroom to monitor any improvement in the targeted behavior after the 2D Animated Social Story intervention sessions. The result from the baseline and maintenance sessions was then compared to find any changes of the student's behavior.

Target Behaviors Identification

The participants were not videotaped during the baseline, intervention and maintenance period. This was the request from their parents and the school principal to conceal the children's privacy. As a substitution to video recording, observation notes were taken during the intervention period.

Through the observation and interviews with the participants' teachers and class helpers, certain aberrant behavior was identified. The observations for the baseline were conducted during their class time for 1 week for the duration of 4 to 5 hours each session, while each participant was engaged in their regular classroom routine. The interventions were executed for one week with each participant interacting with the 2D Animated Social Stories under the guidance of the researcher for 20 to 30 minutes. The maintenance period were carried out for two weeks after the intervention period for approximately 4 to 5 hours daily.

There were five target behaviors for the three different 2D Animated Social Stories. The target behavior for the first story, "Snack Time" was to initiate conversation or interact with their friends during their snack time and to hold a decent conversation by asking for more snacks or drink. Second story, "Talking at School" was to train the children to keep quiet during teaching and learning period in school, to raise their hands if they have something to say or request from the teacher or class helper. Lastly, "Lunch at Classroom" was targeted to teach the children to keep quiet while waiting for their lunch to be served.

Copyright © 2011, IGI Global. Copying or distributing in print or electronic forms without written permission of IGI Global is prohibited.

Figure 3. The sequences of "Snack Time" social story

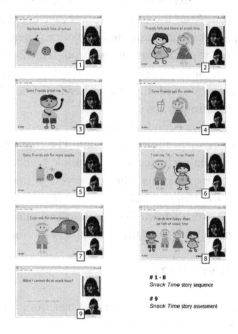

Social Stories

Three 2D Animated Social Stories were designed to address the target behaviors of the participants. Each story was taken from previously published paper, which adhered to Gray's guidelines, the author of Social Story. The original social stories were presented in formal instructions and were read to the children for a period of time. All the three Stories were adapted in the 2D animated prototype and were constructed using Adobe Flash CS3 and ActionScript3.0. The stories were briefly discussed below.

1. Snack Time

The first story, "Snack Time" was adapted from Crozier and Tincani (2007), "Effects of Social Stories on Pro-social Behavior of Preschool Children with Autism Spectrum Disorders". Crozier and Tincani tested the stories on three ASD children. The "Snack Time" story was selected as it was applicable to the situation at the local school. It was written based on a structured approach under the suggested ratio of 1 directive sentence to 2-5 descriptive or perspective sentences. The result showed

Copyright © 2011, IGI Global. Copying or distributing in print or electronic forms without written permission of IGI Global is prohibited.

Figure 4. The sequences of "Talking at School" social story

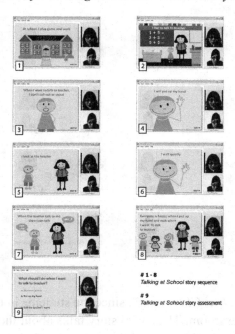

 # 1 - 8
Talking at School story sequence

 # 9
Talking at School story assessment

an improvement in their behavior but at a different degree. The interface for 'Snack Time' 2D Animated Social Story is illustrated in Figure 3.

2. Talking At School

Second social story, titled "Talking at School" was taken from Crozier and Tincani (2005), "Using Modified Social Story to Decrease Disruptive Behavior of a Child with Autism". There was no modification to the original story since it was suitable and applicable to the local scenes. This story stressed on the appropriate conduct in class to reduce interference during lesson. The result of the study should demonstrate a reduction in some disruptive behavior after the intervention.

The interface for 'Talking at School' 2D Animated Social Story as illustrated in Figure 4.

3. Lunch at Classroom

The third social story was obtained from Crozier and Sileo (2005), "*Encouraging Positive Behavior with Social Stories. An Intervention for Children with Autism Spectrum Disorders*" with the social story titled, "*Lunch at Cafeteria*". This story was adapted into the 2D prototype to reflect the situation at the local school and

Copyright © 2011, IGI Global. Copying or distributing in print or electronic forms without written permission of IGI Global is prohibited.

Figure 5 - The sequences of "Lunch at Classroom" social story

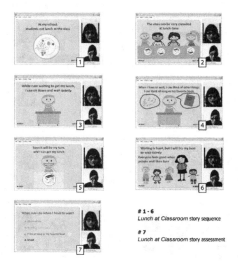

was modified to *"Lunch at Classroom"*, since the students in the local school have their lunch in their classroom. The social story talks about the etiquette of waiting up for food; to stay calm and patient while waiting for their turn to be served. This story had not been tested on the children with autism; however, the story does follow the guidelines set by the Social Story author, Gray. The interface for 'Lunch at Classroom' 2D Animated Social Story is illustrated in Figure 5.

RESULTS

The preliminary evaluation results were discussed in the section below based on clinical observation of the participants. The results were analyzed and hypothesize according to each participant's response to each social story that he went through. The correctness of answering each social story's assessment was also discussed.

1. Snack Time Social Story

During the observation in the baseline phase, participant 1 and 3 never asked for additional snacks from their teachers or peers. After the intervention, participant 1 showed a more proactive behavior by requesting snacks from his friends and was willing to share his snacks with others, with or without verbal prompts. Participant 1 had also shown generalization of behavior from the increased interaction with his

Copyright © 2011, IGI Global. Copying or distributing in print or electronic forms without written permission of IGI Global is prohibited.

peers and would invite his friends to sit down with him. Before the intervention, participant 1 would isolate himself from his peers.

As for participant 3, he showed a slight improvement in this target behavior and would request the teacher to get snacks for him instead of just waiting to be offered some. There was a noticeable increase in interaction for participant 3 as he was seen holding his friend's hand and would have short chat with them while walking in the hall. Before the intervention, participant 3 appeared to be aloof and did not know how to initiate short conversation with his peers.

Participant 2 has problems sharing the same interests with his peers. After going through the treatment, he was able to share story books with his friends and would request for additional snacks from the teacher or class helper.

2. Talking at School Social Story

All the participants exhibited disruptive behavior during class sessions in their own respective ways. Participant 1 would speak out loudly during lesson time; participant 2 would talk to himself and roam about while participant 3 appeared to be restless. He would go outside the classroom or walk towards the computers across the room to play with it during the classroom learning session.

During the maintenance probe, all the 3 participants managed to behave themselves by keeping quiet while the lesson was going on. There were times when they would raise their hands to get the teacher's attention. They have cultivated a sense of respect for other people's belonging and would ask permission before doing or taking something. There was lesser interference in the class.

3. Lunch at Classroom Social Story

All the 3 participants would be noisy before lunch was served. After going through the intervention, the participants would behave by keeping quiet before getting their lunch. Participant 1 would actually entertain himself by singing softly to himself; do coloring activities or reading story books while waiting for his lunch, and participant 3 would also do drawing and coloring activities. This indicated a satisfactory improvement as a whole.

4. Result of Assessment (Quiz Section)

For each session, three complete rounds of intervention were carried out. In each round, the set of the three 2D Animated Social Stories were delivered.

Participant 1 could only answer one question out of three in the first round. However, he managed to answer all the questions correctly after the second and

Copyright © 2011, IGI Global. Copying or distributing in print or electronic forms without written permission of IGI Global is prohibited.

Figure 6. Social behavior changes before and after 2-D animated social story intervention for participant 1 -3

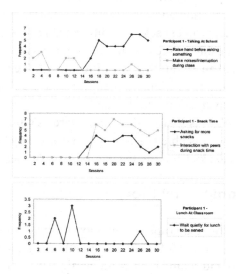

third round. Participant 1 exhibited an interesting trait when he was playing with pair matching puzzle which belongs to the classroom. Every time he successfully matched a pair, he would call out "next" repeatedly until the 4 pairs were done. Then, he would say "quiz" and repeated the names of the 4 pairs of puzzle. After he had correctly named all the four pairs, he would clap his hands and said "well done". He was actually reciting the steps from the 2D animated social story. This proves to show that the tool was engaging and gave a lasting impression by providing a conducive learning environment to these children. Participant 1 showed a burst of effervescence every time he received the "clapping hand" animation and was motivated to continue on.

As for participant 2, he could only answer 1 out of 3 questions throughout the 3 rounds in the first session. He might be distracted by his peers and failed to pay attention to the social story. In the second session, he showed slight improvement and could successfully attempt all the questions in the last round.

Participant 3 showed a greater interest in computer but he found it unchallenging and was quick to get bored with the animated social story once he had mastered it. He could answer all the assessments questions correctly with some assistance in the language area as his English literacy skill was below average. During the last session, he was totally distracted from the story and requested for a different computer program.

Copyright © 2011, IGI Global. Copying or distributing in print or electronic forms without written permission of IGI Global is prohibited.

Figure 7. Social behavior changes before and after 2-D animated social story intervention for participant 1 -3

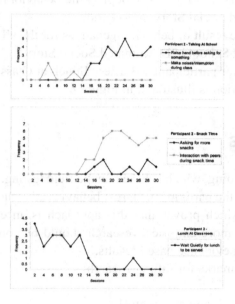

Figure 8. Social behavior changes before and after 2-D animated social story intervention for participant 1 -3

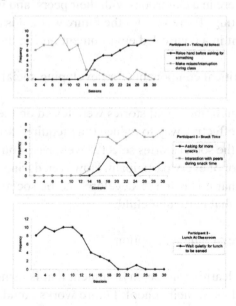

Copyright © 2011, IGI Global. Copying or distributing in print or electronic forms without written permission of IGI Global is prohibited.

The results for the 3 participants who underwent the "Snack Time" 2D Animated Social Story are plotted in Figure 6. It depicts the behavioral changes before and after the 2D Animated Social Story intervention.

Figure 7 shows the result of behavioral changes for the all the participants who attempted "Talking at School" 2D Animated Social Story.

The chart results for participant 1-3 after "Lunch at Classroom" 2D Animated Social Story intervention is illustrated in Figure 8.

FUTURE WORKS

In the lights of the finding, which is based on the field testing, the result has shown a positive increase in the participants' target behavior after the 2D animated Social Story intervention, which proves that this approach is an effective intervention technique. However, more empirical research should be conducted to produce a more concrete and an evidence based results.

There are some remarks for future research:

• more accurate experimental control

The current research was lacking accurate experimental control. During the testing, the participants were in a classroom with their peers, and were often distracted by them during the testing. Therefore, for the future work, it is advisable to conduct an accurate experiment in a controlled environment during the testing.

• examining the critical components for developing social stories

In the current research, the social stories were tested on the three different participants. This was an effective way to reduce time required for the development of the social stories, and the social stories selected were based on its generic nature to meet the target behavior of every participant. However, during and after the testing, the researcher found that it is better to develop specific social story tailored to the interests and needs of that particular child.

• To add on feature of language option

The students were learning in the environment that is using different language in their homes as well as in their school. Future works could include a feature of language option to meet the needs of each child specifically.

Copyright © 2011, IGI Global. Copying or distributing in print or electronic forms without written permission of IGI Global is prohibited.

It is suggested by Sansosti et al (2004) that the implementation of social stories on a continuous basis is necessary to achieve the desired result. It is relatively difficult, time-consuming and costly to create a 2D animated social story as it requires information technology expertise specifically from the multimedia stream. Thus, these affect the possibility of a continuous production of subsequent social stories tailored to specific needs and the practicality of this approach is in question. Further research should emphasize on this area to include the creation of a tool or application which provides ready-made templates for creating a 2D-animated social stories to make the deployment possible.

CONCLUSION

As ASD cases are on the rise each year, remedial action has to be developed to provide adequate support for ASD diagnosed children to learn social communication of neuro-typicals within an inclusive environment. Social Stories is an old and effective ways in teaching children with ASD by describing social situations to help them cope and to resolve related cognitive confusion. To increase the efficacy of Social Stories, computer presented Social Stories had been tested and it produced a positive outcome. As advancement to the computer presented social story, the researcher had implemented a prototype to test the effectiveness of the 2-D animated Social Stories, which offers a dynamic source of learning. 2D animated social story is proven to be effective in changing the social behavior of children with ASD. Comparing with traditional paper-based social story, the participant would only manage to project good social behavior changes after the two doses of interventions and must be triggered by verbal prompts.

However, in 2D animated social story, transferable literacy occurred naturally when the participant successfully applied the knowledge learnt in their daily activities after the first intervention without verbal prompts. Social stories enacted in 2D animation are more appealing and engaging especially for the children as they are visual learners and this could in turn accelerate their learning process and stimulate their curiosity in exploring exciting ideas.

REFERENCES

American Psychiatric Association. (2000). *Diagnostic and statistical manual for mental disorders* (4th ed.-text revision), (pp. 70-71). Washington, DC: American Psychiatric Association.

Copyright © 2011, IGI Global. Copying or distributing in print or electronic forms without written permission of IGI Global is prohibited.

Attwood, T. (2006). *The complete guide to Asperger's syndrome*. London, UK: Jessica Kingsley Publisher.

Autism Society. (2008). *What causes autism*. Retrieved October 5, 2009, from http://www.autism- society.org/ site/ PageServer?pagename= about_whatcauses

Bauminger, N. (2002). The facilitation of social-emotional understanding and social interaction in high-functioning children with autism: Intervention outcomes. *Journal of Autism and Developmental Disorders, 32*(4), 283–298. doi:10.1023/A:1016378718278

Bregman, J. D. (2005). Definitions and characteristics of the spectrum. In Zager, D. B. (Ed.), *Autism spectrum disorders: Identification, education and treatment* (3rd ed., pp. 3–46). Routledge.

Capps, L., Kehres, J., & Sigman, M. (1998). Conversational abilities among children with autism and children with developmental delays. *Autism: The International Journal of Research and Practice, 2*(4), 325–344.

Cheng, Y., Moore, D., McGrath, P., & Fan, Y. (2005). Collaborative virtual environment technology for people with autism. In *Proceedings of the Fifth IEEE International Conference on Advanced Learning Technologies, ICALT'05,* (pp. 247-248). Washington, DC: IEEE Computer Society.

Crozier, S., & Sileo, N. M. (2005). Encouraging positive behavior with social stories. *Teaching Exceptional Children, 37*(6), 26–31.

Crozier, S., & Tincani, M. (2007). Effects of social stories on prosocial of preschool children with autism spectrum disorders. *Journal of Autism and Developmental Disorders, 37*, 1803–1814. doi:10.1007/s10803-006-0315-7

Crozier, S., & Tincani, M. J. (2005). Using a modified social story to decrease disruptive behavior of a child with autism. *Focus on Autism and Other Developmental Disabilities, 20*(3), 150–157. doi:10.1177/10883576050200030301

Dawson, G., Rogers, S., Munson, J., Smith, M., Winter, J., Greenson, J., et al. Varley, J. (2010). Randomized, controlled trial of an intervention for toddlers with autism: The early start Denver model. *Pediatrics, 125*, e17-e23. Retrieved May 6, 2010, from http://pediatrics. aappublications.org/ cgi/ content/ abstract/ peds.2009-0958v1

Del Valle, P. R., McEachern, A. G., & Chambers, H. D. (2001). Using social stories with autistic children. *Journal of Poetry Therapy, 14*(4), 187–197. doi:10.1023/A:1017564711160

Copyright © 2011, IGI Global. Copying or distributing in print or electronic forms without written permission of IGI Global is prohibited.

Dixon, D. R., Garcia, M. J., Granpeesheh, D., & Tarbox, J. (2009). Differential diagnosis in autism spectrum disorders. In Matson, J. L. (Ed.), *Applied behavior analysis for children with autism spectrum disorders* (pp. 83–108). New York, NY: Springer. doi:10.1007/978-1-4419-0088-3_5

Elzouki, S. Y. A., Fabri, M., & Moore, D. J. (2007). Teaching severely autistic children to recognise emotions: Finding a methodology. In D. Ramduny-Ellis & D. Rachovides (Eds.), *Proceedings of the 21st British Computer Society Human Computer Interaction Group Conference: Vol. 2. Human Computer Interaction 2007*, (pp. 137-140). Lancaster University, UK: British Computer Society.

Evans, R. (n.d.). Asperger's syndrome – is there real cure for it? *Comeunity: Children's Disabilities and Special Needs,* 1996-2009. Retrieved December 1, 2009, from http://www.comeunity.com/ disability/ autism/ aspergers syndrome.html

Fombonne, E. (2003). Modern views of autism. *Canadian Journal of Psychiatry*, *48*(8), 503–505.

Gabbert, C. (2010). *Using social stories to teach kids with Asperger's disorder*. Bright hub, The Hub for Bright Minds. Retrieved May 7, 2010, from http://www.brighthub.com/ education/ special/ articles/ 29487.aspx

Hagiwara, T., & Myles, B. S. (1999). A multimedia social story intervention: Teaching skills to children with autism. *Focus on Autism and Other Developmental Disabilities*, *14*(2), 82–95. doi:10.1177/108835769901400203

Heffner, G. J. (2002). Social stories: An introduction. *BBB Autism.* Retrieved December 17, 2009, from http://www.bbbautism.com/ pdf/ article_27_ Social_ Stories.pdf

Heimann, M., Nelson, K. E., Tjus, T., & Gillberg, C. (1995). Increasing reading and communication skills in children with autism through an interactive multi-media computer program. *Journal of Autism and Developmental Disorders*, *25*(5), 459–480. doi:10.1007/BF02178294

Heward, W. L. (2006). *Exceptional children: An introduction to special education*. Wisconsin: Pearson Allyn Bacon Prentice Hall.

Hirsch, D. (2009). *Autism spectrum disorders*. WebMD Medical Reference. Retrieved October 06, 2009, from http://www.webmd.com/ brain/ autism/ autism- spectrum-disorders? page=2

Holmes, B. (2009, December 05). Treat autism early. *New Scientist, 2737*, 7.

Copyright © 2011, IGI Global. Copying or distributing in print or electronic forms without written permission of IGI Global is prohibited.

Johnson, S. (2008, October 17). There are 5 different types of autism disorders. *ezinearticles.com.* Retrieved August 30, 2009, from http://ezinearticles.com/?There-Are-5 -Different- Types-of-Autism- Disorders& id=1592117

Kalb, C. (2009, January 16). Autism: Kids with autism love this software. *Newsweek.* Retrieved from http://www.newsweek.com/ id/179952

Loomis, J. W. (2008). *Staying in the game: Providing social opportunities for children and adolescents with autism spectrum disorder and other developmental disabilities.* Shawnee Mission, KS: Autism Asperger Publishing Company.

Mancil, G. R., Haydon, T., & Whitby, P. (2009). Differentiated effects of paper and computer-assisted social stories™ on inappropriate behavior in children with autism. *Focus on Autism and Other Developmental Disabilities, 20*(10), 1–11.

Matson, J. L., & Neal, D. (2009). History and overview. In Matson, J. L. (Ed.), *Applied behavior analysis for children with autism spectrum disorders* (pp. 1–13). New York, NY/ Dordrecht, The Netherlands/ Heidelberg, Germany/ London, UK: Springer. doi:10.1007/978-1-4419-0088-3_1

National Autistic Society. (2008). *Picture symbols: For professional and students.* Retrieved October 30, 2009, from http://www.nas. org.uk/ nas/ jsp/ polopoly. jsp?d= 297&a= 3642

Parsons, S., Beardon, L., Neale, H. R., Reynard, G., Eastgate, R., Wilson, J. R., et al. Hopkins, E. (2000). Development of social skills amongst adults with Asperger's syndrome using virtual environments: The AS interactive project. In P. Sharkey, A. Cesarani, L. Pugnetti & A. Rizzo (Eds.), *3rd International Conference of Disability, Virtual Reality and Associated Technology. 2000 ICDVRAT* (pp. 163-170). Alghero, Italy: University of Reading.

Roger, M. F., & Myles, B. S. (2001). Using social stories and comic strip conversations to interpret social situations for an adolescent with Asperger syndrome. *Intervention in School and Clinic, 36*(5), 310–313. doi:10.1177/105345120103600510

Rutten, A., Cobb, S., Neale, H., Kerr, S., Leonard, A., Parsons, S., & Mitchell, P. (2003). The AS interactive project: Single-user and collaborative virtual environment for people with high-functioning autistic spectrum disorders. *The Journal of Visualization and Computer Animation, 14*(5), 233–241. doi:10.1002/vis.320

Sansosti, F. J., & Powell-Smith, K. A. (2008). Using computer-presented social stories and video models to increase the social communication skills of children with high-functioning autism spectrum disorders. *Journal of Positive Behavior Interventions, 10*(3), 162–178. doi:10.1177/1098300708316259

Copyright © 2011, IGI Global. Copying or distributing in print or electronic forms without written permission of IGI Global is prohibited.

Sansosti, F. J., Powell-Smith, K. A., & Kincaid, D. (2004). A research synthesis of social story intervention for children with autism spectrum disorders. *Focus on Autism and Other Developmental Disabilities, 19*(4), 194–204. doi:10.1177/1088 3576040190040101

Schneider, N., & Goldstein, H. (2009). Using social stories and visual schedules to improve socially appropriate behaviors in children with autism. *Journal of Positive Behavior Interventions, 20*(10), 1–12.

Scurlock, M. (2008). *Using social stories with children with Asperger syndrome.* Unpublished Master's thesis, Ohio University, Athens, Ohio, United States.

Sigafoos, J., Schlosser, R. W., O'Reilly, M. F., & Lancioni, G. E. (2009). Communication. In Matson, J. L. (Ed.), *Applied behavior analysis for children with autism spectrum disorders* (pp. 109–127). New York, NY: Springer. doi:10.1007/978-1-4419-0088-3_6

Sparks, B. F., Friedman, S. D., Shaw, D. W., Aylward, E. H., Echelard, D., & Artru, A. A. (2002). Brain structural abnormalities in young children with autism spectrum disorder. *Neurology, 59*, 184–192.

Tartaro, A. (2007). Authorable virtual peers for children with autism. In *CHI '07 extended abstracts on Human factors in computing system, Conference on Human Factors in Computing Systems* (pp. 1677-1680). New York, NY: ACM.

Tartaro, A., & Cassell, J. (2008). Playing with virtual peers: Bootstrapping contingent discourse in children with autism. In *Proceedings of the Eighth International Conference for the Learning Sciences: Vol. 2. International Conference on Learning Sciences* (pp. 382-389). Utrecht, The Netherlands: International Society of the Learning Sciences.

Thiemann, K. S., & Goldstein, H. (2001). Social stories, written text cues, and video feedback: Effects on social communication of children with autism. *Journal of Applied Behavior Analysis, 34*(4), 425–446. doi:10.1901/jaba.2001.34-425

Wallin, J. M. (n.d.). Social stories: An introduction to social stories. *polyxo.com, teaching children with autism,* 2001-2004. Retrieved December 17, 2009, from http://www.polyxo.com/ socialstories/ introduction.html

Weiss, M. J., LaRue, R. H., & Newcomer, A. (2009). Social skills and autism: Understanding and addressing the deficits. In Matson, J. L. (Ed.), *Applied behavior analysis for children with autism spectrum disorders* (pp. 129–144). New York, NY/ Dordrecht, The Netherlands/ Heidelberg, Germany/ London, UK: Springer. doi:10.1007/978-1-4419-0088-3_7

Copyright © 2011, IGI Global. Copying or distributing in print or electronic forms without written permission of IGI Global is prohibited.

ADDITIONAL READING

Asperger, H. (1944/1991). "Autistic psychopathy" in childhood (U. Frith, Trans., Annot.). In U. Frith (Ed.), *Autism and asperger syndrome* (pp. 37–92). New York, NY: Cambridge University Press. (Original work published 1944)

Bernad-Ripoll, S. (2007, Summer). Using a self-as-model video combined with social stories™ to help a child with asperger syndrome understand emotions. *Focus on Autism and Other Developmental Disabilities, 22*(2), 100–106. doi:10.1177/10 883576070220020101

Grandin, T. (1996). *Thinking in pictures: And other reports from my life with autism (Vintage Series)*. USA: Vintage Books.

Kuoch, H., & Mirenda, P. (2003, Winter). Social Story interventions for young children with autism spectrum disorders. *Focus on Autism and Other Developmental Disabilities, 18*(4), 219–227. doi:10.1177/10883576030180040301

KEY TERMS AND DEFINITIONS

Asperger Syndrome: A type of ASD with high functioning features.
Baseline Phase: Duration of participant's behaviors before the intervention.
Intervention Phase: Duration of the testing of the prototype.
Maintenance Phase: Duration of participant's behaviors after the intervention.
Social Skill: Skills necessary to initiate and responses to social interaction and communication in everyday living situation.
Social Story: An intervention to help children with ASD learns social skills, first introduced by Carol Gray in 1991.

Copyright © 2011, IGI Global. Copying or distributing in print or electronic forms without written permission of IGI Global is prohibited.

Chapter 2
3D Assistive Technologies and Advantageous Themes for Collaboration and Blended Learning of Users with Disabilities

Georgios Dafoulas
Middlesex University, UK

Noha Saleeb
Middlesex University, UK

ABSTRACT

The significance of newly emergent 3D virtual worlds to different genres of users is currently a controversial subject in deliberation. Users range from education pursuers, business contenders, and social seekers to technology enhancers and many more who comprise both users with normal abilities in physical life and those with different disabilities. This study aims to derive and critically analyze, using grounded theory, advantageous and disadvantageous themes, and their sub concepts of providing e-learning through 3D Virtual Learning Environments (VLEs), like Second Life, to disabled users. Hence providing evidence that 3DVLEs not only support traditional physical learning, but also offer e-learning opportunities unavailable through 2D VLEs (like Moodle, Blackboard), and offer learning opportunities unavailable through traditional physical education. Furthermore, to

DOI: 10.4018/978-1-60960-541-4.ch002

Copyright ©2011, IGI Global. Copying or distributing in print or electronic forms without written permission of IGI Global is prohibited.

achieve full potential from the above-mentioned derived concepts, architectural and accessibility design requirements of 3D educational facilities proposed by different categories of disabled students to accommodate for their needs, are demonstrated.

INTRODUCTION

The ultimate goal of this research is to analyze factors enhancing disabled students' blended learning experiences comprising of both face-to-face and online courses. The research focuses on the investigation of:

1. Educational prospects that can help achieve maximum assimilation, achievement and enjoyment from e-learning within 3D Virtual Learning environments such as Second Life,
2. Finding the effect of 3D virtual architectural design elements of learning spaces on students and their e-learning experience.

The driver for emphasising on the above areas is recognising the design characteristics of the learning space as one of the vital aspects recognised in affecting students' physical learning. This would hence allow reaching best practices in virtual architectural design of 3D educational building facilities. Subsequently it would most definitely help increase the accessibility of the learning space and make it more suitable and desirable for the benefit of students and augmenting their e-learning experience within virtual worlds.

This research applies to multiple sectors of disabled students in higher education e.g. large universities (under-graduate and post graduate student), community colleges, adult education and ongoing researchers. This study is also not specific to Second Life but rather general to 3D Virtual worlds in general since the psychological impact of the design of a 3D virtual learning space on its users is universal in any virtual world.

Online 3D Virtual Learning Environments (3D VLEs) have been since their onset a receptor for virtual campuses, built by hundreds of universities such as Harvard, Princeton, and Oxford. Innovation in educational techniques within these virtual existences offer e-learning opportunities for all diversities of students in many fields including science, medicine, engineering, business, law, computer science, humanities and many more (Kay, 2009). Such opportunities include experimentation, teleporting between sites, flying, game-based activities, role-play, modeling and co-creation, immersion, critical incident involvement, medical training and many other practices. This has reaped noticeable participation, satisfaction and hence achievement from students (Calongne, 2008). Through 3D VLE online courses, online avatars allow

Copyright © 2011, IGI Global. Copying or distributing in print or electronic forms without written permission of IGI Global is prohibited.

students and their instructors to interact synchronously by audio, text chat and other media presentation techniques (Butler & White, 2008). It thus becomes imperative to utilize the merits and drawbacks of delivery of e-learning within these environments to encourage blended learning. The appearance of digitally inclined generations of students, some of which are confined due to disability and whose refuge to a more able life is through technology, whom Prensky (2001; 2007), Oblinger and Oblinger (2005) refer to as "Digital Natives, "Games Generation" and "Millenials", deems it rational to anticipate that in order to boost future learning, these students will be encouraged to employ the game-like 3D virtual worlds, or VLEs like Second Life, Active Worlds and others to accommodate for new evolving learning style changes. These changes play a vital role in shaping future e-learning since "Today's students are no longer the people our educational system was designed to teach". This pedagogical transformation is considered beneficial even by researchers like Margaryan and Littlejohn (2008) who argue that students are not using technology effectively to support learning, but rather primarily for recreation.

This research helps demonstrating, by practical grounded theory evidence, the presence of three advantageous themes for using 3D VLEs to deliver education to disabled users:

- Proving that 3D VLEs augment and complement traditional learning techniques in physical classrooms to help reach higher educational achievement.
- Proving that 3D VLEs provide additional opportunities and options for e-learning unavailable within 2D Virtual Learning environments such as moodle and Blackboard.
- Proving that 3D VLEs can, furthermore, not only sustain traditional methods of learning but can offer e-learning prospects that are not probable to achieve using conventional real-life methods of education.

Along with this trend appeared creative opportunities for constructing buildings that cross boundaries of reality and delve into the dominion of creativity of the designer. This is because of the fundamental difference between the physical and virtual worlds where there are no constraints on budgets, no engineering natural forces and material strength limitations, no infrastructure requirements, sound, ventilation regulations or even gravity which can be defied to have 3D virtual buildings floating in midair or immersed under the deepest ocean. Such innovative construction techniques have also been used to erect virtual university campuses in 3D VLES to produce a wide variety of designs from realistic depictions or replicas of physically existing campuses, to completely imaginative embodiments.

Copyright © 2011, IGI Global. Copying or distributing in print or electronic forms without written permission of IGI Global is prohibited.

However there is no academically conducted research that directly correlates between the new e-learning blended learning techniques sprouting within 3D VLEs, and the design specifications of the 3D virtual spaces within which this e-learning is taking place, and thus whether these design specifications have an impact on the effectiveness of e-learning in 3D VLEs. One of the factors that have been proven to affect learning in the physical world, the degree of assimilation of knowledge, achievement and enjoyment of students from education, is the architectural design and physical building characteristics of the space in which students learn in which affect accessibility and satisfaction from the space. Such design features include color, texture, dimensions of space, lighting, and ventilation amongst others. On the other hand, sparse study explores the effect of 3D architecture in virtual worlds in general on any genre of users, not just disabled students in 3D VLEs, and their satisfaction and contentment from it. The current research thus focuses, as one of its objectives, on closing this gap by raising the query on and capturing the specific architectural design elements of virtual educational buildings, within 3DVLEs, proposed by students to provide satisfaction and contentment from their e-learning session, hence giving the opportunity to issue recommendations for future learning space enhancement.

Learners are divided into three groups: under-graduate students, post-graduate students, and adult learners and researchers. Data collection techniques include surveys to demonstrate students' perception of the visual qualities of the spaces, preferences and suggestions for a better learning environment. Data analysis focused on in this study involves comparing satisfaction results attained from the identified three groups of learners, subsequently examining the impact that this might have on a student's blended learning experience. Moreover this research can help initiate the development of a framework or recommendations for building codes, for educational facilities within 3D Virtual Environments, to complement existing codes for erecting such facilities in the physical real-life world.

The results of this research disseminate recommendations for possible applications of the technology through the use of a variety of educational scenarios in 3D Virtual Learning Environments. The key contribution is to initiate discussions, trigger debates and offer brainstorming opportunities for students with respect to the use of such assistive technologies in Higher Education. Additionally, this study offers insights in preliminary stages for defining the effect of environmental factors on a disabled student's e-learning experience within 3D Virtual Learning Environments. More specifically the use of 3D VLEs could address issues relating to learning & technology, open educational resources and inclusion.

Copyright © 2011, IGI Global. Copying or distributing in print or electronic forms without written permission of IGI Global is prohibited.

BACKGROUND

Disabilities in 3D Virtual Environments

According to the U.S. Census Bureau, around 17% of the U.S. population, aged 16 and over, lives with some form of disability. Types of disabilities include visual and auditory disabilities like color blindness, low-vision, and complete or partial-blindness, being hard of hearing or completely deaf. The expression also includes cognitive impairments like Autism, Dyslexia, and ADHD, and also psychiatric conditions. Finally, disability can also comprise motor or dexterity impairments like Cerebral Palsy, Repetitive Strain Injury or even paraplegia and quadriplegia (Epstein, 2008). Moreover, according to the World Health Organization, every 5 minutes for example, a child goes blind. This is just one of many disabilities of children who are going to grow up needing special access to education, employment, entertainment, and social engagement. These needs can be provided through 3D virtual worlds like Second Life (SL) as will be shown later. In fact, current demographics show that people with disabilities represent at least 20% of the users of SL (5% higher than their representation in physical world) and spend much more time in SL than avatars who do not identify themselves as disabled in RL (Information Solutions Group, 2008). Testimonials from different disabled users attribute the reasons behind this phenomenon to the fact that a virtual world is a place where they can feel equal because their disability doesn't hold them back from anything like in "real life". For whether they choose for their avatars to use a wheelchair or to be without disability e.g. in SL, they can mingle with others, walk, fly, dance, socialize, work, visit different places whenever they wish with no restrictions or constrains to one place and without being discerned, alienated, pitied or judged by others who do not know of their disabilities (Stein & Waterstone, 2006). In other words, virtual worlds like SL give the freedom for users to be however they wish, and to know each other in ways they would not have without SL, hence adding enjoyment to their lives (Black, 2007; Hickey-Moody & Wood, 2008). As one user states, "it is very inspiring to know that when an obstacle, such as being a paraplegic, may happen to one, that you can still make something of yourself and make life better for other handicapped individuals through exploiting potential not judgment of condition" (Information Solutions Group, 2008).

Within this research, grounded theory will be used as a scientific method to provide evidence for the advantages and disadvantages of using 3D virtual learning environments for delivering education for differently abled people. This will be done by deriving themes and their sub-concepts from existing case studies of universities and educational institutions using Second Life for e-learning.

Copyright © 2011, IGI Global. Copying or distributing in print or electronic forms without written permission of IGI Global is prohibited.

DESIGN OF EDUCATIONAL FACILITIES FOR ACCESSIBILITY IN 3D VIRTUAL ENVIRONMENTS

In the physical world, various design measures are taken to provide appropriate accessibility within buildings for the use of the disabled. For example, the US Disabilities Act ensures that new structures are built so that they are accessible to the disabled. The (UK) DDA - Disabilities Discrimination Act 1995 - also states taking 'reasonable steps' to supply business services or products to disabled persons, including 'online services' (McCullough & Beauchamp, 2009).

However do buildings in 3D virtual worlds, e.g. SL, need to adhere to "real life" principles of accessible design?

As Black and Clark stated, "The "biophysics" of SL are clearly designed in part to surpass the universal human impairments of our physical embodiment" (Black, 2007). This means that people with certain disabilities in the physical world might be without disabilities in the virtual world, or maybe their real life disability causes them no impediment in SL e.g. people with lower body physical mobility problems face no problems dealing with the virtual world using their upper limbs. However people with arm, hand or finger control problems might be able to walk in real life, might find difficulty using keyboard, mouse or navigating in the virtual world and might therefore need features like wide ramps or corridors "in-world" to manipulate their avatar across. The same applies to people who might have specific digital visual impairment only and thus might need certain colors in the background or building textures or fonts (Krueger, Ludwig & Ludwig 2009). Other disabled users, while not suffering from any difficulty inside a virtual world, might feel more comfortable if certain accessibility elements appear "in-world" analogous to what they are used to in the physical world. Also the nature of the 3D digitalized world might exacerbate or improve other aspects of accessibility for the disabled. These aspects need to be investigated as they might change the architectural and accessibility requirements for designing educational learning spaces in 3D VLEs for the disabled.

As mentioned previously, there are endless possibilities for creativity in building in SL and similar virtual worlds. This innovation also includes designing educational facilities and campuses. However there are currently no existing specifications or design codes especially created for building in virtual worlds, analogous to those present in the physical world, that can be used as guidelines for designing 3D virtual educational facilities or even general constructions in 3D VLEs. There is also no research conducted up-to-date depicting students' needs and preferences from design elements of their learning space to enhance their e-learning experience. Even though no avatar in Second Life is actually physically disabled, creating specification guidelines with universal design principles for disabilities in mind has several

Copyright © 2011, IGI Global. Copying or distributing in print or electronic forms without written permission of IGI Global is prohibited.

benefits: (i) It ensures a baseline modality. (ii) If buildings are designed to accommodate users with challenges, the overall experience will be improved for all users. (iii) Virtual environments should be built to consider best practices in interface usability as acknowledgement of respect for others (Smith, 2009).

Currently educational campuses, buildings and learning spaces in 3D VLEs are being designed using one of three approaches:

1. On an ad-hoc basis according to the designer's preferences or best practice experience (with no consideration to specific educational or accessibility needs of students in virtual world buildings).
2. As a blind replica of an existing building in real-life (maybe of the same university e.g. Harvard University – Austin Hall Berkman)
3. Using universal "real-life" documented design codes for constructing similar buildings physically (e.g. Universal Design (UD), developed at North Carolina State University) (Krueger, et al., 2009). E.g. in Virtual Ability island in SL spiral stairs, grass, sand, and deep carpet textures for the ground are avoided because they are difficult to move a wheelchair across, while smoothly leveled and landscaped walkways, ramps with rails and bright high-contrast signs are used by users with visual impairments with beige textured background and tilted downward at roughly 15 degrees from eye level to be at eye level of users with wheel chairs (Zielke, Roome, & Krueger 2009).

However, all three approaches for building, mentioned above, do not guarantee satisfaction of students from the design of their learning spaces since there might be additional factors affecting them during e-learning sessions in 3D VLEs that are different to those in the physical world. Regarding students with disabilities, this issue is further aggravated by the fact that the design of the virtual buildings might also need to cater for accessibility issues for different disabilities. Hence arises the need to uncover the effect of different 3D virtual architectural design elements of the learning space on students' assimilation, participation and enjoyment in general and disabled students in particular.

This research delves into capturing architectural and environmental design elements proposed by disabled students from different categories (under graduates, post-graduates, adult learners and researchers) in order to accommodate for and provide accessibility improvements in 3D educational spaces, so as to achieve the advantageous themes and sub-concepts of delivering education in 3D VLEs derived henceforth, and subsequently enhance their e-learning experience.

Copyright © 2011, IGI Global. Copying or distributing in print or electronic forms without written permission of IGI Global is prohibited.

THEMES AND SUB-CONCEPTS OF DELIVERING EDUCATION IN 3D VIRTUAL LEARNING ENVIRONMENTS

Method

The primary concept of Grounded Theory established by Glaser and Strauss (1967) designates that research, starting with no preset hypothesis or theory, can eventually generate one by examining primary data sources, whether from qualitative empirical data, existing literature or any kind of data (Glaser, 2001; 2002), where the unit of analysis is an incident. From many incidents, a chain of key points can be mined which are then tagged with "codes". These in turn are grouped into "concepts", and from related concepts emerge main "categories" (or themes) (Glaser, 1992). Within this study, our raw source of data (or incidents) was documented literature representing case studies of Second Life colonization or usage by a multitude of educational institutions for e-learning in its diverse types. Key points, each signifying a possible advantage or disadvantage for delivering e-learning in VLEs, were deduced from each documented incident and clustered into three main groups of codes:

1. Those supporting traditional physical education,
2. Those unavailable in and adding to capabilities of 2D virtual learning environments (2D VLEs), and
3. Those unavailable in physical classroom learning.

Components of each code group were then named as 70 concepts, which were in turn grouped into 16 advantageous and disadvantageous categories (themes). A final general hypothesis was devised as a result of the emerging categories (themes). Whilst the low level individually mined key points are not included in this research, following is a description of each theme and its sub concepts, formulated from the key points, showing the division of these concepts into the 3 coding clusters mentioned above.

ADVANTAGEOUS THEMES AND SUB-CONCEPTS OF LEARNING IN 3D VLES

The following fifteen categories, summarized in Figure 1 and 2, are high level advantageous themes of delivering e-learning within 3D VLEs for users with disabilities. Underneath each of them is their sub-concepts derived used grounded theory divided into three categories:

Copyright © 2011, IGI Global. Copying or distributing in print or electronic forms without written permission of IGI Global is prohibited.

Figure 1. Advantageous themes and sub-concepts of using Virtual Worlds to deliver learning for disabled students

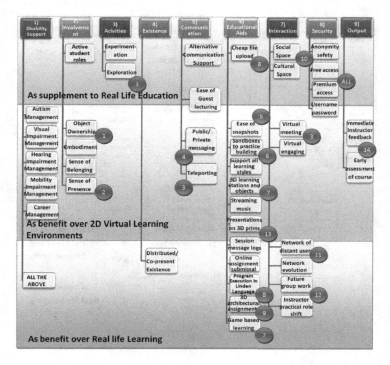

1.   As supplement to real life education
2.   As benefit over 2D virtual learning environments
3.   As benefit over real life learning

The circles in the figures represent the educational institutions in real life that employ these themes and concepts in Second Life shown in Table 1.

Disability Support

Second Life as an example of virtual worlds has taken many considerations into account to reduce accessibility problems for differently challenged users to be able to use the environment easily, offering at the same time therapeutic and educational solutions that are both beneficial over real life learning and 2D virtual learning environments as follows.

Copyright © 2011, IGI Global. Copying or distributing in print or electronic forms without written permission of IGI Global is prohibited.

Figure 2. Advantageous & Disadvantageous themes and sub-concepts of using Virtual Worlds to deliver learning for disabled students

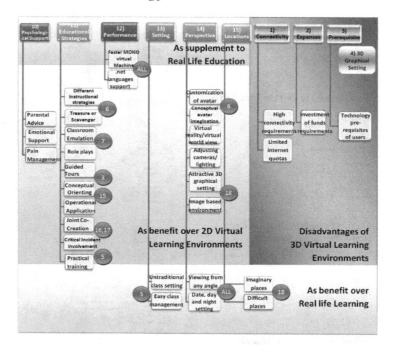

Table 1.

1) Massachusetts Institute of Technology	10) Hong Kong Polytechnic University
2) Trinity University San Antonio	11) Virtual Ability Island
3) Johnson & Wales University	12) Harvard University Law School
4) Bradley University	13) Oxford University
5) University of Kansas	14) Edinburgh University
6) Colorado Technical University	15) University of Houston
7) Texas A & M University	16) University of London
8) University of Florida	17) Kingston University
9) University of Colorado	18) University of Texas

Copyright © 2011, IGI Global. Copying or distributing in print or electronic forms without written permission of IGI Global is prohibited.

Concepts as Benefit over 2D VLES and Real Life Education

- *Autism Management:* audio visual pseudo-immersive stimulus inside virtual worlds could provide a potential communications pathway for both those suffering from autism as well as those close to ones suffering from autism to be able to interact with them (Talamasca, 2009).
- *Visual Impairment Management:* a user interface suitable for usage of blind students in virtual worlds is "Accessible Rich Internet Application" (ARIA) which gives the ability to participate in many virtual world activities. It provides basic navigation, communication, and perception functions using GUI (graphical user interface) elements that are familiar to blind computer users. In Second Life, other accessibility scripting groups also devised "inworld" tools for these special users like scripted canes and guide dogs that can help navigation inside the virtual world by voice or text commands (IBM, 2008). People who are blind tend to assume sequential, route-based strategies for moving around the physical world. Virtual worlds provide great opportunity for allowing people who are blind to explore new spaces, reducing their reliance on guides, and aiding development of more proficient spatial maps and strategies. This is because when exploring virtual spaces, people who are blind use more and different strategies than when exploring real physical spaces, and thus develop accurate spatial illustrations of them (White, Fitzpatrick & McAllister 2008).
- *Hearing Impairment Management:* consideration is made for people with hearing impairment. When presentations are conducted in voice, they can be simultaneously transcribed into print (voice-to-text or V2T) to aid those with hearing disabilities. Sound signals, such as for starting a race, can also be given in a simultaneous visual manner (Joseph, 2007).
- *Mobility Impairment Management:* Scientists in Japan have created a small helmet that enables the wearer to animate a 3D avatar in Second Life so it will perform basic movements just through thought impulses. Future plans will allow avatars to execute more complex movements and gestures, with the ultimate goal of enabling students (with severe paralysis, who are often too depressed to undergo rehabilitation) to communicate and do future business in virtual worlds as readily as fully able people. This device can help all students with upper limb disabilities who have problems with typing e.g. only one hand, one finger, or toes they can control to type. Voice recognition software can also be used to control the computer and overcome these challenges inside virtual worlds (Vivian, 2007).
- *Career Management:* Virtual worlds as a form of improved reality, allows surpassing users' physiological or cognitive challenges. Differently abled

Copyright © 2011, IGI Global. Copying or distributing in print or electronic forms without written permission of IGI Global is prohibited.

students sometimes suffer from discrimination in real life and are forced to drop out of courses which are unable to compromise with certain disabilities. Furthermore many job fields overlook hiring graduates with disabilities for misconception that they are unable to function with their conditions. However there are proven cases of Second life users for example who were able to run whole companies from inside SL, work in consultancy, take up photography etc.

An example of this is a quadriplegic student who set up an exhibition for his art work inside SL at the building that Illinois-based Bradley University have established on Information Island (Cassidy, 2007). Virtual world employment fairs for graduates are also an added asset e.g. those conducted by major organizations like IBM. Another example is an online company, Coraworks, which has currently employed up to 200 graduates with disabilities in jobs ranging from data entry to computer programming to architectural design, and many other computerized jobs (Carey, 2008).

Involvement

In the context of this research, involvement can be defined as student participation, interaction and contribution during a 3D VLE e-learning session. This can be seen noticeably in 3D VLEs, encompassing the ensuing concepts grouped according to the following classification codes.

Concepts as Supplement to Real Life Education

- *Active student roles:* New roles surface as disabled students move from the physical campus or online discussion boards to the virtual world classroom. Learning generally centers on discovery, yet students may feel that they are space confined with a restricted view of their role in the physical classroom. Shifting students from passive roles of survivors and castaways in real-life to the active roles of researchers can be done in 3DVLEs (Calongne, 2008).

Concepts as Benefit over 2D VLEs

- *Object ownership:* The capability to buy or freely acquire personalized accessories, buildings, contraptions etc. in each user's individual "in-world" inventory, gives a feeling of belonging and true existence adding to the allegiance to the virtual world and motivation to return back again and resume activity within the environment (Robbins, 2007).

Copyright © 2011, IGI Global. Copying or distributing in print or electronic forms without written permission of IGI Global is prohibited.

The Second Life (SL) Design Competition organized by Massachusetts Institute of Technology required from each student to design and create his own space for learning and residence, so as to interact and connect with others, is an example of imposing active student roles and object ownership (Nesson, 2007). This can be achieved without requiring much previous knowledge of how to build and create.

- ***Embodiment and sense of belonging:*** The personification of the disabled user in the form of an avatar and the ability to revamp its shape, skin and style, can convert the sentiment of the disabled user towards the space of a virtual world into a sense of belonging to a place (Joseph, 2007).
- ***Sense of presence:*** The ability to communicate, add face gestures and body movements to the avatar, adds to the sense of presence within the scene (Robbins, 2007).

For example, media students at Trinity University San Antonio employ promotional campaigns in SL by exploiting these avatar functionalities to advertise (Michels, 2008).

Activities

Positive actions and behavior undertaken by students in 3D virtual environments can be categorized into the following concepts.

As Supplement to Real Life Education

- ***Experimentation:*** The virtual world opens up opportunities for disabled students that the physical world does not offer, e.g. experimentation with simulated real life difficult science experiments like fertilization, space phenomena, studying minute biological entities or chemical reactions enlarged.
- ***Exploration:*** This also includes exploring new ideas that might be impossible or too dangerous to approach in reality like nuclear explosions (Joseph, 2007).

Johnson & Wales University demonstrates these concepts through BLAST, a scientific ballooning project committed to understanding the origins of the universe. Students work with practicing scientists to translate the complexity of scientific ballooning into SL. They design, build, and operate the balloons (Mason, 2007).

Copyright © 2011, IGI Global. Copying or distributing in print or electronic forms without written permission of IGI Global is prohibited.

Existence

The nature of presence as a user in 3D VLEs differs entirely from real life, enriching the e-learning process via the following concept.

As Benefit Over Real Life Learning

• *Distributed/ co-present existence:* 3D VLEs enable submergence within them. This is due to the fact that they are spaces populated by users, who are themselves both distributed (their physical bodies are spread out all over the world) and co-present (their avatars are in the same space) (Thomas & Brown, 2009).

Communication

Contact methods during e-learning sessions between disabled students and students in general, and transportation between locations, are innovative techniques for delivering education within 3DVLEs, characterized by the consequent concepts coded as follows.

Concepts as Supplement to Real Life Education

• *Alternative communication support:* There are also benefits from using alternative communication support for 3D VLEs via voice in the virtual world, voice over IP, or by means of a conferencing tool (Dickey, 2005).
• *Ease of guest lecturing:* Guest speakers can also be invited in to attend lectures, seminars or conferences without their actual physical presence (Kujawski, 2007).

Concepts as Benefit over Real Life Learning

• *Public and private messaging:* Students with disabilities can communicate via text if they have hearing impairments or voice if they have visual or upper limb motor impairment that prevents them from writing. Using text communication they can ask confidentially whenever they please, without interrupting others, by corresponding with classmates or teacher via private messaging channels, thus overcoming shyness (Calongne, 2008). This is essential in interactive courses such as that conducted by Bradley University to coach its students in the qualitative research methodology field (SimTeach, 2009).

Copyright © 2011, IGI Global. Copying or distributing in print or electronic forms without written permission of IGI Global is prohibited.

- *Teleporting* can be done in seconds between different 3D sites, whether replicas of existing places and countries or representations of historical simulations e.g. "Paris 1900" in SL (Joseph, 2007). This is extremely important for students with disabilities in the "real-life" who are often confined to their place due to their disability and unable to travel, venture or experience different places in the world whether touristic or scientific or even to attend meetings, exams, conferences, perform jobs in remote areas etc. A successful example introduced by Johnson and Wales University was creating "virtual Morocco" to provide an immersive experience that educates about Moroccan culture while enticing students to teleport to it, develop technical prototypes on an unfamiliar platform like SL, and communicate with partners on another continent and across language barriers (Mason, 2007).

Educational Aids

additional methods and objects are available within 3D VLEs to assist delivery of e-learning for students with challenges, including the ensuing concepts grouped as follows.

Concepts as Supplement to Real Life Education

- *Ease of snapshots:* the simplicity of recording pictures/ snapshots within e.g. SL allows for future reference to events in lectures and workshops etc. (Rickenbacker, 2009). For example University of Kansas hosted its first online International Media festival in SL featuring works by art students around the globe, with live interactive lectures. These events required extensive imagery recording as a form of documentation (Lombardi & McCahill, 2004).

Concepts as Benefit over 2D VLES

- *Cheap file upload* is also available for presentations, images etc. only requiring inexpensive payment per file for usage within a 3D VLE (Burton, 2006).
- *Streaming music* can also be used by instructors during live lectures unlike in 2D VLEs (Burton, 2006).
- *Presentations on 3D objects:* Furthermore presentation images and streaming videos can be placed on cubical objects and presented to students in a more interesting manner than 2D environments (Burton, 2006). Professors from Texas A & M University upload photographs, students' work, streaming video, written projects and presentations to conduct Second Life classes, provide tutorials, assign projects and achieve research related to digital visual

Copyright © 2011, IGI Global. Copying or distributing in print or electronic forms without written permission of IGI Global is prohibited.

culture (Kujawski, 2007), e.g. Oxford University's virtual First World War Poetry Digital Archive inside SL dedicated to honoring classical works and poems connected to this era, including audio and video interactive tools and tutorials for students (Elen, 2009).

- *Sandboxes to practice building* are used freely by students and instructors in 3D VLEs like Second Life (Joseph, 2007). Students from Colorado Technical University learn basic virtual world building and texturing skills, develop user-interface prototypes, design usability experiments, and conduct usability evaluations with the help of sandboxes in Second Life. The virtual world classroom becomes an open space version of a usability lab (Calongne, 2008).
- *Supporting all learning styles:* Some people learn best by listening to course content, others by seeing and visualizing, and some using a hands-on approach. In case of students with disabilities more than one learning style may be required to best convey educational concepts and material. In 3D VLEs, a mix of content and activity supports all learning styles: auditory, visual, and kinesthetic (Kujawski, 2007).
- *3D learning stations and objects:* Learning stations "in-world" can be designed to provide content to students who are absent or who need extra time to study and reflect. Students with disabilities can take note cards easily by touching 3D objects, listen to podcasts, or watch streaming video covering lesson material without leaving the vicinity of their home or risking undesirable contact or conflict with others. Although this ability is also obtainable in online course management systems and websites (2D VLEs), the shared nature of an avatar interacting with an object and seeing 3D simulations of the content come to life, is more powerful (Calongne, 2008).

This is exemplified in stations offered by Texas A&M University for students to receive assignments written on note cards along paths on the SL campus (Michels, 2008).

Concepts as Benefit over Real Life Learning

- *Session message logs:* Instant communication messages can be saved as logs for future reference of lectures (Calongne, 2008).
- *Online assignment submission:* Students can also submit assignments in the form of note cards easily to teacher by dropping it over his avatar or profile (Burton, 2006).
- *Program execution in linden language:* Submission of a program assignment can be done in SL Linden scripting language (LSL) to see the program

Copyright © 2011, IGI Global. Copying or distributing in print or electronic forms without written permission of IGI Global is prohibited.

run directly in the environment and working. The advantage is that LSL is easy to learn for its similarity to Java and other programming languages like C# (Icaza, 2008).

Students from University of Florida, for example, created programs represented in 3D using scripting languages like LSL, Java, Python and Lisp (Mason, 2007).

- *3D architectural assignments* can moreover be submitted in a virtual environment as 3D models that can be rotated around or entered inside. Students can create any structure, using built-in tools to construct their ideas as a form of virtual sketching. These 3D objects and models help students express ideas and offer a context for discussion during class projects (Calongne, 2008). Architecture students from University of Colorado are an example of utilizing SL to design buildings (Michels, 2008).
- *Engagement in real world issues* is another experience, undergone by students from University of South Australia. Interacting with their experimental clients through SL provides insight into the real world through virtual work encounters i.e. by experiential learning (Wood, 2009). Furthermore Texas A&M University engages students in SL with significant questions about real-life and virtual associations (Michels, 2008).

Interaction

Additionally, different types of networking options between disabled users are offered in 3DVLEs, characterized by the following concepts.

As Supplement To Real Life Education

- *Social spaces* existing within 3D VLEs provide successful shared communities. These are also *cultural spaces* opening up opportunities to truly engage and communicate with others to learn about different customs, behaviors and ethnicities (Joseph, 2007). This is an option not readily available for students whose disabilities hamper their movement, make them too withdrawn from facing real society, give them difficulties in talking or communicating, or sometimes whose disabilities might be intimidating in real life for others to encourage them to correspond with them. In SL and other virtual worlds all of these inhibitions disappear by communication through avatars.

Copyright © 2011, IGI Global. Copying or distributing in print or electronic forms without written permission of IGI Global is prohibited.

Hong Kong Polytechnic University uses SL to help 1st year students get acquainted with university life and adjust to the transition from high school, offering a variety of interpersonal, learning and self-management ideas to help excel in their undergraduate life (SimTeach, 2009).

As Benefit Over Real Life Learning

- *Networks of distant users* can be created for the sharing of skills and knowledge through blogs, wikis and knowledge repositories that can be opened within a 3D VLE window during active e-learning sessions (Butler & White, 2008).
- *Network evolution and Future group work:* Any network within a 3D VLE can develop and increase in size with time to include people from many backgrounds or collaborative universities (Butler & White, 2008). An example of this is the launch of Virtual Ability Island, an environment in Second Life created by the Alliance Library System (ALS) and Virtual Ability, Inc. (VAI) to help residents with disabilities find fellowship, training and education (Smith, 2009).
- *Instructor practical role shift:* In virtual worlds, the instructor's role shifts from being the "sage on the stage" to being the domain specialist or facilitator who motivates and manages discovery while providing organization, guidance, feedback, and assessment without being the main focus of the session (Calongne, 2008).

A successful implementation at Harvard University (Law School) involved building a court room in SL for students to practice their advocacy skills, but without the intimidation from similar real-life spaces. Under the supervision of their professors, simulations of trials were conducted on Berkman Island in SL. Weekly office hours were also held on SL to discuss material and homework with teachers, or simply socialize with classmates & faculty (Nesson, 2007; Shepherd, 2007).

Security

User identity protection and account safety are vital issues within 3D VLEs, as demonstrated by the following concepts.

Copyright © 2011, IGI Global. Copying or distributing in print or electronic forms without written permission of IGI Global is prohibited.

As Supplement To Real Life Education

- *Anonymity safety*: The sense of safety through anonymity of a user's identity can encourage students to experiment in ways not possible offline (Joseph, 2007). This is especially useful for disabled users who are unable to do certain activities in the physical world due to their disabilities e.g. dancing, rock climbing etc. without uncovering their true identity in "real-life".
- *Username & password*: Requirement of access permissions is similar in 2D and 3D VLEs – both environments necessitate authorization of the participant in the form of a user name and password. Furthermore each educational institution can restrict usage of its premises within a 3D VLE to only specified lists of students thus ensuring security (Robbins, 2007).
- *Free registration* to 3D VLEs is available for normal users e.g. students. Premium (paid) access is only for organizations like universities to purchase lands and build their personalized virtual campuses (Butler & White, 2008).

2. Output

The degree of productivity of courses within 3D VLEs can be assessed through the following concepts.

As Benefit Over 2D Virtual Learning Environments

- *Immediate instructor feedback* within the synchronous class experience in a 3D VLE allows for engaging interaction and expression while drafting ideas and conducting activities (Calongne, 2008).
- *Early assessment of course* can be performed by students since the learning process and measurement instruments are observable. This allows immediate in-course enhancement and spending less time in critically assessing a course after it ends (Calongne, 2008), e.g. The Management School at Edinburgh University UK, relies heavily on instructor feedback and assessment issues for its MBA courses delivered in SL (Nesson, 2007).

Psychological Support

Moral and psychological support provided for both students with disabilities and the people in close contact with them is an important aspect of consideration in virtual worlds. It is manifested in the following concepts.

Copyright © 2011, IGI Global. Copying or distributing in print or electronic forms without written permission of IGI Global is prohibited.

Concepts As Benefit Over 2D VLEs and Real Life Education

- *Parental Advice:* "Contact a Family" is a charitable organization that has an existence in Second Life and is dedicated to helping parents of disabled children access services that can help them deal with their children's disabilities and educate them. Parents are given a lot of useful information at any time of the day, and share experiences with others in similar situations thus providing moral support and exchange of ideas. This is vital for parents who do not have the luxury of leaving the house to attend such events in real life due to supervision of their disabled children (Parker, 2008).
- *Emotional support* is one of the major advantages of immersion inside virtual worlds by disabled students and users in general. An enhanced sense of community, equal environment, disclosure, an outlet for creativity, constructive use of time working with various entities within SL and even just having 24/7 contacts is an extreme moral boost for those who are unable to achieve that in the physical world. It can be considered a form of medical treatment (Yifenghu, 2010; Later & Milena, 2009).
- *Pain Management:* virtual environments are also a good pain management tool. It helps people with disabilities not to "escape into fantasy", but rather "escape from persecution." Therefore by creating a meditative state through focusing on an activity in a virtual world like SL, this can help ease the pain of the disabled user (Epstein, 2008).

Educational Strategies

3D learning environments can provide innovative instructional techniques, methods or archetypes for learning facilitation (Scopes & Lesley, 2009) including:

Concepts as Benefit over 2D VLEs

- *Classroom emulation* allows for re-creation of the physical classroom environment within the 3D world. The advantage of this method is achieving familiarity with the virtual space because of its analogy with the real-life space. This provides disabled students with a sense of connection through the classroom representation (Scopes & Lesley, 2009), as can be observed by the immersion experience of Texas A&M University in SL, teaching reading competency in reality depicted learning spaces (Michels, 2008). Accessibility elements of design can also be added to the classrooms to add to the sense of comfort and familiarity of the learning space to the disabled students, even

Copyright © 2011, IGI Global. Copying or distributing in print or electronic forms without written permission of IGI Global is prohibited.

though their avatars may not be disabled or need the accessibility elements in the virtual world.

- *Game based learning - treasure, scavenger hunts:* With little time and a lot of content to cover, one way to realize effective learning is to use game-based techniques to pique students' interest especially with the resemblance in appearance of 3D VLEs with game settings (Calongne, 2008). Examples of such game metaphors are treasure or scavenger hunts which provide opportunities to explore areas. This could e.g. be used to orient students with how a campus is laid out (Scopes & Lesley, 2009). A software design class from Colorado Technical University, for example, created a 3D game maze and populated it with traps, sensors, flags, a scoreboard, treasures, and other game features, then played the game on the last night of class as a form of testing. These students were so immersed in the learning experience they didn't realize they had accomplished goals of several classes in a single term (Calongne, 2008). This movement-based activity for example would be impossible for students with mobility disabilities to join in "real life".

- *Role play:* enacting or assuming an alternate character to oneself is a widely employed learning technique which can also occur virtually within a 3D VLE. This virtuality might remove some of the traditional hindrances and obstacles of performing face-to-face role plays especially with the presence of disabilities, e.g. it's easier to dress the avatar in a variety of clothes, be placed in the right imaginary situation, be given the right tools and not be shy to participate. This enhances learning because students are encouraged to use all their skills and abilities to impersonate the role play presented to them (Scopes & Lesley, 2009). One example of class role-play represents literature activity in which students enact the courtroom scene from John Steinbeck's Of Mice and Men, to benefit from this social learning environment (Calongne, 2008).

- *Guided Tours* are used to show learners in a 3D synchronous environment the location of items and features within an area. A tour can be led by the instructor or it could be a pre-programmed item the avatar carries with him that takes him on a virtual "guided tour" without the need for a live person. E.g. a tour of countries or historical buildings or battle fields or forts or a tour inside a blood capillary or volcano where the learners appear to be diminished to a tiny size to experience areas they could not otherwise travel to (Scopes & Lesley, 2009), like project "Virtual Morocco" created by Johnson and Wales University described earlier (Mason, 2007).

- *Conceptual Orienting:* learning to create plans, e.g. for business. This entails providing the student with examples and non-examples of a concept and then allowing him to determine the attributes that do and do not apply to the con-

Copyright © 2011, IGI Global. Copying or distributing in print or electronic forms without written permission of IGI Global is prohibited.

cept. The procedure of side-by-side contrast allows a student to identify and apply concepts in a multitude of environments and do a mental comparison through the capability of instantaneously moving from one site to another (Scopes & Lesley, 2009). As an example, University of Houston architecture students build business plans in the SL virtual world and subject their models to the forces of SL's free market (Michels, 2008).

- *Operational Application:* This is "learning by doing" in the virtual environment. Students must follow the regulations and constraints of the physical world to achieve a goal. The facilitator monitors the students and then makes remarks or recommendations. This could be fixing a piece of equipment, trouble shooting a computer network, performing a virtual experiment or repairing a car (Scopes & Lesley, 2009). This can be extremely helpful for hand-on training for students with disabilities who are unable to achieve similar training physically.
- *Joint Co-Creation:* This is when more than one person collaboratively craft items within the 3D world. This procedure teaches teamwork, cooperation and sheds light on benefits and pitfalls of group work (Scopes & Lesley, 2009). This is again vital for disabled users who due to disability might not be able to change location in order to engage in group or team work.

An innovative group work approach adopted by St George's, University of London and Kingston University was presenting paramedic students with critical patient emergency scenarios on the streets "inworld". The students then have to collaborate in synchronous teams taking rapid decisions to check a dummy avatar's vital signs e.g. pulse, and apply preliminary treatment e.g. dressing wounds, oxygen masks, administering drugs, setting GPS in ambulance etc. Their submitted reports in virtual hospital are then mailed to their real-life instructor. This educational approach solves the problem of rarity of critical cases in reality to practice on, and relieves stress from risk of trying out incorrect remedial techniques in reality (Online Nursing, 2008).

- *Critical Incident involvement:* students are positioned into an environment or dilemma comparable to the real situation, where they have to use their previous knowledge to resolve a problem. For example a student can be placed into the heart of a disaster like the aftermath of a hurricane, earthquake, car accident or into a blazing building (Scopes & Lesley, 2009) which is a situation not possible to create in "real life" for students with disabilities.

Copyright © 2011, IGI Global. Copying or distributing in print or electronic forms without written permission of IGI Global is prohibited.

Concepts as Benefit over Real Life Learning:

- *Practical training:* Students get the chance to be given real life situations to train at within a 3D VLE allows them to brainstorm together (Online Nursing, 2008).

University of Kansas teaches medical and nurse training in Second Life, including how to deal with different equipment, studying anatomy of patients and attaching different devices to them. Moreover, physical therapy and occupational therapy students use Second Life to evaluate handicap hazards in virtual homes, recommend improvements and apply changes. The simulation records all steps of the process, which are then sent to the instructor (Skiba, 2007).

Performance

Speed, efficiency, quality of technical connectivity and delivery issues online while using 3D VLEs for e-learning are evident through the presence of the following concepts as a supplement to delivering real life Education.

As Benefit over Real Life Learning

- *Faster MONO virtual machine:* on August 29, 2008, the entire production grid of SL was updated to being able to use the Mono Virtual Machine (VM). The LSL scripting language remains, but executing on the Mono VM gives up to 220 times speed increase, reduced lag and improved stability (Icaza, 2008).
- *Dot-net languages' support:* An additional benefit is that any dot-net language that compiles to the Mono VM can be uploaded to execute in SL. This will enable any program of a student to be seen working immediately by an instructor on submission (Icaza, 2008).

Setting

The importance of the surrounding environmental arrangement and background settings of the spaces, where educational sessions are held within 3D VLEs, constitutes the following concepts as benefit over real-life physical learning conditions.

Copyright © 2011, IGI Global. Copying or distributing in print or electronic forms without written permission of IGI Global is prohibited.

As Benefit over Real Life Learning

- *Untraditional class settings,* including non confinement to having chairs facing forwards, helps revolutionize to capture students' attention by moving freely within the learning environment, putting chairs or sitting in any position without affecting the view (Dickey, 2005). Examples of untraditional classrooms are on display within the Art Department at the University of Kansas featuring a lecture hall, open air studios, a film production area and an interactive gallery of sculpture, animation, game creation and performance arts (Lawrence, 2009).
- *Easy class management* can be attained, for few problems can arise from noisy interruptions of students. This is because communication is either text-based, or even with audio transmissions only one person can talk on the system at a time. Instructors can also block or remove inappropriately behaving students (Burton, 2006).

Perspective

The viewpoint and angles of perception of a user within a virtual 3D space are essential factors signified by the consequent concepts encoded as follows.

As Benefit over 2D Virtual Learning Environments

- *Customization and conceptual imagination of avatar:* As mentioned before, alteration of the personal representative avatar in the virtual world allows for the user's identification with it. Conceptual blending also provides further insight into the role of imagination e.g. using talking animal avatars. One can change his or her gender, race, and even species (Joseph, 2007).

Students from Colorado Technical University commented that "the sense of presence and customization of avatars are high on the list of priorities for learning and participating in virtual world classes", despite the fact that it took time for them to modify their avatars and to master communication, expressing emotion and gesturing (Calongne,2008).

- *Virtual reality versus virtual world view:* The option of changing between virtual reality view (in 1st person by looking through the eyes of the avatar within the environment) or as a virtual world view (in 3rd person by watching the avatar move) can change the feeling of immersion in the environment

Copyright © 2011, IGI Global. Copying or distributing in print or electronic forms without written permission of IGI Global is prohibited.

giving a more dynamic perspective for the student during an e-learning session (Dickey, 2005).

- *Adjusting cameras and lighting:* This can be done by adjusting cameras/lighting etc within the 3D environment to change the angle of perception of the real user within the 3D VLE despite the position and direction of the avatar (Rickenbacker, 2009).
- *Day and night settings* can also be customized within a 3D VLE according to users' preferences e.g. to be dusk, dawn, midday, to help learn in the most idealistic and comfortable surroundings possible (Robbins, 2007). This is a vital option for students with visual disorders who require certain colors or brightness for the background lighting of the environment in order for the interface to be seen comfortably by the "real-life" student. Furthermore, users with physical medical conditions can benefit from the same option, for example a testimonial from inside SL recorded a case of a user with migraines who could only operate comfortably if the background lighting settings were adjusted to midnight.

An example of teaching by adjusting viewpoints inside Second Life can be seen through the virtual historic and contemporary worlds' visit of students, at the University of Texas, inside enlarged replicas of Vincent van Gogh's Starry Night, the cave paintings in Lascaux and Gotham City--the home of Batman (Kujawski, 2007).

- *Attractive 3D graphical setting:* The three-dimensional (3D) graphical settings themselves are very attractive and vivid for users. The dominant content form of a 3D VLE is imagery thus making it an image-based environment (Robbins, 2007) which is suitable for most students with disabilities.

As Benefit over Real Life Learning

- *Viewing and hearing from any position:* Viewing and hearing any part of the learning space from any angle with clarity, regardless of the position of the avatar (even if seated behind the lecturer), eliminates the need, like in real-life, to sit near an instructor to see him properly or find acoustic solutions for hearing a lecture conveniently (Dickey, 2005), which is a suitable solution for students with manual dexterity disabilities. These are disabilities which render them unable to maneuver their position adequately and easily inside the virtual world.

An application of this feature can be seen with Buffalo State College fashion design students (Polvinen, 2007) who manage host fashion shows in SL without have to

Copyright © 2011, IGI Global. Copying or distributing in print or electronic forms without written permission of IGI Global is prohibited.

give consideration to positioning all spectator avatars near the runway for proper viewing.

Locations

There are multitudes of places to visit and learn from in 3D VLEs as benefit over real life learning places.

As Benefit over Real Life Learning

- *Imaginary, dangerous, historical or unreachable places:* Students with disabilities are able to examine and explore a variety of places that are imaginary or difficult to reach or teach in reality e.g. on the top of a mountain, in outer space, bottom of the ocean, representations of historic or extinct civilizations, travelling between continents during the same session thus saving time and money to do so in reality, etc (Joseph, 2007). Texas University, for example, holds classes on a tropical island in Second Life (Michels, 2008).

In an attempt to summarize the above advantageous themes and sub-concepts, the authors have examined each one of them under the prism of different stages in the lifecycle of a person's experience in a virtual world. From the initial creation of a virtual world environment and the design of the user's avatar, to the actions of this avatar specifying its behavior and integration with the entire virtual world community formulated, some clear stages can be identified. The authors perceive the learning experience in a virtual world as a journey that begins with a promise made by the virtual world designers when an environment is designed to serve certain predefined aims and an overall purpose. The promise made is in the form of the SL Island and its contents, and can be described as an allegiance to provide a unique user/learner experience. The users accept the promise by engaging in creating their own avatars and joining this virtual world. When the promise is kept and the learning experience is delivered according to the objectives of the designers as well as the expectations of its users then both needs and the designer aspirations amalgamate in a successful blend.

The three stages identified in this process can be defined as:

A. Conception – at this stage the early ideas of how the learning environment should be and provide, are used to form the virtual world in accordance to any identified requirements and specifications provided. At this stage each user becomes a virtual world entity through his/her avatar and participates in a new learning relationship with everyone else who enters the virtual world

Copyright © 2011, IGI Global. Copying or distributing in print or electronic forms without written permission of IGI Global is prohibited.

and joins the same learning experiences. At this stage the virtual world is still in its infant stage and key concepts are still reconsidered while the dynamics of the learning relationships are defined.

The advantageous themes included in this stage are (i) disability support, (ii) educational aids, (iii) psychological support and (iv) educational strategies (see Table 2).

B.   Action – this second stage is in-wrought with the behavioral patterns of the learners and how these may declare patterns of use for each element designed as part of the virtual world. The action stage is primarily concerned with the behavior expressed by learners in the virtual world as well as selected behavioral patterns that are either expected or encouraged by the designers. In addition, this stage allows room for reassessing the success criteria for the learning experience and prioritizes any changes required for the learning process as well as any relating design issues.

The advantageous themes included in this stage are (i) involvement, (ii) activities, (iii) communication, (iv) interaction, (v) output and (vi) performance (see Table 3).

C.   Fusion – this final stage is analogous to the maturity of the learning relationship in the virtual world. The parameters involved are finalized after experiencing a continuous development of the learning relationship till the point that learners become part of the virtual world and the virtual world itself becomes the learning experience. After this stage the established community does not behave as a group of learning individuals but rather as a set of symbiotic learning entities.

The advantageous themes included in this stage are (i) existence, (ii) security, (iii) setting, (iv) perspective and (v) locations (see Table 4).

From Table 2, it can be deduced that most themes associated with the Conception stage relate to the benefits offered by virtual worlds in comparison to 2D VLE systems. Most efforts attempt to support functionality and usability aspects of the learning environment and improve the learning experience in terms of the capabilities offered to the users/learners.

Table 3 shows the behavioral Action stage, it seems that an equilibrium has been achieved in arranging themes and sub-concepts under the three different categories. Most effort seem to be directed towards establishing an improvement on the learning and educational experiences obtained in real life.

Copyright © 2011, IGI Global. Copying or distributing in print or electronic forms without written permission of IGI Global is prohibited.

Table 2. Conception stage: Themes and sub-concepts

As supplement to real life education	As benefit over 2D VLE	As benefit over real life learning
	Disability Support	

	• Autism Management
	  (+) providing additional communication means
	  (-) using improper stimuli
	• Visual Impairment Management
	  (+) allowing movement based on coordinated directions
	  (-) using the interface becomes the core task
	• Hearing Impairment Management
	  (+) Providing text alternatives
	  (-) Ensuring use of audio is constrained
	• Mobility Impairment Management
	  (+) Allowing mobility
	  (-) Requiring additional devices
	• Career Management
	  (+) Generating career opportunities
	  (-) Leading to potential isolation	

	Educational Aids	

• Ease of Snapshots
  (+) Offering a visual diary
  (-) Filtering which snapshots can be taken is not possible
	- Cheap File Upload
	  (+) Offering an affordable media exchange tool
	  (-) Lacking the incentive to prioritize content
	- Streaming Music
	  (+) Allowing audio stimulation
	  (-) Contradicting the hearing impairment management
	- Presentations on 3D Objects
	  (+) Offering imaginative media
	  (-) Contradicting the hearing impairment management
	- Sandboxes to Practice Building
	  (+) Practicing design skills
	  (-) Controlling the usability evaluation variables is difficult
	- Supporting All Learning Styles
	  (+) Being an adaptable VLE
	  (-) Using mainly VARK model
	- 3D Learning Stations and Objects
	  (+) Catching up with the class
	  (-) Offering route to escape synchronous sessions
		- Session Message Logs
		  (+) Providing a text based diary
		  (-) Lacking ability to backtrack
		- Online Assignment Submission
		  (+) Reducing time delays
		  (-) Supporting formative feedback
		- Program Execution in Linden Language
		  (+) Embedding information in the virtual world
		  (-) Learning unnecessary skills
		- 3D Architectural Assignments
		  (+) Allowing 3D manipulation
		  (-) Shifting from 2D techniques
		- Engagement in Real World Issues
		  (+) Having a reality check
		  (-) Misunderstanding the critical aspects of such work

continued on following page

As shown in the Table 4, the maturity Fusion stage of the virtual world and the 3DVLE seems to deal with all three aspects (life education, life learning and 2D VLE) but with minimum overlapping between the various themes. It seems that distinct themes and sub-concepts deal with specific issues of the learning experience.

Copyright © 2011, IGI Global. Copying or distributing in print or electronic forms without written permission of IGI Global is prohibited.

Table 2. continued

As supple-ment to real life education	As benefit over 2D VLE	As benefit over real life learning
	Psychological Support	
	- Parental Advice (+) Allowing access to additional support means (-) Challenging the traditional pathways for such support - Emotional Support (+) Getting community support (-) Antagonizing other means for such support - Pain Management (+) Maintaining a realistic view of the situation (-) Detaching from the real world	
	Educational Strategies	
	- Classroom Emulation (+) Recreating learning spaces (-) Loosing the respect for the environment - Game Based Learning (+) Offering a more informal setting (-) Adopting game like behavior - Role Play (+) Allowing to overcome communication barriers (-) Blaring the original roles - Guided Tours (+) Providing induction support (-) Removing the joy of exploration - Conceptual Orienting (+) Supporting conceptual modeling (-) Understanding how concepts affect real life architecture design - Operational Application (+) Assessing practical skills (-) Lacking real life impact appreciation - Joint Co-Creation (+) Establishing peer support (-) Collaborating must always be synchronous - Critical Incident Involvement (+) Practicing relevant skills (-) Viewing scenario as a game	- Practical training (+) Practicing necessary skills (-) Resorting primarily on peer support

DISADVANTAGEOUS THEMES AND SUB-CONCEPTS OF LEARNING IN 3D VLES

Contrary to the preceding assertions elaborated so far within this research, the following four categories are the perceived high level disadvantageous themes of delivering e-learning within 3DVLEs derived using the grounded theory methods described earlier.

Copyright © 2011, IGI Global. Copying or distributing in print or electronic forms without written permission of IGI Global is prohibited.

Table 3. Action stage: Themes and sub-concepts

As supplement to real life education	As benefit over 2D VLE	As benefit over real life learning
Involvement		
- Active student roles (+) Increasing engagement (+) Supporting hyperkinetic persons	- Object ownership (+) Creating an interface identity (-) Intimidating learning curve - Embodiment and Sense of Belonging (+) Establishing a typical presence (-) Shifting between the avatar and real life presence - Sense of Presence (+) Belonging to the community (-) Accepting the virtual reality of the SL community	
Activities		
• Experimentation (+) Increasing the boundaries of feasible actions (-) Obtaining only the virtual reality aspect of senses • Exploration (+) Allowing to broaden experiential horizons (-) Feeling the effects of the aftermath after logging off		
Communication		
• Alternative Communication Support (+) Establishing a support network (-) Shifting between real life and SL support means • Ease of Guest Lecturing (+) Increasing the knowledge base on offer (-) Blaring the boundaries of the constructivist paradigm		• Public and Private Messaging (+) Communicating in private (-) Challenging to maintain focus • Teleporting (+) Seamless boundary free environment (-) Affecting synchronous sessions

continued on following page

Connectivity Problems

An apparent problem experienced by users of virtual worlds like Second Life is the lag in service or "rezzing" (appearance of items inside the virtual world). Smooth online server connections with 3D VLEs are not always available since they necessitate:

Copyright © 2011, IGI Global. Copying or distributing in print or electronic forms without written permission of IGI Global is prohibited.

Table 3. continued

As supplement to real life education	As benefit over 2D VLE	As benefit over real life learning
Interaction		

• Social Spaces
    (+) Engaging with peers and the wider community
    (-) Opening up to dangers of social networking
		• Networks of Distant Users
		    (+) Accessing resources and different perspectives
		    (-) Clashing priorities and agendas
		• Network Evolution and Future Group Work
		    (+) Allowing the enlargement of the class
		    (-) Maintaining a network of SL friends
		• Instructor Practical Role Shift
		    (+) Having the lecturer as a helper
		    (-) Fading notion of respect

Output		

	• Immediate Instructor Feedback
	    (+) Reducing delay & vague support
	    (-) Lacking opportunity to reflect
	• Early Assessment of Course
	    (+) Providing formative feedback
	    (-) Making early assumptions	

Performance		

• Faster MONO Virtual Machine
    (+) Supporting technology
    (-) Proprietor based platform
• Do-net Languages' Support
    (+) Supporting technology
    (-) Proprietor based platform		

- ***High connectivity requirements:*** Dial-up access is inadequate for connectivity with online 3D virtual worlds like Second Life (Butler & White, 2008).
- ***Limited internet quotas:*** For practical and financial reasons, universities commonly limit student internet access by imposing quotas. Access to virtual worlds for synchronous classes, or extended periods required for creating educational models, such as virtual landscaping and orientation to Second Life, can quickly drain standard access quotas (Butler & White, 2008).

Copyright © 2011, IGI Global. Copying or distributing in print or electronic forms without written permission of IGI Global is prohibited.

Table 4. Fusion stage: Themes and sub-concepts

As supplement to real life education	As benefit over 2D VLE	As benefit over real life learning
Existence		
		- Distributed/ Co-present Existence (+) Submerging within the VLE (-) Confusing reality
Security		
• Anonymity Safety (+) Allowing anonymous contributions (-) Maintaining control of sessions • Username & Password (+) Allowing a secure environment (-) Limiting access to institutional users • Free Registration (+) Allowing free access (-) Being crowded by random, casual users		
Setting		
		• Untraditional Class Settings (+) Allowing unconventional learning and creativity (-) Requiring a steep learning curve • Easy Class Management (+) Controlling class activities (-) Maintaining asynchronous class management

continued on following page

Expenses

Financial requirements to setup and maintain an existence on a 3D VLE can be quite high. Involvement in Second Life, for example, requires a modest investment of funds by the university to establish an ongoing base of operation and premium account to assist with distribution of 'in world' currency. Staff and students however are not required to make a monetary investment. Return from this investment may be measured in terms of learning experience afforded to students and professional development of staff in the skills and pedagogy associated with the technology (Butler & White, 2008).

Copyright © 2011, IGI Global. Copying or distributing in print or electronic forms without written permission of IGI Global is prohibited.

Table 4. continued

Perspective		

	• Customization and Conceptual Imagination of Avatar
	  (+) Personalizing the look and feel
	  (-) Moving away from reality
	• Virtual Reality Versus Virtual World View
	  (+) Enabling users to achieve the unthinkable
	  (-) Confusing the real and virtual
	• Adjusting Cameras and Lighting
	  (+) Customizing the interface
	  (-) Differentiating own experience of the environment
	• Day and Night Settings
	  (+) Choosing own settings
	  (-) Moving away from reality
	• Attractive 3D Graphical Setting
	  (+) Using familiar gaming interfaces
	  (-) Focusing too much on interface
		• Viewing and hearing from any position
		  (+) Allowing truly customizable experience
		  (-) Overlapping of avatars

Locations		

		• Imaginary, dangerous, historical or unreachable places
		  (+) Allowing experiences not possible in real life
		  (-) Obtaining designer's perception of settings

Prerequisites

Previous technological knowledge of users can be an asset for using a 3D VLE easily. Students familiar with 3D gaming environments do not need much orientation to utilize 3D VLEs unlike novice users to technology. Also, the text-based nature of 3D VLES sometimes does not favor every student's learning style and physical abilities especially if there are manual dexterity problems, since text typing requires that its participants have fast fingers. This is further aggravated by what educators refer to as loss of face-face contact between instructors and students, which is important for visual learners in particular. However, many online learners are familiar with the principles of an alternative online social environment, one that is not text-based but instead predominately visual – e.g. the immersive, interactive online game environments which lessens from the gravity of the previously mentioned disadvantages (Lombardi & McCahill, 2004).

Copyright © 2011, IGI Global. Copying or distributing in print or electronic forms without written permission of IGI Global is prohibited.

3D Graphical Setting

As mentioned earlier, the dominant content form of a 3D virtual learning environment is imagery thus making it an image-based environment (Robbins, 2007). This renders it unsuitable for students with visual disabilities who require customized interfaces in order to operate inside virtual worlds. An example of an interface is "Radegast Metaverse Client", which is a text-based alternative for accessing Second Life. It is proving to be very useful for people with disabilities because of speech plugins and keyboard enhancements (Radegast, 2010).

ARCHITECTURAL REQUIREMENTS PROPOSED FOR DESIGN OF EDUCATIONAL FACILITIES FOR THE DISABLED

Method

In order to achieve best results from the above explicated advantages for delivering e-learning in 3D VLEs for disabled students, the environment must be subjected to the best possible design criteria that can ensure maximum accessibility, satisfaction and contentment of users from the environment to achieve a successful e-learning experience.

This study is part of an ongoing research to determine the optimum architectural design elements of educational facilities that can be used to realize highest participation, assimilation and enjoyment of students during their e-learning sessions in the 3D virtual learning space. The current study focuses on depicting the most desirable architectural design features suggested by students with disabilities to be utilized within their 3D learning spaces.

This was achieved by adopting a quantitative research approach comprising of a survey questionnaires containing open ended questions (Alarafi, 2008). The partaking sample of users consisted of 50 online participants all using Second Life as a 3D VLE and all having one or more type of disability. These were divided into the following categories which correspond to the different clusters of users utilising 3D virtual university campuses for e-learning sessions in general: 14% undergraduate students, 33% graduate students, and 53% adult learners and researchers. The purpose of the study was explained to them in an online general invitation to Second life educational lists, groups and educators' lists.

The open-ended questions were:

- What interior design aspects would you recommend in your 3D learning space? How do they make you feel (optional)?

Copyright © 2011, IGI Global. Copying or distributing in print or electronic forms without written permission of IGI Global is prohibited.

- What interior design aspects do you dislike most in 3D learning spaces? How do they make you feel (optional)?
- What exterior design aspects would you recommend in your 3D learning space? How do they make you feel (optional)?
- What exterior design aspects do you dislike most in 3D learning spaces? How do they make you feel (optional)?

The open ended questions were used to allow students to think freely with no inhibitions on their desires, thus opening up points for discussion that we as researchers might overlook and not specifically asked about within closed options questions.

RESULTS

Quantitative results were calculated from the conducted questionnaire described above. The resulting propositions offered by students and researchers, to enhance the interior and exterior design of learning spaces within 3D VLE university campuses, were grouped into 10 major categories as follows:

1. The architectural style (e.g. modern, classic, gothic) and shape of the building (e.g. circular, square, use of columns etc.)
2. Wall design, finishing and colours
3. External environment elements of design
4. Seating arrangements and shapes
5. Window styles, shapes and lighting intensity
6. Internal space design factors (e.g. dimensions)
7. Roof and ceiling design, finishing and colours
8. Floor design, finishing and colours
9. Circulation design specifications (e.g. stairs, corridor width etc.)
10. Entrance design (e.g. width, height, shape, doors, ease of accessibility etc.)

The above 10 categories represent all the design features of a 3D virtual educational building that are of interest to the disabled categories of students to provide satisfaction and contentment during an e-learning session within a 3D learning space. These are illustrated in the above Figure 3 which portrays the top 30 architectural design characteristics proposed or requested by students from all age groups to be present in their ideal 3D virtual learning environment (representing 65% of total suggested votes and features). As can be seen, the top 30 propositions are divided into 8 major categories, the highest achieving were those related to lighting, walls, internal circulation and environmental elements; whilst shape of space, floors, roofs,

Copyright © 2011, IGI Global. Copying or distributing in print or electronic forms without written permission of IGI Global is prohibited.

Figure 3. Highest 30 recommended architectural features of a learning space proposed by disabled learners

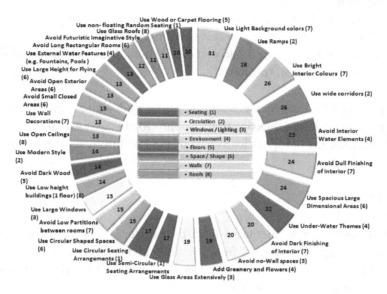

seating arrangements were less in demand, and those related to building entrance and style were non-existent within the highest 30 characteristics (although existing in the list of major categories). This can be attributed to the fact that the elements of space most seen directly at student's eye level are the lighting, walls, surrounding environment (e.g. water elements, greenery etc.), and also presence of accessibility elements like ramps, wide corridors, elevators have an impact on them and therefore demanded most despite their avatars being without disability in SL; whilst floors, ceilings and seats are below and above direct eye perspective, hence perceived and required less by students. As for building entrance and style, since these are outside the immediate learning space that the students take their e-learning session in and do not affect their manipulation "in-world", they are probably not remembered as essential categories for design by students.

On an individual element's basis, the following could be noticed. The highest recommended characteristic was presence of light interior colors, followed by spaciousness, ramps and usage of one floor single space building. This indicates that users with disabilities are highly conscious of usability requirements for design of their learning spaces above any other design requirements. As for building style, simple modern and plain classic styles were most preferred with no over decoration or imagination so as not to cause distraction for learners. Semi-circular or circular seating arrangements (along with circular shaped spaces) also seemed most agreeable for students. An unexpected finding was the fact that students recommended

Copyright © 2011, IGI Global. Copying or distributing in print or electronic forms without written permission of IGI Global is prohibited.

abundance of greenery, flowers and water elements (e.g. fountains, sea etc.) but surrounding their learning space more than inside of it, again so as not to cause distraction among them but rather comfort surrounding them.

In general, the fact that over 500 votes comprising almost 100 different design features in total were recommended by students i.e. almost 10 suggestions per student is definitive evidence that architectural design of the virtual learning space is important in disabled students' opinions.

RECOMMENDATIONS

The major problematic issue faced during this research was the scarcity of locating participants eligible for answering the survey used. Future recommendations can include conducting focus groups and individual interviews in a more qualitative approach to the research to delve into specific issues regarding requirements and needs of disabled students from the design of their learning spaces.

FUTURE RESEARCH

Since this study is part of an ongoing research to define best design practices for educational facilities within 3D virtual learning environments suitable for users with disabilities, the following strategic goals are subject to future research:

- Defining the propositions of students with disabilities based on the following categorizations: gender, type of disability, ethnicity, and field of education
- Measuring the effect of individual design elements of the 3D virtual learning space on the understanding, assimilation, participation and enjoyment of the disabled students during e-learning sessions
- Conducting interviews with 3D design professionals to depict their contribution towards the same goal of enhancing educational space design.

CONCLUSION

So far we have seen numerous pieces of research presenting virtual worlds as the means to support users with disabilities and the mechanism to overcome the obstacles of geographic dispersion, location and distance. In our work we have emphasized on the importance of 3DVLE applications in enhancing the learning experience of disabled students. In an attempt to integrate our work with previous

Copyright © 2011, IGI Global. Copying or distributing in print or electronic forms without written permission of IGI Global is prohibited.

research in virtual teams, tele-work and outsourcing we would recommend that 3DVLE applications should attempt to align (i) the solutions provided by virtual worlds in addressing learning needs along with (ii) the ones available for supporting mobility problems. The key factor is that 3DVLE may provide adequate support both for online learning and distance education activities as well as eliminating any obstacles relating to mobility difficulties. The potential benefits are numerous and span across various fields, offering possibilities even for virtual work and virtual businesses. A few years ago Mollman (2007) reported for CNN several cases where virtual worlds have provided clear benefits for the disabled. More specifically David Stone, a Harvard University scholar, argues that SL "offers the opportunity to those who are disabled to be productive members of the world economy by doing very useful work". Several examples, as seen earlier, have been presented where SL applications have offered work satisfaction, intellectual stimulation and professional as well as personal relationships. Blurring the line between real world and virtual worlds means that people with disabilities may experience the ability to contribute, the freedom and worth. After reviewing our current practices in SL and the existing virtual world we have established for some of our students, we are reviewing the priorities we have identified for the design of virtual world environments as well as the learning activities supported by SL. The authors' initial aim was to investigate the way architectural features as well as other environment factors may affect the learning experience provided by a 3DVLE. Following the recent findings of our investigation we have identified the following concerns that are likely to affect our research decisions in the immediate future. We envisage that design principles of 3DVLE applications will evolve so they can accommodate the needs of all user groups without heavily customizing their interfaces. This would allow us to provide a harmonized set of learning activities available to all members of our student cohorts, therefore providing a homogeneous learning experience. Furthermore the ability to design a learning environment, where any mobility or usability obstacles are dealt with prior to the engagement of the learners, should succeed in supporting disabled learners' engagement and integration.

REFERENCES

Alarifi, S. A. (2008). *An exploratory study of higher education virtual campuses in Second Life*. Nottingham, UK: University of Nottingham.

Black, K. (2007). *Flying with disability in Second Life*. Retrieved January 15, 2010, from https://lists.secondlife.com/ pipermail/ educators/ 2007-May/ 009309.html

Copyright © 2011, IGI Global. Copying or distributing in print or electronic forms without written permission of IGI Global is prohibited.

Burton, A. (2006). *Giving a Powerpoint presentation in Second Life*. Retrieved January 19, 2010, from http://oreilly.com/ pub/h/5239

Butler, D., & White, J. (2008). A slice of second life: Academics, support staff and students navigating a changing landscape, Hello! Where are you in the landscape of educational technology? In *Proceedings of ascilite*, Melbourne.

Calongne, C. M. (2008). Educational frontiers: Learning in a virtual world. *EDUCAUSE Review, 43*(5).

Carey, T. (2008). *Real life employment through Second Life*. Retrieved March 20, 2010, from http://disabilityvoicespace.org/ dnn/ Articles/ Education Employment/ Real Life Employment Through Second Life/ tabid/ 89/ Default.aspx

Cassidy, M. (2007). Flying with disability in second life. *Jesuit Communications Australia, 17*(8).

Dickey, M. D. (2005). Brave new (interactive) worlds: A review of the design affordances and constraints of two 3D virtual worlds as interactive learning environments. *Interactive Learning Environments, 13*, 121–137. doi:10.1080/10494820500173714

Elen, R. (2009). *Oxford University's virtual first World War site opens in Second Life*. Retrieved January 20, 2010, from http://brideswell.com/ content/ uncategorized/ oxford- universitys- virtual- first- world- war- site- opens- in- second- life/.

Epstein, F. (2008). Second Life is my wheelchair. *The Metaverse Journal*. Retrieved April 1, 2010, from http://www.metaverse journal.com/ 2008/ 09/ 19/ second- life- is- my- wheel chair/

Glaser, B. G. (1992). *Emergence vs forcing: Basics of grounded theory*. Mill Valley, CA: Sociology Press.

Glaser, B. G. (2001). *The grounded theory perspective: Conceptualization contrasted with description*. Mill Valley, CA: Sociology Press.

Glaser, B. G. (2002). *Private conversations in Paris*. Mill Valley, CA: Sociology Press.

Glaser, B. G., & Strauss, A. L. (1967). *The discovery of grounded theory: Strategies for qualitative research*. Aldine.

Hickey-Moody, A., & Wood, D. (2008). *Imagining otherwise: Deleuze, disability & Second Life. ANZCA08 Conference*. Wellington: Power and Place.

IBM. (2008). Virtual worlds user interface for the blind. Retrieved April 10, 2010, from http://services. alphaworks. ibm.com/ virtual worlds/

Copyright © 2011, IGI Global. Copying or distributing in print or electronic forms without written permission of IGI Global is prohibited.

Icaza, M. D. (2008). *Scripting with mono*. Mono-Project. Retrieved January 20, 2010, from http://www.mono- project.com/ Scripting_ With_ Mono

Information Solutions Group. (2008). *Disabled gamers comprise 20% of casual video game audience*. Retrieved September 28, 2009, from http://www.infosolutions group.com/ press_ release_ E.htm

Joseph, B. (2007). *Global Kids, Inc's best practices in using virtual worlds for education*. Second Life Education Workshop 2007, Part of the Second Life Community Convention, (pp. 7-14). Chicago, IL: WordPress.

Kay, J. (2009). *Educational uses of Second Life*. Retrieved March 3, 2009, from http://sleducation. wikispaces.com/ educational uses

Krueger, A., Ludwig, A., & Ludwig, D. (2009). *Universal design: Including everyone in virtual world design. Journal of Virtual Worlds Research- Universal Design, 2(3)*. Technology, Economy, and Standards.

Kujawski, J. (2007). *Learning isn't second notch in second life*. Texas A&M University College of Education and Human Development. Retrieved March 16, 2010, from http://tlac.tamu. edu/ articles/ learning_ isn_t_ second_ notch_in_ second_ life

Later, L., & Milena, D. (2009). *Proposal for the creation of a disability liasion*. Retrieved March 15, 2010, from http://jira.second life.com/ browse/ MISC-2867

Lawrence, K. (2009). Kansas University department of art enters the virtual world on Second Life. Retrieved January 17, 2010, from http://www.infozine.com/ news/ stories/ op/ stories View/ sid/32117/

Lombardi, J., & McCahill, M. P. (2004). Enabling social dimensions of learning through a persistent, unified, massively multi-user, and self-organizing virtual environment. *Proceedings of the Second International Conference on Creating, Connecting and Collaborating through Computing*, (pp. 166-172). Washington DC: IEEE.

Margaryan, A., & Littlejohn, A. (2008). *Are digital natives a myth or reality? Students' use of technologies for learning*. Retrieved December 16, 2009 from http:// www.academy. gcal.ac.uk/ anoush/ documents/ Digital Natives Myth Or Reality Margaryan And Little john- draft- 11208.pdf

Mason, H. (2007). *Experiential education in Second Life*. Second Life Education Workshop 2007, Part of Second Life Community Convention, (pp.14-19). Chicago, IL: WordPress.

Copyright © 2011, IGI Global. Copying or distributing in print or electronic forms without written permission of IGI Global is prohibited.

McCullough, C., & Beauchamp, M. (2009). *Proposal for the creation of a disability liasion*. Retrieved February 15, 2010, from http://jira.second life.com/ browse/ MISC-2867.

Michels, P. (2008). *Universities use Second Life to teach complex concepts*. Retrieved January 21, 2010, from http://www.govtech.com/ gt/252550? topic=118264

Mollman, S. (2007). *Online a virtual business option for disabled*. Retrieved January 25, 2010, from http://edition.cnn.com/ 2007/BUSINESS/ 07/10/ virtual. disabled/ index.html

Nesson, R. (2007). *Virtual worlds*. Harvard Extension School. Retrieved March 15, 2010, from http://www.eecs.harvard.edu/ ~nesson/e4/

Oblinger, D., & Oblinger, J. (2005). Is it age or IT: First steps towards understanding the net generation? In Oblinger, D., & Oblinger, J. (Eds.), *Educating the Net generation* (pp. 2.1–2.20). Boulder, CO: EDUCAUSE.

Online Nursing. (2008). *First paramedic course to use Second Life*. Retrieved January 25, 2009, from http://www.your nursing.com/ 2008/10/16/ first-paramedic-course-to-use- second-life/

Parker, Q. (2008). *Second Life: Disability charity sets up virtual advice service*. Society Guardian.

Polvinen, E. (2007). *Teaching fashion in a virtual environment*. Retrieved January 2, 2010, from http://fitsl.wordpress.com/ 2007/12/05/ elaine-polvinen- teaching-fashion- in-a-virtual- environment/

Prenksy, M. (2001). Digital natives, digital immigrants. *Horizon, 9*(5), 1–6. doi:10.1108/10748120110424816

Prensky, M. (2007). *How to teach with technology: Keeping both teachers and students comfortable in an era of exponential change. Emerging Technology for Learning, 2(1)*. BEC.

Radegast Metaverse Client. (2010). Retrieved April 10, 2010, from http://radegast-client.org/wp/

Rickenbacker, D. (2009). *Some hints on taking pictures in Second Life*. Retrieved January 2, 2010, from http://drickenbacker. wordpress.com/ 2007/08/27/ some-hints- on-taking- pictures-in- second-life/

Copyright © 2011, IGI Global. Copying or distributing in print or electronic forms without written permission of IGI Global is prohibited.

Robbins, S. (2007). *A futurist's view of Second Life education: A developing taxonomy of digital spaces*. Second Life Education Workshop 2007, Part of the Second Life Community Convention, (pp. 27-34). Chicago, IL: WordPress.

Scopes, A., & Lesley, J. M. (2009). *Learning archetypes as tools of cybergogy for a 3D educational landscape: A structure for e-teaching in Second Life*. Unpublished Master's thesis, University of Southampton, School of Education.

Shepherd, J. (2007). It's a world of possibilities. *The Guardian*.

SimTeach. (2009). *Institutions and organizations in SL*. Retrieved October 15, 2009, from http://simteach.com/ wiki/index. php?title=Institutions_and_ organizations_in_ sl#universities.2c_ colleges_.26_ schools

Skiba, D. (2007). Nursing education 2.0: Second Life. *Nursing Education Perspectives*, *28*, 156–158.

Smith, K. (2009). *Disability and virtual worlds: Universal life*. Retrieved February 15, 2010, from http://www.headstar.com/ eablive/?p=366

Stein, M. A., & Waterstone, M. (2006). Disability, disparate impact and class actions. *Duke Law Journal*, *56*, 861–922.

Talamasca, A. (2009). *Proposal for the creation of a disability liaison*. Retrieved April 5, 2010, from http://jira.second life.com/ browse/ MISC-2867

Thomas, D., & Brown, J. S. (2009). Why virtual worlds can matter. *International Journal of Media and Learning*, *1*(1).

Vivian, K. (2007). *Disability aid: Brain-computer interface for Second Life*. Retrieved March 30, 2010, from http://dove-lane.com/ blog/?p=186

White, G. R., Fitzpatrick, G., & McAllister, G. (2008). Toward accessible 3D virtual environments for the blind and visually impaired. In *Proceedings of the 3rd international Conference on Digital interactive Media in Entertainment and Arts*, (pp.134-141). Athens, Greece.

Wood, D. (2009). Experiential learning through real world placements undertaken in 3D virtual world spaces, same places, different spaces. *Proceedings of ascilite*. Auckland.

Yifenghu, Z. (2010). Second Life & disability. *New Media Square*. Retrieved April 10, 2010, from http://yifenghu. wordpress.com/ 2010/02/01/ secondlife disability/

Copyright © 2011, IGI Global. Copying or distributing in print or electronic forms without written permission of IGI Global is prohibited.

Zielke, M., Roome, T., & Krueger, A. (2009). A composite adult learning model for virtual world residents with disabilities: A case study of the virtual ability Second Life island. Pedagogy, education and innovation in 3-D virtual worlds. *Journal of Virtual Worlds Research, 2*(1).

ADDITIONAL READING

Abrahams, P. (2006). Second Life class action, Abrahams accessibility. Retrieved April 1, 2010, from http://www.it director.com/ blogs/ Abrahams_ Accessibility/ 2006/11/ second_ life_ class_ action.html

Abrahams, P. (2007). Second life is now too important not to be accessible. Retrieved March 5, 2010, from http://www.it director.com/ blogs/ Abrahams_ Accessibility/ 2007/12/ second_ life_ is_ now_ too_ important_n_.html

Annable, G., Goggin, G., & Stienstra, D. (2007). Accessibility, disability, and inclusion in information technologies: Introduction. *The Information Society:an International Journal, 23*(3), 145–147.

Bruce Lindsay Maguire v Sydney Organising Committee for the Olympic Games (2000). No. H 99/115, *in the Human Rights and Equal Opportunity Commission Disability Discrimination Act 1992, 24 August 2000 1-25.*

Cassidy, M. (2007). Flying with disability in Second Life - Eureka Street. Retrieved January 20, 2010, from http://www.eurekastreet. com.au/ article. aspx? aeid=2787

Deleuze, G. (1988). *Spinoza: practical philosophy* (p. 28). (Hurley, R., Trans.). San Francisco: City Light Books. (Original work published 1972)

Deleuze, G., & Guattari, F. (1983). *Anti-oedipus: capitalism and schizophrenia. R. Hurley, M. Seem & H. R. Lane, Trans.* London: Athlone. (Original work published 1972)

Deleuze, G., & Guattari, F. (1987). *A thousand plateaus: capitalism & schizophrenia.* Minneapolis: University of Minnesota Press.

Deleuze, G., & Guattari, F. (1996). *What is philosophy?* London: Verso Publishers.

Fruchterman, J. (2007). Beneblog: technology meets society: *Brighton Beach brainstorm.* Retrieved February 17, 2010 from http://benetech. blogspot.com/ 2007/11/ brighton- beach- brain storm.html

Copyright © 2011, IGI Global. Copying or distributing in print or electronic forms without written permission of IGI Global is prohibited.

Goggin, G., & Newell, C. (2007). The business of digital disability. *The Information Society: an International Journal, 23*(3), 159–168.

Mitcham, C. (1995). Ethics into design. In R. Buchanan, R. & V. Margolin, V. (Eds.). *Discovering design: explorations in design studies.* (pp. 173-189). Chicago: The University of Chicago Press.

Nietzsche, F. (1978). *Thus spoke Zarathustra* (Kaufmann, W., Trans.). New York: Penguin Books. (Original work published 1886)

Nietzsche, F. (1990). *Beyond good and evil: prelude to a philosophy of the future.* London: Penguin Classics. (Original work published 1973)

Nomensa, (2006). United nations global audit of web accessibility. Retrieved November 16, 2009, from http://www.nomensa.com/ resources/ research/ united- nations global- audit- of- accessibility.html

Oliver, M. (2007). Exclusion & community in second life. Retrieved December 4, 2010, from http://learning from social worlds. wordpress.com/ exclusion community- in- second- life/

Putnam, M. (2005). Developing a framework for political disability identity. *Journal of Disability Policy Studies, 16*(3), 188–204. doi:10.1177/10442073050160030601

Qi, S. (2007). Experts debate how accessible virtual worlds are to the disabled. Retrieved December 4, 2010, from http://www.slnn.com/ index.php? SCREEN= article&about= accessibility- in-a-3d- world

Red Cardinal, (2006). eGovernment accessibility report: a study into the accessibility and coding standards of key Irish Government & political web*sites.*

Spinoza, B. (2001). *Ethics.* England: Wadsworth. (Original work published 1677)

Stein, M. A., & Waterstone, M. (2006). Disability, disparate impact and class actions. *Duke Law Journal, 56*, 861–922.

Stein, R. (2007). Online avatars are helping the disabled fight back. Retrieved January 23, 2010, from http://www.nashuatelegraph.com/ apps/pbcs.dll/ article?AID=/ 20071125/ HEALTH/ 311250005/-1/ health

The Times. (2007). Is this a real life, is this just fantasy? Retrieved December 15, 2009, from http://women. timesonline. co.uk/ tol/life_and_style/ women/ body_and_ soul/ article1557980.ece

Copyright © 2011, IGI Global. Copying or distributing in print or electronic forms without written permission of IGI Global is prohibited.

Tremain, S. (2006). On the Government of disability: Foucault, power, and the subject of impairment. In Davis, L. J. (Ed.), *The disability studies reader* (pp. 185–196). New York, London: Routledge.

UK Disability Rights Commission. (2005). Making websites accessible—new guidance planned, Retrieved from http://www.accessibility 101.org.uk/ drc.htm

United Nations. (1948). Universal declaration of human rights. Retrieved November 17, 2009, from http://www.un.org/ Overview/rights.html World Wide Web Consortium: Web Content Accessibility Guidelines 1.0 1999.

KEY TERMS AND DEFINITIONS

2D Virtual Learning Environment: An online software system with a website interface containing tools to support learning.

3D Virtual Learning Environment: An online environment that can be used for learning, created in 3 Dimension where users can move, build, communicate using created 3D characters.

Attention Deficit Disorder (ADHD): A condition (mostly in boys) characterized by behavioral and learning disorders.

Architectural Design Guidelines: These are the different codes, specifications and rules used to design a building.

Autism: An abnormal absorption with the self marked by communication disorders and short attention span and inability to treat others as people.

Avatar: A 3D character which the user creates to login and use a 3D virtual environment.

Cerebral Palsy: A loss of motor control with involuntary spasms caused by permanent brain damage present at birth.

Dyslexia: A learning disability that manifests itself as a difficulty with reading decoding, reading comprehension and/or reading fluency.

In-World: A term meaning being logged into the 3D virtual world.

Rezzing: A term referring to the process of appearance or loading of objects inside a 3D virtual environment.

Second Life: An online software which allows creation of a virtual environment.

Copyright © 2011, IGI Global. Copying or distributing in print or electronic forms without written permission of IGI Global is prohibited.

Chapter 3
A Face Based Real Time Communication for Physically and Speech Disabled People

Ong Chin Ann
Swinburne University of Technology, Malaysia

Marlene Valerie Lu
Swinburne University of Technology, Malaysia

Lau Bee Theng
Swinburne University of Technology, Malaysia

ABSTRACT

The main purpose of this research is to enhance the communication of the disabled community. The authors of this chapter propose an enhanced interpersonal-human interaction for people with special needs, especially those with physical and communication disabilities. The proposed model comprises of automated real time behaviour monitoring, designed and implemented with the ubiquitous and affordable concept in mind to suit the underprivileged. In this chapter, the authors present the prototype which encapsulates an automated facial expression recognition system for monitoring the disabled, equipped with a feature to send Short Messaging System (SMS) for notification purposes. The authors adapted the Viola-Jones face detection algorithm at the face detection stage and implemented template matching technique for the expression classification and recognition stage. They tested their model with a few users and achieved satisfactory results. The enhanced real time behaviour

DOI: 10.4018/978-1-60960-541-4.ch003

Copyright ©2011, IGI Global. Copying or distributing in print or electronic forms without written permission of IGI Global is prohibited.

monitoring system is an assistive tool to improve the quality of life for the disabled by assisting them anytime and anywhere when needed. They can do their own tasks more independently without constantly being monitored physically or accompanied by their care takers, teachers, or even parents. The rest of this chapter is organized as follows. The background of the facial expression recognition system is reviewed in Section 2. Section 3 is the description and explanations of the conceptual model of facial expression recognition. Evaluation of the proposed system is in Section 4. Results and findings on the testing are laid out in Section 5, and the final section concludes the chapter.

INTRODUCTION

Communication is a social process of exchanging information from one entity to another in verbal and non-verbal form. It defines our existence and it is an important instrument that connects people together. It comes naturally as a raw skill embedded in most people at birth and we acquired the ways of communication through cognitive learning. Communication is the basis, which drives the process of development in all the fields (Manohar, 2008) and it is the very core of our civilisation. The ability to communicate allows us to express emotion, feelings, convey our thoughts and ideas as well as to relate our experiences. It plays an important role in the dissemination of information and sharing of knowledge especially in the academic arena. Research has found that human started to learn how to communicate with each other since they are born not only through spoken and written languages but also body gesture, posture, facial expression and eye contacts (Busso, et al., 2004; Cohen, Grag & Huang, 2000).

Communication skill might come as a natural ability in majority of people. However, there are some people inflicted with some form of physical defects which affect their ability to communicate. One of the more severe disabilities is known as "cerebral palsy", a congenital disorder at birth which causes abnormality in their motor system. It affects their muscle movement and coordination, learning and speech abilities. Their malfunctioned motor system causes an uncontrollable and involuntary movement. They are unable to control their oral-facial muscles, thus affects their ability to perform facial expression appropriately.

Many assistive tools or formally termed as Alternative and Augmentative Communication (AAC) has been developed and employed to assist people with impaired communication skills. The term encompasses the whole combination of methods used for communication such as text to speech system, pointing gestures, facial expression and body language. Although these AACs have been widely used to assist the disabled, but it is not potentially effective because most AACs are text

Copyright © 2011, IGI Global. Copying or distributing in print or electronic forms without written permission of IGI Global is prohibited.

Figure 1. Examples of alternative and augmentative communication (AAC) tools

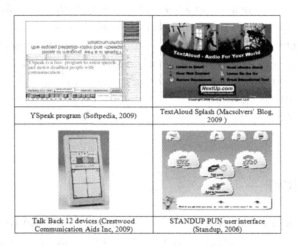

YSpeak program (Softpedia, 2009)	TextAloud Splash (Macsolvers' Blog, 2009)
Talk Back 12 devices (Crestwood Communication Aids Inc, 2009)	STANDUP PUN user interface (Standup, 2006)

to speech and touch screen based applications, which are unsuitable for those with severe physical abilities. There are many kinds of AACs tools available in the market which is shown in Figure 1.

From the limitation of the existing tools reviewed (Novita, 2006; Macsolvers, 2009; Standup, 2006; Universiteit van Amsterdam, 2008; Crestwood, 2009; ScienceDaily, 2008), there is still a pressing need for more effective and efficient tools to alleviate this problem. One the possible methods is to implement a facial expression recognition system to predict or determine the emotional state of a disabled person through his expression projected on his face. The implementation of such method can be made possible through biometrics information systems. According to Gregory and Simon (2008), biometrics information system can be employed as a means to detect and classify the physiological aspect of a person in real time. Franco and Treves (2001) further support the notion that facial expression can be used for human computer interaction and usability enhancement.

Based on the problem statements deliberated above, we propose an improved real time behaviour monitoring application for the disabled by employing real time biometric information i.e. the facial expression recognition system. The aim to create a model that is capable of detecting user's emotion without engaging any physical action from the users. To increase the usability and interactivity of the tool, the emotion detected by the system will be sent to the care-taker's mobile phone in the form of SMS.

Copyright © 2011, IGI Global. Copying or distributing in print or electronic forms without written permission of IGI Global is prohibited.

FACIAL EXPRESSION

Facial expressions recognition is an ability to recognize people by their facial characteristic and differentiate it with one another. Human is born with the ability to recognize other people easily by identifying their facial features such as shape, appearance, skin texture and skin complexion. Other than that, humans also have the ability to express, interpret and differentiate facial expressions. The regular recurring ones are happiness, anger, disgust, fear, surprise and sad (Ekman & Friesen, 1978). The six facial emotions stated above are important and play a major role in expressing emotion as well as recognising facial expression (Busso, et al, 2004).

In real life, inter personal human interaction are performed not only using speech or spoken language, but also non verbal cues for example hand gesture, body gesture, facial expression and tone of the voice. All these cues are sometimes being used for expressing feeling and give feedback (Busso, et al, 2004; Cohen, et al., 2000). We can see how human interact with each other using non-verbal cues everyday. For example a child cries in front of his mother because he is not happy or dissatisfied with something. Other people might interpret it differently thinking that the child might be in pain.

Facial expression interaction is relevant mainly for community social life, teacher and student interaction, credibility in difference contexts, medicine and so on. Besides, facial expression recognition is useful for designing new interactive devices which offers the possibility of new ways for human computer interaction - HCI (Franco & Treves, 2001). Cohen, et al. (2000) conducted survey on their users and noticed that they have been through traditionally HCI consists of the keyboard, mouse, joystick, trackballs, data gloves and touch screen monitors. The interaction can be improved and enhanced by introducing facial expression recognition that requires no direct contact from the user.

Facial Expression Recognition System (FER) has been a topic for research since Ekman and Friesen (1978) who pioneered this research and worked from the psychology perspective. In the past 20 years, many researchers have tried to adopt their idea and make improvement, innovation and modification on facial expression recognition by introducing different techniques, mainly concentrated on the improvement in term of accuracy, efficiency, mobility, and speed (Kotsia & Pitas, 2007). With all the enhancements on techniques for facial detection and recognition, the development of the facial expression recognition has also improved (Zhan & Zhou, 2007). The most active researches in computer vision and pattern recognition is face recognition in forensic identification, access control, user interface design (Wang, Plataniotis & Venetsanopoulos, 2005), emotion analysis, interactive video, indexing and retrieval of image and video database, image understanding and synthetic face animation (Zhan & Zhou, 2007).

Copyright © 2011, IGI Global. Copying or distributing in print or electronic forms without written permission of IGI Global is prohibited.

In real world, humans are able to read complex communication where the synthesis of verbal and non-verbal communication is used to express feelings and opinions. Human can interpret and generate major facial expressions but a computer is not built with any facial recognition ability unless through the use of some software. It is even more complicated for the computer to interpret irregular facial expression, especially from those suffering from cerebral palsy. Due to their disorder, they do not have the ability to reflect their emotions like a normal typical person. Thus, a more natural and naive method has to be employed for the system to work by a manual labelling of the image captured with the emotion of the user.

FACIAL EXPRESSION RECOGNITION

The same concept of inter-human interaction can be applied for human-computer interaction in facial expression recognition. A computer uses microphone and camera to "see" and "hear" human expressions and learns to recognize it (Cohen, et al., 2000). The human face is captured by the camera attached to a computer and the captured images is stored for processing with some methods to recognize the identity and emotion of a user based on the features achieved. With automated facial expression recognition, the subjects do not need to operate the computer device or performing any actions in order to get a task done. Besides, facial expression recognition method has been recommended by many researchers to be a good technique to interpret a person's emotion if compared with other recognition methods such as speech (Zhan & Zhou, 2007; Pantic & Patras, 2006; Lau, 2009).

There are myriads of attempts and research done to produce computer algorithms that serve as models to automate human face recognition function. One of the widely applied systems is known as Facial Action Coding System (FACS). Facial Action Coding System (FACS) was initiated by Ekman and Friesen (1978). It involves the analysis of facial muscle anatomy. It detects the changes to the facial muscle, the contraction and relaxation of a group of muscles to produce certain facial expression. Due to the method employed, it is not suitable to be used by a disabled person namely "Cerebral Palsy" candidates as they have difficulty controlling their muscles and their facial expressions are non-typical. Apart from that, Cohen, Sebe, Garg, Chen, and Huang (2003) stated that FACS processes were very time consuming and tedious.

Another technique is the Skin Color Model that extracts the skin colour from any region of the image as a matching based to detect the face. It will not be accurate if it is taken from other region like legs, arms, and neck appear in the image or video (Singh et. al., 2003). It is also easily affected by the lighting condition and camera settings.

Copyright © 2011, IGI Global. Copying or distributing in print or electronic forms without written permission of IGI Global is prohibited.

There are other numerous methods developed over the years with their own technique and accuracy. We have chosen to integrate the Viola and Jones Face detection algorithm alongside template matching technique into our image processing engine.

Viola-Jones algorithm is one of the most widely used techniques for face detection and template matching is also the proven effective algorithm for facial expression classification and matching. Viola-Jones algorithm was used by Barlett, Littlewort, Fasel, and Movellan (2003) in their research to perform real time face detection and facial expression recognition process. Shan, Gong, and McOwan (2005) employed template matching techniques to perform person-independent facial expression recognition. They obtained recognition accuracy of 79.1% for 7-class recognition and 84.5% recognition accuracy for 6-class recognition. Refer to the Appendix for a summary of techniques and algorithms used in automatic facial expression recognition system.

We adopted Viola-Jones Face Detection algorithm (2004) and used the default Haar cascade for human face searching because this algorithm is considered the most common and useful algorithm in the field of facial expression recognition research (Cho et al, 2009; Brubaker et al, 2008; Zhan et al, 2006; Datcu and Rothkrantz, 2007; Bartlett, et al, 2003).

As for template matching, it had been a conventional method for object detection and pattern recognition especially facial features at the early stage of face recognition research (Chai, et al, 2009). The advantage of template matching for our proposed prototype is that it is simple, easy to implement, and does not take so much time and memory. We tried on other algorithm such as Support Vector Machine (SVM) as well as Principal Component Analysis (PCA) as both techniques is widely used and recommended by researchers (Dubuisson, et al., 2002; Chen and Huang, 2002; Bartlett, et al, 2003; Littlewort, et al., 2007; Ashraf et al, 2009) but we found that the expression training using these techniques is processor intensive and is consuming memory.

PROTOTYPE MODELLING

Generally, automated facial expression recognition system involves three major steps or stages. There are the face detection stage, feature extraction stage as well as expression recognition and classification stage (Zhang, Lyons, Schuster, & Akamatsu, 1998; Chibelushi & Bourel, 2002; Zhan et al, 2006). Figure 2 shows two major processes in an automated facial expression recognition system. The blue arrows indicate the process of expression recognition while red arrows indicate the training process of expression recognition. When performing expression recognition, a camera is used to capture the subject's face in video sequence and these video sequences or

Copyright © 2011, IGI Global. Copying or distributing in print or electronic forms without written permission of IGI Global is prohibited.

Table 1. Summary of techniques and algorithms in automatic facial expression recognition system

Processes	Techniques and Algorithms	Integrated by
Face Detection	Viola and Jones Face Detection Algorithm	Cho, Mirzaei, Oberg, and Kastner (2009); Brubaker, Wu, Sun, Mullin, and Rehg (2008); Zhan, Li, Ogunbona, and Safaei (2006); Datcu and Rothkrantz, (2007); Bartlett, et al (2003); Viola and Jones (2004);
	Motion History Image (MHI)	Davis (2001); Valstar, Pantic and Patras (2004);
	Skin Color Model	Singh, Chauhan, Vatsa, and Singh (2003); Kovac, Peer, and Solina (2003)
	Convolution Neural Network (CNN)	Fasel (2002); Matsugu, Mori, Mitari, and Kaneda (2003); Graves, Fernandez, and Schmidhuber (2007);
Feature Extraction	Principal Component Analysis (PCA)	Dubuisson, Davoine, and Masson (2002); Chen and Huang (2002);
	Gabor Features, Filters and Wavelet	Zhan et al (2006); Tian, Kanade and Cohn (2002); Bartlett, et al (2003); Zhan and Zhou (2007);
	Optical Flow	Donato, et al (1999); Aires, Santana, and Medeiros (2008); Riaz, Mayer, Wimmer, Beetz, & Radig (2009); Su, Hsieh, and Huang (2007)
	Active Appearance Model (AAM)	Zhan and Zhou (2007); Datcu and Rothkrantz (2007); Tang and Deng (2007)
Emotion Recognition and Classification	Facial Action Coding System (FACS)	Zhang and Ji (2005); Ashraf et al, (2009)
	Template Matching	Shan, et al. (2005); Chai, Rizon, Woo, and Tan (2009); Xie and Lam (2009)
	Neural Network (Feed forward and Back propagation)	Ma and Khorasani (2004); Tian, et al. (2002); Franco and Treves (2001);
	Hidden Markov Model (HMM)	Cohen, et al (2003); Zhan and Zhou (2007)
	Linear Discriminant Analysis (LDA)	Lyons, Budynek, Plante, and Akamatsu (2000); Price and Gee (2005)
	Support Vector Machine (SVM)	Bartlett, et al (2003); Littlewort, Bartlett and Lee, (2007); Ashraf et al (2009)
	Dynamic Bayesian Network (DBN)	Cohen, et al (2003); Zhang and Ji (2005); Sebe et. al (2007)

images are used as input to perform the face detection. Once the subject's face is detected, his or her face or region of interest is extracted and temporary stored. The initial emotion of the subject is known after the last process which consist of the comparison and matching using the features extracted and the templates which are stored in the system database. Usually an automated facial expression recognition system needs to be trained before it can be used to recognize and classify human emotion. The process of face detection and features extraction in training stage is

Copyright © 2011, IGI Global. Copying or distributing in print or electronic forms without written permission of IGI Global is prohibited.

Figure 2. Facial expression recognition system

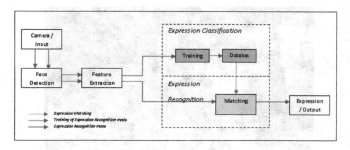

the similar to the expression recognition process but the extracted features is used as training data for classifying subject's expression.

By implementing automated facial expression recognition system, we proposed a real time behavior monitoring for physical and communication disabled which is shown in Figure 3. The automated facial expression recognition system is mounted on the disabled wheelchair for expression recognition purposes. The system will detect the disabled face, extract the face and perform emotion or expression recognition. Critical or preset abnormal expression recognized will trigger notification module via Short Messaging System (SMS) gateway to notify the parents, teachers and the care taker for the disabled.

Figure 3. Real time behavior monitoring system

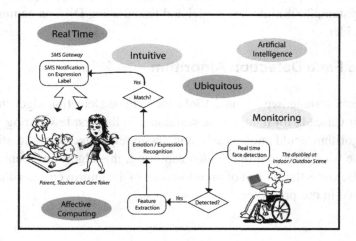

Copyright © 2011, IGI Global. Copying or distributing in print or electronic forms without written permission of IGI Global is prohibited.

Figure 4. Face detection using Viola-Jones algorithm in still image

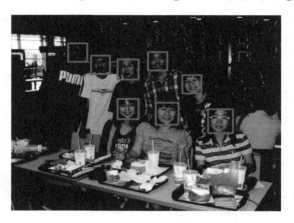

Software and Hardware Specifications

Our proposed automated behaviour monitoring model is built and tested on mobile machine with Intel Core 2 Duo Processor T6600 (2.2 GHz), 2GB DDR3 SD RAM and using 2 MP build in camera for the image capturing process running on PAL standard or 25 frames per second. In the implementation process, we develop our model using Microsoft Visual Studio 2008 C++ Version 9.0.21022.8 RTM with Microsoft .NET Framework Version 3.5 SP1 plug-ins. OpenCV 1.1 (Bradski, & Kaehler, 2008) was used as an assistive library in developing this model either in both face detection stage, feature extraction as well as facial expression training and recognition processes. While for Short Messaging System (SMS) notification, we employed SMS Gateway Development Kit for GSM Modem Type Q24-U-SGDK18 (Mobitek System, 2008) into our model and tested using DiGi as communication service provider.

Real Time Face Detection Algorithm

In face detection stage, we adopted Viola-Jones Face Detection algorithm (2004) and the Haar Cascade for human face searching. In the first few testing, we found that this algorithm could successfully and accurately detect faces in still images but when we tried it on real time video capturing, this algorithm seem to be less intelligent. Below is the snippet of pseudo-codes of the improved algorithm for face detection used in our prototype.

Copyright © 2011, IGI Global. Copying or distributing in print or electronic forms without written permission of IGI Global is prohibited.

Figure 5. Misdetection of face using Viola-Jones face detection algorithm in real time video capturing

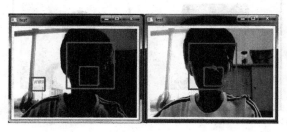

```
INITIALIZE face
WHILE face is equal
    GET face
    IF face is detected
        DRAW region of interest in image
    END IF
END WHILE
```

In Figure 4, we can see the result of Viola-Jones algorithm on still image. All the faces have been detected in still image and drawn with blue square boxes while the same algorithm did not work properly in real time video capturing which is shown in Figure 5. There are multiples detection indicated by the square blue boxes including an object that is not part of the face. This shows an inaccurate detection mechanism and will affect the viability of the facial expression recognition system.

Along the testing period, we found the causes and ways to solve this problem; at the same time we improved the detection accuracy. The Viola-Jones face detection algorithm scan through the whole image or frame using haar cascade classifier and return the face found regardless of the image size. We solve this problem by preset the video frame or resolution to 320 X 240 and minimum face detection or region of interest (ROI) of 100 X 100 pixels. With this scale, the distance between the subject and the camera has to be within 30cm to 60cm which is shown in Figure 6. Hence, small or unwanted objects are no longer detected as it is out of the preset range.

Other than misdetection problem, we also discovered another problem which affected our recognition result. Although the area of the detection or region of interest had been defined, the inconsistent light source is another factor that led to a failure in the detection process. To resolve this issue, we tested on several lighting conditions and tried to gauge the optimum condition suitable for the detection pro-

Copyright © 2011, IGI Global. Copying or distributing in print or electronic forms without written permission of IGI Global is prohibited.

Figure 6. Face detection range

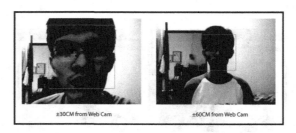

cess. Then we calculated average brightness value of the optimum lighting condition frame using HSV model (Bezryadin, Bourov, & Ilinih, 2007). When performing facial expression training or recognition, we standardized every captured frame by adjusting the average brightness to the optimum lighting condition value.

Figure 7 shows the result after brightness adjustment or brightness standardization based on the control value or optimum lighting condition. The image on the left is the original frame captured in real time using web cam while the image on the right has been edited to the level of brightness required. By implementing the brightness standardization or adjustment, we not only enhanced the original Viola-Jones face detection algorithm but also increased the recognition rate which will be discussed later under Facial Expression Recognition and Classification sub section.

Facial Feature Extraction Algorithm

Feature extraction is performed once the subject's face is correctly detected. In general, feature extraction can be performed in two approaches: Global feature extraction (Holistically) and local feature extraction. (Fasel & Luettin, 2003; Whitehill, 2006). In our model, we chose global features extraction as it does not consume so much computation time and power when performing facial expression recognition. We added a few image processing processes while performing feature extraction process to further increase the chances of recognition. Refer to the sample pseudo-codes below for an overview of the entire process.

Figure 7. Brightness adjustment

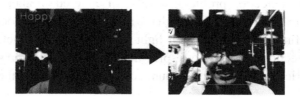

Copyright © 2011, IGI Global. Copying or distributing in print or electronic forms without written permission of IGI Global is prohibited.

Figure 8. Image processing in feature extraction process

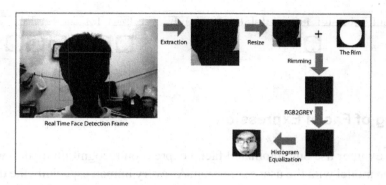

```
IF region of interest is drawn
    EXTRACT region of interest
    RESIZE extracted image
    ADD rim into extracted image
    SET grayscale to extracted image
    SET histogram equalization to extracted image
END IF
```

When the region of interest is detected, it will be extracted and will undergo several levels of modification and filtering. First, we resize the extracted image to 64 × 64 pixels resolution and set it as the standard image size to avoid mismatch or inconsistent template size in recognition process later. We tested it with other resolution such as 128 × 128 pixels but the outcome is similar with the previous resolution and it actually consumed more memory and took more time to process the image. When we tried on smaller resolution, 32 × 32 pixels, we found that the result was not as good as 64 × 64 pixels. Hence we set 64 × 64 Pixels as the standard extracted image size. After the image extraction, we trimmed the resized image to eliminate unwanted area. Then we convert the image from RGB to Greyscale and apply histogram equalization to obtain higher contrast and to increase the intensity of the image. The main purpose of executing all those processes is to reduce system memory usage and processing time when performing facial expression recognition. On top of that, it will simplify the comparison process especially in expression recognition process. The whole processes involved in feature extraction process can be seen in Figure 8.

At the end of the feature extraction process, the histogram equalized image will be used as a template for comparison purposes during the facial expression recognition process. It will be referred to as trained sets.

Copyright © 2011, IGI Global. Copying or distributing in print or electronic forms without written permission of IGI Global is prohibited.

Figure 9. Neutral expression training set storing process

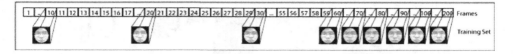

Training of Facial Expression

Before we run or use our automated facial expression recognition model, we need to feed the model with the user expression. As every human especially the disabled has different ways of expressing their emotions, our model requires the users to train the system to recognize their expression before using it. The procedures for the training function are expressed below.

```
INITIALIZE count
INITIALIZE number of train set
INITIALIZE train frame
FOR each of train frame
CALL face detection
     CALL feature extraction and image processing
IF count modules number of train set is equal to 0
     CALL feature extraction and image processing
     SAVE processed image
END IF
INCREAMENT count
END FOR
```

The purpose of the facial expression training process is to capture and store expression template for matching purposes. During the training session, our model captured 200 frames on each label or expression and stored only 20 frames where each frame is taken after every 10 frames interval. We have tried with fewer samples for each expression but the recognition accuracy seemed to drop compared with 20 samples per expression. Hence, we set a standard of 20 samples per expression, which will be stored in a template.

The attributes of the stored templates are 64 pixels × 64 pixels in resolution, trimmed, and histogram equalized to greyscale image which can be seen in Figure 9. Up to date, we have tested and trained 10 expressions or labels and the outcome in term of speed of storing is satisfactory. All the 20 trained images stored in the

Copyright © 2011, IGI Global. Copying or distributing in print or electronic forms without written permission of IGI Global is prohibited.

template will be used to match the real time captured image during the expression recognition phase.

Facial Expression Recognition and Classification

In this final stage, we executed the automated facial expression recognition in real time with the entire enhanced Viola-Jones face detection algorithm. The real time captured image went through similar processes as in the training stage to obtain the histogram equalized image and it will be used to compare with the stored template images through template matching process. Before deciding this algorithm, we tried other algorithm such as Support Vector Machine (SVM) as well as Principal Component Analysis (PCA). Although both techniques are widely used and recommended by researchers (Dubuisson, et al., 2002; Chen & Huang, 2003; Bartlett, et al, 2003; Littlewort, et al., 2007; Ashraf et al, 2009), we found that performing expression training using these techniques required heavy processing power. By training 7 expressions, the system using SVM technique created 60 Megabytes of trained file while our proposed model only created 0.4 Megabytes of trained templates for the same number of expressions. Loading such a large trained file will be put a heavy load on the computer and will slow down the computer's processing speed. Hence we decided to adopt template matching algorithm for expression recognition, which is described below in methodological order.

```
INITIALIZE white pixel
INITIALIZE expression label
INITIALIZE frame capture from camera
IF frame is captured
     CALL face detection
     CALL feature extraction and image processing
FOR each expression label
     FOR each sample
          SUBSTRACT sample image from processed image
          SET histogram equalization to processed image
          SET range filter to processed image
          COMPUTE number of white pixel in processed image

IF number of white pixel in processed image is less than white
pixel
SET white pixel equal to number of white pixel in processed im-
age
               SET expression label equal to sample image label
```

Copyright © 2011, IGI Global. Copying or distributing in print or electronic forms without written permission of IGI Global is prohibited.

Figure 10. Real time extracted face image and stored template face image matching

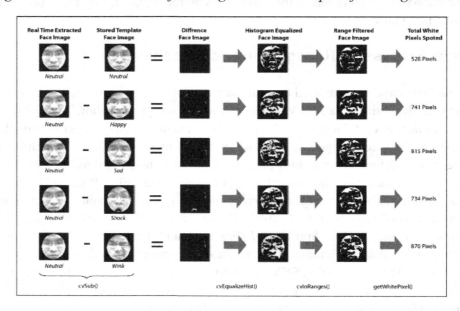

```
            END IF
        END FOR
END FOR
END IF
```

During the matching process, we applied several waves of processing which included image subtraction, another round of histogram equalization and image filtering. We assumed that all the expressions and labels have been fed into the model and the user was sitting within the detection range recommended when performing the facial expression recognition process. The real time captured frame went through the face detection stage followed by the feature extraction stage. The extracted image or processed image will then be used as input of facial expression recognition stage.

Figure 10 illustrated the facial expression recognition process in our model by matching the real time extracted face image with the images stored in the template. Each processed image was compared with every expression stored in the template. Each expression had 20 sample images and there were 5 expressions. Thus, each processed image had to be compared with 100 image templates.

For every sample matching process, our model performed image subtraction by subtracting the pixel value in the stored image template from the processed image to obtain the difference between both images. After that, histogram equalization is

Copyright © 2011, IGI Global. Copying or distributing in print or electronic forms without written permission of IGI Global is prohibited.

Figure 11. Interface of proposed automated facial expression recognition model with personalization module

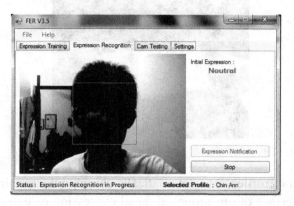

applied to the subtracted image so that the contrast and intensity can be distinguished clearly. Then we applied range filtering on the histogram equalized image to convert the image into dual tone color mode consisting of black and white pixels. The area populated with black pixels indicated no changes to the image while white pixel represented the difference between the input image and the image template. Finally our model calculated the total of white pixels and will select the image with the smallest amount of white pixels. Then it returned the emotional state labeled on the image.

Personalizing of User

To make our model more efficient and dynamic, we propose an additional feature called personalizing user's profile to cater for multiple users. It creates multiple user profiles and stores their expressions in their respective profile.

```
CASE of user task
    ADD Profile          : SAVE new profile
    GET profile          : SELECT profile
    REMOVE profile       : ERASE profile
END CASE
```

This feature is useful, increases the efficiency of the model and it saves time. The users are not required to keep retraining our model. The model will save the profile or the trained sets of first time user and retrieved in when needed. The model will automatically detect the user if it could find a match of the facial image from the

Copyright © 2011, IGI Global. Copying or distributing in print or electronic forms without written permission of IGI Global is prohibited.

Figure 12. Type Q24-U-SGDK18 GSM Modem

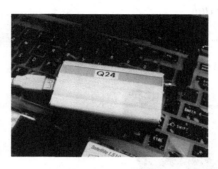

saved templates or profiles, thus automatically skipping the training stage. Figure 11 shows the interface of our proposed facial expression recognition model with personalization module.

Critical Expression Notification

As an enhancement to the facial recognition model, we added Short Messaging System (SMS) notification feature via SMS gateway into our model to notify the care taker, teacher and parent for unusual or critical expression such as anger, sad or shock. We employed SMS Gateway Development Kit for GSM Modem Type Q24-U-SGDK18 (Mobitek System, 2008) into our model which is shown in Figure 12.

```
GET initial expression label
FOR each expression label
IF initial expression label is checked
    SENT sms
END IF
    END FOR
```

Figure 13. Critical expression notification flow chart

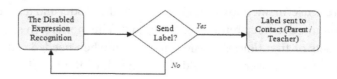

Copyright © 2011, IGI Global. Copying or distributing in print or electronic forms without written permission of IGI Global is prohibited.

User can choose to enable or disable this feature and the user is required to enter his contact number for the notification to work. As shown in Figure 13, when performing facial expression recognition, our model triggered the modem to send subject's initial expression which is marked as "send" to the preset contacts and notify the subject's parent, teacher or caretaker on their critical expression to get immediate attention. Through this, the disabled can be monitored remotely without a close supervision from the care-taker.

EVALUATION

We employed a heuristic approach through multiple sessions of evaluations and testings during the development of our prototype. The evaluations are done on the face detection rates and accuracy, numbers of samples in the template and time required for the training as well as the accuracy of the expression recognition process. A systematic approach is adopted into the testing process. Unit or module testing is done after the completion of each component. Testings were carried out on the face detection, recognition accuracy, response speed of our model, and real time field testing. For face detection module, we tested on an individual under different settings such as indoor environment, outdoor environment, day time as well as night time. For recognition accuracy, we tested on five different users during day time and indoor with white or plain background. We trained our model with 7 expressions for each user and each expression contained 20 sample images. While for response speed, we tested on the same users to examine our model's training time and matching time by training our model with 2 set of expressions per user. Set 1 with 20 samples stored per expression and set 2 with 10 samples stored per expression. For the field testing, we tested with a child who was suffering from physical and communication disabilities. Although we faced some problems and limitations, we managed to solve the major problems.

Face Detection

In the initial stage, we found that Viola-Jones face detection algorithm has some limitation and misdetection especially on the lighting issue. We tried a few ways to solve this problem and fortunately we managed to overcome this problem by adding in auto brightness adjustment based on HSV color model (Bezryadin, et al., 2007). We set a control value or optimum brightness value into our model and it increased or decreased the brightness of the image to the acceptable level before performing face detection. By adding the additional features, our face detection rate has increased from 75% to 95% which is shown in Table 2.

Copyright © 2011, IGI Global. Copying or distributing in print or electronic forms without written permission of IGI Global is prohibited.

Table 2. Face detection frequency under different environments

Brightness Adjustment Environment		Before (%)	After (%)	Increment (%)
Indoor	Day Time	85	100	15
	Night Time	70	95	25
Outdoor	Day Time	85	95	10
	Night time	60	90	30
Overall Face Detection Frequency		**75**	**95**	**20**

Figure 14 shows the same images captured by webcam in real time. The image on left side was the original image but the face was not detected while image on the right was the brightened image and the face was successfully detected. Base on HSV color model, the average brightness value of the original image is 120 which is considered dark image and the image on the right had been adjusted to 200. It might be the appropriate value for this sample but after testing this setting with other sample images under different light intensity, the images were over-exposed. Therefore, we set the brightness value to the average level of 160.

After multiple testings, we obtained a satisfactory face detection accuracy using this setting under different lighting condition and environment such as indoor, outdoor, day and also night time which is shown in Figure 15. As mentioned before, a good quality of face detection result could increase recognition rates in the later process. The testings conducted proved that the enhancement on Viola-Jones face detection algorithm with automated brightness adjustment could help increase the recognition rate in our model.

Recognition Accuracy

Upon completion of our model, we conducted a mini testing on our model's expression recognition accuracy. We invited 5 normal people to participate in this mini test and have achieved satisfactory outcome when tested on 7 common expression

Figure 14. Brightness adjustment does increase face detection rate and accuracy

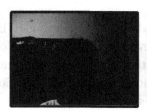 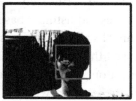

Copyright © 2011, IGI Global. Copying or distributing in print or electronic forms without written permission of IGI Global is prohibited.

Figure 15. Findings of automated brightness adjustment and face detection

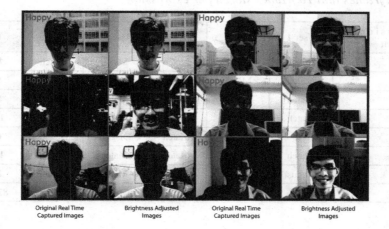

| Original Real Time Captured Images | Brightness Adjusted Images | Original Real Time Captured Images | Brightness Adjusted Images |

which were neutral, happy, sad, surprise, anger, disgust and confuse. We performed this test indoor during the day time with plain background or a wall, 160 brightness value and 20 sample frames per expression. The result is laid out on Table 3 with 91.4% of the overall expression recognition accuracy. We marked "Match" if our model returned the correct label by our participants and a red label indicated incorrect recognition.

As mentioned in the previous section, we captured 200 frames during the training stage and we stored 10% of the captured frames. To improve the efficiency of the training stage, we tried to reduce the captured frames to 100 frames and 10 frames were stored as the image templates. We found that the overall recognition

Table 3. First mini test matching result of facial expression recognition with 200 train frames and 20 frames stored per expression.

Expression / Participant	User 1	User 2	User 3	User 4	User 5	Total
Neutral	Match	Match	Match	Match	Match	**100%**
Happy	Match	Match	Match	Match	Match	**100%**
Sad	Confuse	Match	Match	Match	Match	**80%**
Surprise	Match	Match	Match	Match	Match	**100%**
Anger	Disgust	Match	Surprise	Match	Match	**60%**
Disgust	Match	Match	Match	Match	Match	**100%**
Confuse	Match	Match	Match	Match	Match	**100%**
Total	**71.4%**	**100%**	**85.7%**	**100%**	**100%**	**91.42%**

Copyright © 2011, IGI Global. Copying or distributing in print or electronic forms without written permission of IGI Global is prohibited.

Table 4. Second mini test matching result of facial expression recognition with 100 captured frames and 10 frames stored per expression.

Expression / Participant	User 1	User 2	User 3	User 4	User 5	Total
Neutral	Sad	Match	Match	Match	Match	**80%**
Happy	Match	Match	Match	Disgust	Match	**80%**
Sad	Match	Neutral	Match	Match	Match	**80%**
Surprise	Match	Match	Match	Match	Match	**100%**
Anger	Sad	Match	Match	Disgust	Match	**60%**
Disgust	Match	Match	Match	Match	Match	**100%**
Confuse	Disgust	Match	Match	Match	Match	**80%**
Total	**57.1%**	**85.7%**	**100%**	**71.4%**	**100%**	**82.84%**

accuracy has dropped to 82.84% from the first mini test which was 91.42%. Refer to Table 4.

Response Speed

While performing the two mini tests, we monitored and recorded the time for training as well as template matching to compare the processing speed of our model which is shown in Figure 16.

Table 5 shows the results for the two tests conducted. In the first mini test, the average time consumption for training was 22.56 seconds and for template matching was 50 milliseconds. While for the second mini test, the average time consump-

Figure 16. Time consumption for training and template matching for mini test one

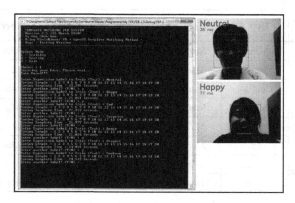

Copyright © 2011, IGI Global. Copying or distributing in print or electronic forms without written permission of IGI Global is prohibited.

Table 5. Time consumption for expression training and testing session

Tests Users	Test 1		Test 2	
	Avg. Train Time per Expression (Seconds)	Avg. Test Time (Milliseconds)	Avg. Train Time per Expression (Seconds)	Avg. Test Time (Milliseconds)
User 1	22.28	49	12.78	27.5
User 2	22.18	51.5	12.35	29.5
User 3	22.47	51.5	11.13	27
User 4	22.88	50.5	11.87	25.5
User 5	23.00	47.5	11.62	26.5
Average	**22.56**	**50**	**11.95**	**27.2**

tion for training was 11.95 seconds and average time consumption for template matching was 27.2 milliseconds.

From the result of the experimental testings conducted, the number of frames captured during the training phase will have a domino effect on other components as well. It will reduce the time required to execute the facial expression recognition component and at the same time reduced the recognition accuracy.

The results in both our testing showed the time for expression training and testing session for test 2 has been reduced by 47.03% and 45.6% respectively. But at the same time, the recognition accuracy suffered a decreased from 91.42% in test 1 to 82.84% in test 2.

Another test was conducted to determine the duration for the expression notification to reach the care-taker's mobile phone. We have tested it under normal weather condition by using DiGi as communication operator and the notification arrived within 15 seconds. There are multiple factors that will affect the delivery; the weather condition and the throughput. We did not manage to test this feature under those conditions specified.

Field Test

During the field testing, we tested our model with a cerebral palsy patient labelled as Student A, who suffered from physical and communication disabilities. Student A did not have the ability to walk and had difficulty holding an object with his hands. He had impaired communication skills and his speech was incomprehensible.

The setup of our model for Student A was different from the other users we tested previously. We tested 5 basic expressions with the student which include neutral, anger, happy, sad and surprise expressions. In the expression training phase, we configured our model to extract 5 out of 50 frames captured and saved them in the

Copyright © 2011, IGI Global. Copying or distributing in print or electronic forms without written permission of IGI Global is prohibited.

Figure 17. Cerebral palsy patient field testing result

Images	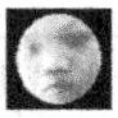	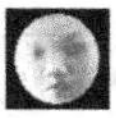	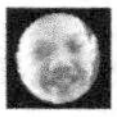	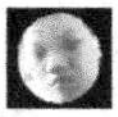	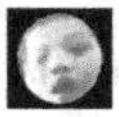	Overall Matching (%)
Expressions	Neutral	Angry	Happy	Sad	Shock / Surprise	
Matching (%)	100	80	100	60	100	88

dataset for expression recognition matching process later. The reduced frame rates were due to inconsistency of the facial pattern while performing expression training.

We performed 1 set of expression training consisting of 5 expressions and 5 rounds of expression recognition during our field testing. We achieved an 88% of overall matching result while performing expression recognition with Student Refer to Figure 17 for the result. This has proven that our proposed model as an assistive communication tool is effective for physically and speech disabled patients.

FINDINGS

From the testings and observations conducted, we discovered a few potholes. In the face detection stage, we found that the original Viola-Jones face detection algorithm has a few limitations. It is affected by the lighting condition and it produced multiple face detections on similar area which led to misdetection. We have tried various ways to overcome this problem and we managed to solve it by adding an automated brightness adjustment features into an image before performing Viola-Jones face detection algorithm. With the added feature, our model could detect human face regardless of the environment and the lighting condition.

When training the user expression, users have to be consistent with their expression as our model is using pattern recognition or template matching method to perform facial expression recognition. This means that our model only returns the nearest expression matched.

In our second mini testing, our model returned the label "Disgust" while the subject is expressing a happy emotion which is shown in Figure 18. Initially we thought that our model did not work well and misrecognized the subject emotion. But when we explored further into the subject's trained set, we found that the misrecognition was caused by the incorrect or inappropriate training conducted.

Based on Figure 18, we can see a set of happy expressions and a set of disgusted expressions. The first frames of both emotions reflect almost similar expressions.

Copyright © 2011, IGI Global. Copying or distributing in print or electronic forms without written permission of IGI Global is prohibited.

Figure 18. Incorrect training causing misrecognition

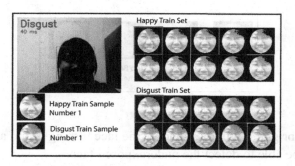

When the real time captured imaged is compared with the stored template, it returned an incorrect result. The model detected a disgusted emotion while the participant was actually feeling happy. Thus, it is important that the training phase should be conducted accurately to obtain a valid result.

In term of processing and respond speed, our proposed model could respond within 100 milliseconds to our user in template matching stage. For recognition accuracy, our proposed model could achieve 91.42% accurate rate in distinguishing 7 types of expressions for the same person conducted in the mini test and **88%** of recognition accuracy in the field test with our targeted user. Through our testings, we found that by collecting more samples per expression, it will increase the accuracy when performing expression recognition. At the same time, it will increase the duration required for the training and recognition phase.

CONSTRAINTS

In the face detection stage, we have enhanced the detection rate and accuracy by adding the auto brightness adjustment base on HSV colour model into the naïve Viola-Jones face detection algorithm. However, in some cases, our model still failed to detect human face in certain conditions as shown in Figure 19. When the

Figure 19. Backlight is too strong

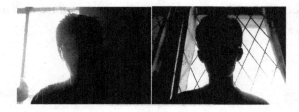

Copyright © 2011, IGI Global. Copying or distributing in print or electronic forms without written permission of IGI Global is prohibited.

Figure 20. Face detection and extraction

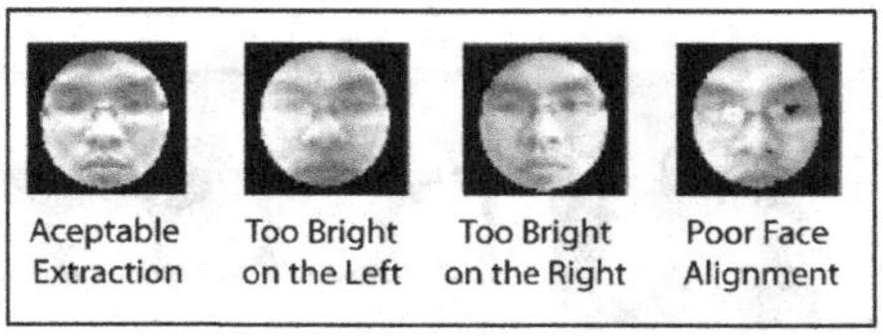

backlight is too bright, it will overshadow the face turning it into a silhouette. The model will not be able to detect the underexposed face.

The second constraint on detection stage is the distance between the subject's face and the web cam. As we have preset our video or capture frame resolution to 320 × 240 pixels and minimum detection area is 100 × 100 pixels, the subject's head must be within 30 cm to 60 cm from the webcam. Otherwise our proposed model will fail to detect the face. It is important that the captured image and the extracted image have to be in good quality. We use the term "good quality" to indicate a proper alignment between the face and the camera in an upright position with proper lighting as shown in Figure 20. A poor face detection will reduce the recognition accuracy. Hence, users have to perform expression recognition in a controlled environment with suitable lighting.

In training stage, our model required a time frame of 20.024 seconds to 24.137 seconds to store a set of expression which consisted of 20 images extracted from 200 frames captured. Our users complained that the duration of the training time is too long. But to achieve a higher accuracy of recognition rate (91.42%), we have to capture at least 200 frames.

For critical expression notification via SMS, the delivery of the notification is affected by the weather condition, communication operators as well as their connection speed.

Up to date, we did not find any critical constraint for expression recognition stage as long as the input for facial expression training is properly conducted; we believe our model could obtain higher recognition accuracy than 91.42%. One issue that is worth discussing and taken into consideration is that certain people may appear indifferent. For example some people might feel sad even though their face showed

Figure 21. One face pattern may represent many expressions, Sad on the left; Neutral on the right

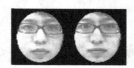

Copyright © 2011, IGI Global. Copying or distributing in print or electronic forms without written permission of IGI Global is prohibited.

a neutral look which is shown in Figure 21. This is beyond our model's ability to distinguish from one expression to another because the facial pattern is the same.

FUTURE WORKS AND IMPROVEMENT

After a series of evaluations and continuous testing and probing on our proposed model, we have identified several limitations on a few stages.

The first unforseen issue emerged when we did the training session with a cerebral palsy boy who could not prop his head up and position his face directly in front of the camera. His head was constantly tilted to the right. The face detection mechanism failed to detect his face completely. Further exploration is required to improve the face detection mechanism taking this into consideration to give a wider angle of flexibility. There are rooms for improvements to increase the facial expression recognition rates. We are delving into ways to improve the quality of the face detection result as it will have a direct impact on the expression recognition process.

Other than that, we going to fine tune some settings when performing image processing in features extraction stage. With that, we hope we could refine the quality of the extracted face images for later processes. In the training stage, we will do more research specifically on how we could shorten the training time and reduce the number of templates within a train set while maintaining the recognition rate.

CONCLUSION

Communication is the very essence of our daily lives. The inability to communicate will hamper us from moving forward as an individual and as a community, robbing us from a normal life. Humans have tried ways to communicate since the beginning of time and communication has evolved throughout ages. It is a complex process triggering many senses and it comes naturally to most of us. Unfortunately there is a small group of people with physical and communication disabilities since birth. To assist these people in their communication needs, we propose an improved real time behaviour monitoring application for the disabled by employing a real time facial expression recognition system and Short Messaging System (SMS) to send notification to the third party for monitoring purposes. Our proposed automated real time behaviour monitoring has been designed and implemented with the ubiquitous and affordable concept in mind which suits the underprivileged who suffers from both physical and communication disabilities. In facial expression recognition system, we employed Viola-Jones face detection algorithm which is commonly used by researchers to detect the subject face and apply template matching methods for

Copyright © 2011, IGI Global. Copying or distributing in print or electronic forms without written permission of IGI Global is prohibited.

expression classification and recognition. The emotional state of the inflicted party will be sent to the care-taker in a form of SMS. From the testing result of our proposed model, the face detection rate was approximately 95% under different lighting condition and environment. At the same time, we achieved 82.84% to 91.42% recognition accuracy on average when conducting expression recognition testing. The processing speed for the expression training took 11.95 seconds to 22.56 seconds per expression and 27.5 milliseconds to 50 milliseconds for expression recognition process. While developing and testing our model, we identified the limitation of using naïve Viola-Jones face detection algorithm and the way to overcome this problem. Besides that, we discovered that by using template matching method for recognition, some expressions cannot be distinguished by the machine if the facial expression of one emotion has close similarities with the other. This would be another domain for further research on how a machine could distinguish different emotional state but reflected with the same facial expression. Apart from that, we are going to enhance and improve a few modules on our model especially the face detection stage as well as the feature extraction stage to increase the recognition accuracy. With the enhanced real time behaviour monitoring system, it could make the disabled life easier and assist them anytime and anywhere when needed. They can do their own tasks more independently without being physically monitored or accompanied by their care taker, teacher or even parent.

ACKNOWLEDGMENT

The author would like to thanks Noris, Valeria, N., Mandasari, V., Tran, C.T., Jain, N., Sim, S., Lau, T.C., Wee, S., as well as Liew, J. for participating in the proposed model testing as well as allowing the author to use their photos in Figure 4, Figure 17, Figure 18 and Figure 21.

REFERENCES

Aires, K. R., Santana, A. M., & Medeiros, A. A. D. (2008). Optical flow using color information: Preliminary results. *Proceedings of the 2008 ACM Symposium on Applied Computing.* Fortaleza, Ceara, Brazil: ACM.

Ashraf, A. B., Lucey, S., Cohn, J. F., Chen, T., Ambadar, Z., Prkachin, K. M., & Solomon, P. E. (2009). The painful face–pain expression recognition using active appearance models. *Image and Vision Computing, 27*(12), 1788–1796. doi:10.1016/j.imavis.2009.05.007

Copyright © 2011, IGI Global. Copying or distributing in print or electronic forms without written permission of IGI Global is prohibited.

Bartlett, M. S., Littlewort, G., Fasel, I., & Movellan, J. R. (2003). Real time face detection and facial expression recognition: Development and applications to human computer interaction. *Computer Vision and Pattern Recognition Workshop, 5,* 53.

Berhad, M. I. M. O. S. (2008). *National biometrics technology roadmap.* Ministry of Science, Technology and Innovation, Malaysia. Retrieved December 31, 2009 from http://www.mosti. gov.my/ mosti/ images/ stories/ DICT/ policy/ Biometrics% 20Technology% 20Roadmap% 20Public% 20Version.pdf

Bezryadin, S., Bourov, P., & Ilinih, D. (2007). *Brightness calculation in digital image processing.* Technologies for Digital Fulfillment, KWI International Inc. Retrieved March 25, 2010, from http://www.kweii.com/site/color_theory/2007_LV/ BrightnessCalculation.pdf

Bradski, G., & Kaehler, A. (2008). *Learning OpenCV: Computer vision with the OpenCV library.* O'Reilly Media, Inc. ISBN: 9780596516130

Brubaker, S. C., Wu, J., Sun, J., Mullin, M. D., & Rehg, J. M. (2008). Fast asymmetric learning for cascade face detection. *IEEE Transactions on Pattern Analysis and Machine Intelligence, 30,* 369–382. doi:10.1109/TPAMI.2007.1181

Busso, C., Deng, Z., Yildirim, S., & Bulut, M. Lee, C. M., Kazemzadeh, A., ... Narayanan, S. (2004). *Analysis of emotion recognition using facial expression, speech and multimodal information.* International Conference on Multimodal Interfaces.

Chai, T. Y., Rizon, M., Woo, S. S., & Tan, C. S. (2009). Facial features for template matching based face recognition. *American Journal of Applied Sciences, 6*(11), 1897–1901. doi:10.3844/ajassp.2009.1897.1901

Chen, X., & Huang, T. (2003). Facial expression recognition: A clustering-based approach. *Pattern Recognition Letters, 24,* 1295–1302. doi:10.1016/S0167-8655(02)00371-9

Chibelushi, C. C., & Bourel, F. (2002). *Facial expression recognition: A brief tutorial overview.* University of Edinburgh, UK. Retrieved February 4, 2010, from http://homepages.inf.ed.ac.uk/rbf/CVonline/LOCAL_COPIES/CHIBELUSHI1/ CCC_FB_FacExprRecCVonline.pdf

Cho, J., Mirzaei, S., Oberg, J., & Kastner, R. (2009). *FPGA-based face detection system using Haar classifiers.* International Symposium on Field Programmable Gate Arrays.

Cohen, I., Grag, A., & Huang, T. S. (2000). *Emotion recognition from facial expression using multilevel HMM.* Neural Information Processing Systems.

Copyright © 2011, IGI Global. Copying or distributing in print or electronic forms without written permission of IGI Global is prohibited.

Cohen, I., Sebe, N., Garg, A., Chen, L. S., & Huang, T. S. (2003). Facial expression recognition from video sequences: Temporal and static modeling. *Computer Vision and Image Understanding, 91*, 160–187. doi:10.1016/S1077-3142(03)00081-X

Crestwood Communication Aids Inc. (2009). *Product: Talk Back12*. Retrieved October 14, 2009 from http://www.communicationaids.com/talkback12.htm

Datcu, D., & Rothkrantz, L. (2007). Facial expression recognition in still picture and video using active appearance models: A comparison approach. *ACM International Conference Proceeding Series, 285.*

Davis, J. W. (2001). *Hierarchical motion history images for recognizing human motion*. IEEE Workshop on Detection and Recognition of Events in Video, (pp. 39-46).

Donato, G., Bartlett, M. S., Hager, J. C., Ekman, P., & Sejnowski, T. J. (1999). Classifying facial action. *Advances in Neural Information Processing Systems, 8.*

Dubuisson, S., Davoine, F., & Masson, M. (2002). A solution for facial expression representation and recognition. *Signal Processing Image Communication, 17*, 657–673. doi:10.1016/S0923-5965(02)00076-0

Ekman, P., & Friesen, W. V. (1978). *Facial action coding system: Investigator's guide*. Palo Alto, CA: Consulting Psychologists Press.

Fasel, B. (2002). Multiscale facial expression recognition using convolutional neural networks. In *Proceedings of the Third Indian Conference on Computer Vision, Graphics and Image Processing (ICVGIP 2002).*

Fasel, B., & Luettin, B. (2003). Automatic facial expression analysis: A survey. *Pattern Recognition, 36*, 259–275. doi:10.1016/S0031-3203(02)00052-3

Franco, L., & Treves, A. (2001). *A neural network facial expression recognition system using unsupervised local processing*. Image and Signal Processing and Analysis.

Graves, A., Fernandez, S., & Schmidhuber, S. (2007). Multi-dimensional recurrent neural networks. *Proceedings of the 17th International Conference on Artificial Neural Networks* (pp. 549-558). Porto, Portugal: Springer-Verlag

Gregory, P., & Simon, M. A. (2008). *Biometrics for dummies*. Wiley Publishing, Inc.

Kotsia, I., & Pitas, I. (2007). Facial expression recognition in image sequences using geometric deformation features and support vector machines. *IEEE Transactions on Image Processing, 16*(1), 172–187. doi:10.1109/TIP.2006.884954

Copyright © 2011, IGI Global. Copying or distributing in print or electronic forms without written permission of IGI Global is prohibited.

Kovac, J., Peer, P., & Solina, F. (2003). Human skin colour clustering for face detection. In B. Zajc (Ed.), *EUROCON 2003—International Conference on Computer as a Tool*, Ljubljana, Slovenia, Sept. 2003.

Lau, B. T. (2009). Portable real time needs expression for people with communication disabilities. In D. Versick (Ed.), *Communication in computer and Information Science: Intelligent interactive assistance and mobile multimedia computing* (pp. 85-95). International Conference, Rostock-Warnemunde, Germany, Nov 2009. Berlin/Heidelberg, Germany: Springer-Verlag.

Lin,D. T.(2006). Facial expression classification using PCA and hierarchical radial basis function network.

Littlewort, G. C., Bartlett, M. S., & Lee, K. (2007). *Faces of pain: Automated measurement of spontaneous facial expressions of genuine and posed pain*. International Conference on Multimodal Interfaces. Oral session 1: Spontaneous behaviour (pp. 15-21).

Lyons, M., Budynek, J., Plante, A., & Akamatsu, S. (2000). Classifying facial attributes using a 2-D gabor wavelet representation and discriminant analysis. In *Proceedings of the 4th international conference on automatic face and gesture recognition*, (pp. 202–207).

Ma, L., & Khorasani, K. (2004). Facial expression recognition using constructive feed forward neural networks. *IEEE Transactions on Systems, Man, and Cybernetics, Part B, 34*(3). Macsolvers' Blog. (2009). *Testing the text to speech function*. Retrieved October 12, 2009 from http://macsolvers.wordpress.com/2009/03/24/text2speech/

Manohar, U. (2008). Why is communication important? *Buzzle.com*. Retrieved November 3, 2009, from http://www.buzzle.com/articles/why-is-communication-important.html

Matsugu, M., Mori, K., Mitari, Y., & Kaneda, Y. (2003). Subject independent facial expression recognition with robust face detection using a convolutional neural network. *Neural Networks, 16*, 555–559. doi:10.1016/S0893-6080(03)00115-1

Mobitek System. (2008). *SMS gateway development kit*. Mobitek System. Retrieved February 24, 2010, from http://www.mobitek.com.my/SMS_Gateway/SMS%20Gateway.html

Novita Children's Services. (2006). *Alternative and augmentative communication* (AAC). Retrieved October 23, 2009 from http://www.novita.org.au/Content.aspx?p=64

Copyright © 2011, IGI Global. Copying or distributing in print or electronic forms without written permission of IGI Global is prohibited.

Pantic, M., & Patras, I. (2006). Dynamics of facial expression: Recognition of facial actions and their temporal segments from face profile image sequences. *IEEE Transactions on Systems, Man and Cybernetics—Part B, 36*(2).

Price, J. R., & Gee, T. F. (2005). Face recognition using direct, weighted linear discriminant analysis and modular subspaces. *Pattern Recognition, 38*, 209–219. doi:10.1016/S0031-3203(04)00273-0

Riaz, Z., Mayer, C., Wimmer, M., Beetz, M., & Radig, B. (2009). A model based approach for expression invariant face recognition. In Tistarelli, M., & Nixon, M. S. (Eds.), *Advances in biometrics: Third International Conferences* (pp. 289–298). Alghero, Italy: Springer Berlin. doi:10.1007/978-3-642-01793-3_30

ScienceDaily. (2008). *Facial expression recognition software developed.*

Sebe, N., Lew, M. S., Sun, Y., Cohen, I., Gevers, T., & Huang, T. S. (2007). Authentic facial expression analysis. *Image and Vision Computing, 25*(12), 1856–1863. doi:10.1016/j.imavis.2005.12.021

Shan, C., Gong, S., & McOwan, P. W. (2005). *Robust facial expression recognition using local binary patterns.* IEEE International Conference, Image Processing, 2005. ICIP 2005.

Singh, S. K., Chauhan, D. S., Vatsa, M., & Singh, R. (2003). A robust skin color based face detection algorithm. *Tamkang Journal of Science and Engineering, 6*(4), 227–234.

Softpedia. (2009). *Y speak.* Retrieved October 20, 2009, from http://mac.softpedia.com/progScreenshots/Y-Speak-Screenshot-10550.html

Standup. (2006). *The STANDUP system.* Retrieved October 12, 2009 from http://www.csd.abdn.ac.uk/research/standup/software.php

Su, M. C., Hsieh, Y. J., & Huang, D. Y. (2007). Facial expression recognition using optical flow without complex feature extraction. *WSEAS Transactions on Computers, 6*(5), 763–770.

Tang, F., & Deng, B. (2007). *Facial expression recognition using AAM and local facial features.* Third International Conference Natural Computation, 2007. ICNC 2007. (p. 632).

Tian, Y., Kanade, T., & Cohn, J. F. (2002). *Evaluation of Gabor wavelet based facial action unit recognition in image sequences of increasing complexity.* Fifth IEEE International Conference, (pp. 229–234).

Copyright © 2011, IGI Global. Copying or distributing in print or electronic forms without written permission of IGI Global is prohibited.

Universiteit van Amsterdam. (2008). *eMotion: Emotion recognition software.* Retrieved October 12, 2009, from http://www.visual-recognition.nl/eMotion.html

Valstar, M., Pantic, M., & Patras, I. (2004). *Motion history for facial action detection in video.* International Conference on Systems, Man and Cybernetics.

Viola, P., & Jones, M. J. (2004). Robust real-time face detection. *International Journal of Computer Vision, January 10, 52*(2), 137-154.

Wang, J., Plataniotis, K. N., & Venetsanopoulos, A. N. (2005). Selecting discriminate eigenfaces for face recognition. *Pattern Recognition Letters, 26,* 1470–1482. doi:10.1016/j.patrec.2004.11.029

Whitehill, J. R. (2006). *Automatic real-time facial expression recognition for signed language translation.*

Xie, X., & Lam, K. M. (2009). Facial expression recognition based on shape and texture. *Pattern Recognition, 42*(5), 1003–1011. doi:10.1016/j.patcog.2008.08.034

Zhan, C., Li, W., Ogunbona, P., & Safaei, F. (2006). A real-time facial expression recognition system for online games. *ACM International Conference Proceeding Series, 207.*

Zhan, Y., & Zhou, G. (2007). Facial expression recognition based on hybrid features and fusing discrete HMM. In Shumaker, R. (Ed.), *Virtual reality, HCII 2007, (LNCS 4563)* (pp. 408–417). Berlin/ Heidelberg, Germany: Springer-Verlag.

Zhang, Y., & Ji, Q. (2005). Active and dynamic information fusion for facial expression understanding from image sequence. *Pattern Analysis and Machine Intelligence, 27.*

Zhang, Z., Lyons, M., Schuster, M., & Akamatsu, S. (1998). *Comparison between geometry-based and Gabor-wavelets-based facial expression recognition using multi-layer perceptron.* Third IEEE International Conference, (pp. 454–459).

ADDITIONAL READING

Agrawal, N., Cosgriff, R., & Mudur, R. (2009). Mood detection: Implementing a facial expression recognition system. *Stanford University.* Retrieved 31 January 2010, from http://www.stanford.edu/class/cs229/proj2009/AgrawalCosgriffMudur.pdf

Huang, X. & Lin, Y. (2008). A vision-based hybrid method for facial expression recognition. *1st international conference on Ambient media and systems*

Copyright © 2011, IGI Global. Copying or distributing in print or electronic forms without written permission of IGI Global is prohibited.

Jemaa, Y.B. & Khanfir, S. (2009). Automatic local Gabor features extraction for face recognition. *International Journal of Computer Science and Information Security, Vol. 3*, No. 1.

Zhao, Y., Shen, X., Georganas, N. D., & Petriu, E. M. (2009). Part-based PCA for Facial Feature Extraction and Classification. *Haptic Audio visual Environments and Games, 2009*. HAVE 2009. IEEE International Workshop. 99 – 104.

KEY TERMS AND DEFINITIONS

Assistive Communication Tools: Tools used to assist physical and communication disabled peoples to communicate or interact with the others.

Biometrics: A method of verifying a person's identify by analysing a unique physical attribute of the individual for example fingerprints, face, DNA, etc.

Computer Vision: A process of taking a live raster image that represented as a matrix of numeric values and interpreting it into higher level data abstractions and symbolic objects such as humans, limbs, faces, props, poses, gestures, etc.

Facial Expression Recognition System: A tool used to identify and recognize human expression or emotion by providing human face image.

Image: Processing: Involve complex calculation and transformation of image(s) into another form, size, model and channel for example RGB, HSV, Greyscale and Black and White.

Template Matching: Involving the process matching between two or more images at the same time generate matching result.

Viola-Jones Face Detection: A common face detection algorithm used by researchers to search human's face pattern within an image.

Copyright © 2011, IGI Global. Copying or distributing in print or electronic forms without written permission of IGI Global is prohibited.

Chapter 4

A Novel Application of Information Communication Technology to Assist Visually Impaired People

Tee Zhi Heng
The University of Nottingham Malaysia Campus, Malaysia

Ang Li Minn
The University of Nottingham Malaysia Campus, Malaysia

Seng Kah Phooi
The University of Nottingham Malaysia Campus, Malaysia

ABSTRACT

This chapter presents a novel application for wireless technology to assist visually impaired people. As an alternative to the medical model of rehabilitation, the information explosion era provides the foundation for a technological solution to lead the visually impaired to more independent lives in the community by minimizing the obstacles of living. A "SmartGuide" caregiver monitoring system is built as a standalone portable handheld device linked. The objective of this system is to assist blind and low vision people to walk around independently especially in dynamic changing environments. Navigation assistance is accomplished by providing speech guidance on how to move to a particular location. The system delivers dynamic environmental information to lead the visually impaired to more independent lives in the community by minimizing the obstacles of living. Information of changing

DOI: 10.4018/978-1-60960-541-4.ch004

Copyright ©2011, IGI Global. Copying or distributing in print or electronic forms without written permission of IGI Global is prohibited.

environments such as road blockage, road closure, and intelligent navigation aids is provided to the user in order to guide the user safely to his or her destination. This system also includes a camera sensor network to enhance monitoring capabilities for an extra level of security and reliability.

INTRODUCTION

Visual impairment can be quantified in terms of the remaining visual acuity and visual field. Visual acuity is expressed as a fraction of full acuity (Pun, Roth, Bologna, Moustakas, & Tzovaras, 2007). A visual acuity of 1/10 means that a sight handicapped person has only 10% visual acuteness or clearness if compared to a normal sighted person. Visual field or sometimes field of view refers to the physical objects and light sources in the external world that impinge the retina (Wikipedia, 2008a), in other words, the total area in which objects can be seen in the side vision when the eye is focused on a central point. A normally sighted person has a visual field of 60 degrees.

Visual impairment can result from damage at any time in the life cycle of human beings. There are four levels of visual function, normal vision, moderate visual impairment, severe visual impairment and blindness. Severe visual impairment leads to a person being totally blind. Less severe cases cause a person to have partial vision loss that cannot be corrected called low vision. Total blindness means no remaining visual perception at all. Genetic and developmental anomalies can cause visually impairment from birth. Visual impairment may also occur during adulthood when many diseases and genetic patterns manifest themselves. According to the World Health Organization (WHO, 2009) fact sheet, there are 314 million visually impaired people worldwide, where 45 million of them are blind. Still according to WHO, 87% of the world's visually impaired people live in developing countries (WHO, 2009).

The goal of this project is to develop an intelligent wireless assistive system to assist the visually impaired to walk around independently and safely especially in an indoor environment. This project proposes a system which utilizes the advancement of the current Information Communication Technology (ICT), for e-inclusion in current transportation systems and indoor environment to tap new digital opportunities for the inclusion of visually impaired people. Navigation aids are accomplished by providing speech guidance on how to move from one location to another. Public transportation systems like airports, bus terminals and mass rapid transport stations would be made more accessible to this segment of society. They would be able to travel in unfamiliar indoor locations successfully and have a workable strategy for self-familiarization within complex changing environments.

Copyright © 2011, IGI Global. Copying or distributing in print or electronic forms without written permission of IGI Global is prohibited.

BACKGROUND

A typical guidance system consists of three components: Input Component, Processing Component and Output Component. The input component includes information sources to be used by the system which is normally made up by analog/digital sensors, instructions and raw data. The processing component is made up by one or more microcontrollers that utilized the data obtained from the input components to further process the data. Data is processed by using a pre programmed algorithm to calculate further subsequent actions and maintain proper heading. The output component is the component that directly affects the system's velocity and heading. For example, engine control unit, and actuators that will affect the system's overall course.

Several researchers have proposed technological solutions using RFID and GPS technology to assist visually impaired people (D'Atri et al., 2007; Chang, et al., 2005; Ran, Helal & Moore, 2004; BrailleNote, n.d.; Cardin, Thalmann & Vexo, 2007). Amongst the assistive systems which have been reported are SESAMONET (D'Atri et al., 2007), iCane (Chang, et al., 2005), Drishti (Ran, Helal & Moore, 2004), BrailleNote (n.d.) GPS and Werable Systems(Cardin, Thalmann & Vexo, 2007).

The research on assistive technology is finding a way to reduce the barriers of the lives of visually impaired people and to enrich their lives with more accessibility. By utilizing current GPS, RFID and speech recognition technology, reliable, intuitive and intelligent assistive systems can be developed. Table 1 is a summary of the various interactive assistive technologies discussed previously.

In this chapter, we present a wireless assistive system using a combination of RFID technology, dead reckoning module (DRM) with a wireless sensor network backbone for improved localization indoors and outdoors. The system is also designed to be light in weight. An important part of the system is the camera sensor network where caregivers can monitor the user in real time adding an extra layer of security to the system. A comparison of the above discussed interactive assistive technologies can be summarized as in Table 1.

SESAMONET

The SESAMONET (Secure and Safety Mobility Network) system (D'Atri et al., 2007) is developed by the European Joint Research Centre and University of Rome's RFID labs of Sapienza. The system uses RFID technology for user localization and tracking. SESAMONET use a grid of RFID tags which are burrowed in the ground around a depth of 4cm. The tags are wrapped in ceramic cells and embedded at 65cm intervals. An RFID reader is attached to a cane to obtain the tag ID as the

Copyright © 2011, IGI Global. Copying or distributing in print or electronic forms without written permission of IGI Global is prohibited.

Table 1. Comparison of assistive technologies

	SmartGuide	SESAMONET	iCane	Drishti	BrailleNote GPS	Wearable Systems
Localization Method	RFID	RFID	RFID	Differential GPS	GPS	Sonar
Localization Data Storage	Server Database	RFID Tag + Mobile Database	Mobile Static Database	-	-	-
Information Source	Server Database	Replenishing PDA Mobile Database with main source in external server	Local PDA Mobile Database	GIS Database in an external server	Trekker 2.0 GPS Map	PDA
Information Behavior	Static and Dynamic	Static and Dynamic	Static	Static and Dynamic	Dynamic	-
Server Connectivity	Wireless Sensor Network	Any Internet Connection (Wifi / GPRS etc.)	-	WIFI (802.11b)	Internet Connection	-
Usage	Indoor & Outdoor, Restricted Area	Indoor & Outdoor Not restricted	Indoor & Outdoor, Restricted Area	Outdoor only, Area Not Restricted	Outdoor only, Area Not Restricted	Indoor & Outdoor
Device Components Used	SmartGuide Reader, Smart Guide Tracker, Wireless Sensor Network, Server, Microphone	RFID Reader Cane, RFID tag grid, Bluetooth headset, PDA, Server	RFID Reader Cane, RFID tag grid, Bluetooth headset, PDA	DGPS Receiver, Wifi Radio, Wearable Computer, Server	-	PDA, Sonar Sensor, Vibrators
Drawbacks	RFID tags needs to be predefined.	Definitive characteristic causes failure during deviations from path	Old static information might be hazardous in changing environments	Heavy, Can only operate in outdoors	Unable to operate indoors	No Navigation

cane moves over the tag. This information is sent to a PDA where software looks up the navigation data for the tag ID in the data server. The data server holds the database containing all the information used for navigation. The server also has an interface for client data synchronization which automatically updates data on the client side whenever the user approaches a new tag. The navigation data is converted to speech using text-to-speech synthesis and it's sent back to the user via Bluetooth through a Bluetooth headset.

The main barrier in the successful performance of 'SESAMONET' is logistical issues. The system is only available provided the user is on the RFID embedded pavement. Furthermore, the layout and the maintenance of the RFID embedded

Copyright © 2011, IGI Global. Copying or distributing in print or electronic forms without written permission of IGI Global is prohibited.

path can be labour and material intensive. There is also a problem where the user wandered away from the track (RFID Microchip Network) and cannot find an RFID transponder to get back on to the track.

iCane

The iCane (Chang, et al., 2005) system is developed by Tsung-Hsiang Chng of National Taiwan University. The 'iCane' is based on a walking stick which is capable of giving navigational help to user in terms of locating nearby services. It features an individual personal map in order to assist revisiting places of interest easily.

The system functions similarly to SESAMONET. The system utilizes RFID technology for person localization, a PDA to store navigation data and Bluetooth headset as human voice interface. RFID tags are placed on tactile pathways to be read by the RFID reader on the cane. Unlike SESAMONET, iCane utilizes a local database map installed in the PDA in order words; it has a static data source.

The accuracy of the system is proportional to the density of the RFID network. The RFID tags are categorized by storing significant lower nibbles as an indicator of different tactile paving. The tile type is differentiated by the least significant bits (LSB) of the tag ID.

The iCane lags behind SESAMONET as it utilizes a static navigation data source which is unable to handle dynamically changing environments. Since the control is static, there are risks of user navigation in a newly changed area with the old data set; a situation where the physical situation mismatches with the logical situation depicted in the data base. This can be of an enormous danger if the user is guided in a wrong direction in a wrong environment.

Drishti

Drishti (Ran, et al., 2004) which is an integrated navigation system for visually impaired people uses the Global Positioning System (GPS) and Geographical Information System (GIS) technologies. It is designed to be used within the university premises and contains a GIS dataset of the university. This contains geographically referenced information for both static and dynamic environments and is referred to as a spatial database. A differential GPS receiver in the wearable device determines the localization of the user by obtaining the (x,y,z) coordinates. After localization is performed, the spatial database is accessible through a wireless network to a wearable device that is carried by the visually impaired person. Drishti uses the IEEE 802.11b protocol to connect with its GIS server. Drishti is an assistive device which is operable in dynamically changing environments and can optimize routes

Copyright © 2011, IGI Global. Copying or distributing in print or electronic forms without written permission of IGI Global is prohibited.

for navigation when there is an unforeseen obstacle in the path. Like SESAMONET, Drishti gives assistance to the user by means of speech.

Drishti may be considered as the first reliable assistive technology system which is capable to provide navigation assistance for the visually impaired people in dynamically changing environments. However, there are two limitations with this system. First, the prototype weighs eight pounds. Second, the degradation of the RF signals inside buildings degrades the accuracy of the GPS localization.

BrailleNote GPS

The BrailleNote (n.d.) is an assistive device which is on the market since 2005. The BrailleNote is a commercial product with various functions to offer that comes in a small and compact package. The BrailleNote GPS uses the GPS satellites to relay information about user's position and nearby points of interest. The user can easily program personalized travel routes and locations as well as use the thousands of points supplied by the system. BrailleNote GPS provides direction to head or whose driveway the user is crossing, and even which location the user is currently at. The BrailleNote uses the new generation GPS maps which maps larger territories and are divided into regional maps for more convenience. Multiple-maps can be activated and stored in BrailleNote's memory. The Trekker 3.0 also expands the sources of geographical information with the capability to integrate complementary points of interest coming from other users, or databases downloadable from the Web. The 'VoiceNote GPS' is a more advanced version which uses the TTS method to convey speech information to the user. The 'BrailleNote' suffers the same shortfall as Dristhi. The GPS's accuracy is the limitation within indoor environments.

Wearable Systems

Wearable Systems (Cardin, et al., 2007) is a system designed to aid visually impaired people focusing on obstacle detection especially obstacles at shoulder height. The system utilizes sonar sensors to sense dynamic obstacles surrounding the environment and feeding the information through a sensing interface. In other words, the system will serve as an extension of the user's body functions. The major drawback of the system is that it does not provide guidance to the user for travelling.

SMARTGUIDE SYSTEM DESIGN

The SmartGuide System is designed to provide navigation instructions and information for the visually impaired people in real time with minimal weight (<1kg). The

Copyright © 2011, IGI Global. Copying or distributing in print or electronic forms without written permission of IGI Global is prohibited.

Figure 1. System overview

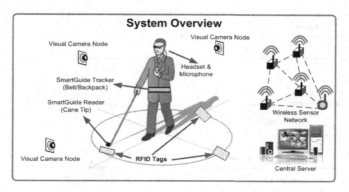

system has a main purpose of assisting and monitoring the visually impaired people to roam freely in an indoor environment. The system consists of four core layers which are the hardware layer (SmartGuide Tracker and Reader), wireless sensor network layer (Crossbow WSN), speech layer (user interface speech components) and software layer (Centralize sever and intelligent management software) as shown in Figure 1. Details of the various layers can be referred to subsections 3.1 to 3.4. RFID, dead reckoning, standalone microcontrollers, speech recognition, speech synthesis and ZigBee technologies is used in the system to achieve navigation and guidance objectives.

The system utilizes RFID tags as its indoor geographical information provider in order to achieve indoor localization. In other words, programmed RFID tags are placed strategically to mark points of interests in an indoor environment. By virtually connecting all the RFID tags, a 3D map is formed. RFID tags make up waypoints (the tags that the user must travel through) which is used during real time navigation to reach the requested destination. The speech layer acts as the main human interface of the system. Commands are given in speech to increase the user friendliness of the system. The hardware layer utilizes various technology and sensors to achieve the localization, navigation and extraction of positional data. The Wireless Sensor Network (WSN) layer acts as the data transportation backbone of the system. Data transfer between the hardware and software layer can be achieved to increase system stability. Throughout the navigation process the user's position will be monitored there will be real-time and fault-tolerant data communication between all the four layers.

The navigation starts with the hardware and speech layer where the user first requests a destination by talking into the microphone. The speech layer will handle the request by performing speech recognition, digitizing the speech into machine understandable command. At the same time, the hardware layer which consists of

Copyright © 2011, IGI Global. Copying or distributing in print or electronic forms without written permission of IGI Global is prohibited.

Figure 2. SmartGuide component layers interaction summary

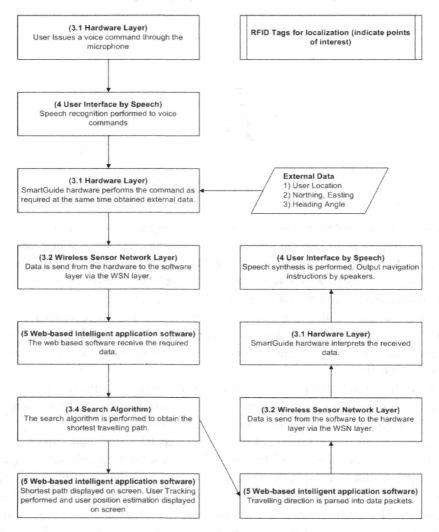

the SmartGuide devices obtained the user's current location. The current location of the user is obtained at the same time the requested destination is digitized into machine understandable command. These data are then relayed to the central server where to software layer is located via the wireless sensor network layer. The software layer on the central server then performs further processing, utilizing an algorithm to obtain the shortest travel path to the requested destination. The shortest path is a string of way points calculated by the system's algorithm which the user has to travel. Figure 2 is a summary of the interaction between the various layer components.

Copyright © 2011, IGI Global. Copying or distributing in print or electronic forms without written permission of IGI Global is prohibited.

Figure 4: The 3D coordinates of a floor plan

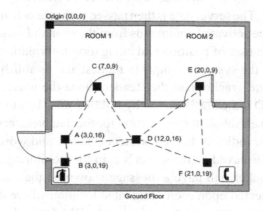

Hardware Layer

The SmartGuide device consists of two parts. One part is attached to the cane (Smart-Guide Reader) and the other part is attached to the person (SmartGuide Tracker). By splitting the hardware into two parts, the SmartGuide Reader is designed to be as compact as possible to increase portability and mobility. Core processing modules and interfacing modules are being installed on the SmartGuide Tracker which will be housed on a belt or a backpack of the user. The use of a belt/backpack system ensures ease of travelling. The two parts communicate wirelessly using Bluetooth technology. Fig. 4.5 shows the block diagram of the SmartGuide Reader and Tracker. Fig. 4.6 shows the SmartGuide Hardware Prototype with the RFID Tags.

The SmartGuide Reader uses various technology and sensors to achieve the localization, navigation and extraction of positioning data. A combination of RFID technology, Global Positioning System (GPS) and Dead Reckoning Module (DRM) tracking are used. The core processor for the system is a PIC Microcontroller. Bluetooth modules are used to replace the physical wires between the RFID Reader attached to the cane and the PIC microcontroller attached to the person. After the data extraction and measurement from the digital compass, GPS and DRM, the data are wirelessly transmitted to the host server via a wireless sensor mote. The host server will locate the current position and sends back the necessary speech information for user guidance and navigation.

The SmartGuide device uses the RFID tags as localization points which are located on the floor in different areas. The RFID reader reads the tag ID from the RFID tags and the DRM which consists of gyroscopes and accelerometers is utilized to complement the positioning method by providing the position between those discrete points. After the data has been sent to the central server, acknowledgement

Copyright © 2011, IGI Global. Copying or distributing in print or electronic forms without written permission of IGI Global is prohibited.

of position and localization will be done by the server from the corresponding data entry in the database. The server data is then passed to the speech module. The speech module accepts voice activated commands from the user and generates synthesized speech to inform the user of position and navigation information.

Upon power up, the system attempts to request and establish the wireless connectivity between the Tracker and the Reader. Once the wireless connectivity is established, the LED indicator is shown by lighting on. The next step is to turn on the wireless mote to establish the connection for the database server. Once the GUI on the software layer indicates that the system is active and working, the positions of the user will be displayed on the server's map for monitoring. At the same time, the SmartGuide Tracker will have a message shown on the LCD to indicate that the RFID Tag is detected upon each designated location where the tags are fixed.

RFID data reading compass data reading and DRM data collection is performed within the Mote interrupt service routine and these data will be sent over to the mote when requested by the mote through the interrupt. The mote will request this information periodically in the interval of few seconds. Once the reader detects an RFID Tag, the tag id is sent to the server via wireless mote. The correct position will be determined according to the RFID tag and necessary speech information is delivered to the user in voice form. Assistive data will be sent back to the SmartGuide Tracker in the form of bytes. The PIC saves the assistive data and sends them to the speech processor to be spoken out as words.

The main loop of the 'SmartGuide' system program consists of all the functions to be performed by all the various modules upon receiving the mote ISR. Crucial and important data parsing actions and data collection is done. The operating system can be seen in Figure 3.

Wireless Sensor Network Layer

The wireless sensor network (WSN) provides remote database and server connectivity with ease. Data such as navigation requests and instructions are relayed on the fly between the hardware and software layer. The Crossbow Wireless Sensor Network is selected as the core hardware for data transportation for the SmartGuide system.

In general, the architecture of Crossbow Wireless Sensor Network via nodes in connection with outside applications (server, PC, cell phone etc.), has three folds:

2.1.1 Node - Acquires data from associate data acquisition board and forwards the data upstream to the base station.

2.1.2 Gateway - Aggregates data from the network; Provides connection to outside applications (PC, PDA, server etc.).

Copyright © 2011, IGI Global. Copying or distributing in print or electronic forms without written permission of IGI Global is prohibited.

Figure 3. SmartGuide operating system flow

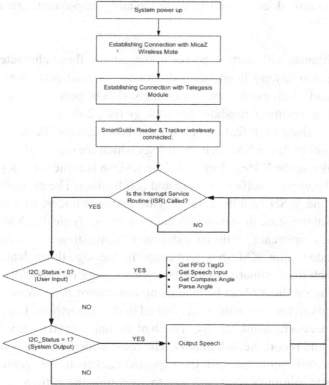

2.1.3 Router - Extends network coverage; Re-routes in case of node failure or network congestion.

Wireless sensor networks have attracted a wide interest from industry due to their diversity of applications. Sensor networks are pervasive by nature; the number of nodes in a network is nearly boundless. Therefore, a key to realizing this potential is multi-hop mesh networking, which enables scalability and reliability. A mesh network is really a generic name for a class of networked embedded systems that share several characteristics including:

2.1.4 Multi-Hop - Capability of sending messages peer-to-peer to a base station, thereby enabling scalable range extension.

2.1.5 Self-Configuring - Capable of network formation without human intervention.

2.1.6 Self-Healing - Capable of adding and removing network nodes automatically without having to reset the network.

Copyright © 2011, IGI Global. Copying or distributing in print or electronic forms without written permission of IGI Global is prohibited.

2.1.7 Dynamic Routing - Capable of adaptively determining the route based on dynamic network conditions (e.g., link quality, hop-count, gradient, or other metric).

When combined with battery power management, these characteristics allow sensor networks to be long-lived, easily deployed, and resilient to the unpredictable wireless channel. With mesh networking, the vision of pervasive and fine-grained sensing becomes reality (Crossbow Technology Inc., 2007a).

Crossbow defines a full featured multi-hop, ad-hoc, networking protocol called *XMesh*. Nodes or motes in XMesh terminology which are wirelessly connected with each other make up the XMesh Network. The XMesh is a true mesh topology (peer-to-peer) which supports self-organizing and self healing. The multi-hop technique supported by the WSN enables data relaying between nodes, maximizing signal coverage area at the same time provides fault tolerance. Typically, XMesh can route data from nodes "upstream" to the base station or "downstream" to individual nodes. If there is a node failure, XMesh will re-route the message through alternative path in order to reach the destination (Crossbow Technology Inc., 2007b).

Data routing on the XMesh is done using the *Any-to-Base Routing Algorithm*. XMesh expands all the available routes linked to the destination. The first goal is to measure the success rate/link quality of each of the links. Each mote will monitor its neighbouring and report the link quality. The route with better link quality ensures higher ratio probability to transmit the expected packets to the receiver node. The second goal is to minimize total path cost to determine the optimal route. The term "cost" is a measure of distance based on hop count, transmission and retries and reconfiguration over time. Figure 4 illustrates the Any-to-Base Routing Algorithm. In this case, the node cost is 40 which is the link cost plus the parent cost.

Crossbow WSN is an ideal solution for SmartGuide system as it provides intelligent, reliable networking with significant fault tolerance. The system is used to assist visually impaired people; thus any fault or delay in message transmission is not wanted and might cause safety issues. On the other hand, the ease of integration and low power consumption makes the Crossbow solution a good choice for the system.

Tag Mapping

The RFID tags must first be defined or mapped before assistive navigation supported can be provided. The tags scattered around in an area marks the points of interests and way points in a real world environment. The tags are mapped using conventional 3D right-handed Cartesian coordinate system to provide straightforward representation of a real world 3D space. The X, Y, Z coordinates is based on orthographic projection, where the +X coordinates points to the right, the +Y position points up

Copyright © 2011, IGI Global. Copying or distributing in print or electronic forms without written permission of IGI Global is prohibited.

and the +Z position points to the viewer. For easier data processing the coordinates in the systems are all set to be in the first octant where all the (X, Y, Z) coordinates are in positive values. In other words, the origin will be the northwest point in the floor plan. This will then give us the coordinates of points A to F respectively as shown in Figure 4. As all the discrete points are located at the ground floor, they all have a Y coordinate of 0.

All these data are stored in a MySql database hosted on the server (software layer) in the "tagmap" table. This information is essential in order for the search algorithm to be performed. The database also stores additional information such as the "Stair Tag" and "Adjacent Tag" parameters. The Stair Tag parameter holds information whether it is a tag that can provide access to different levels (tag positioned at stairs, escalators or elevators).

The adjacent tag property is required parameter in order to perform the search algorithm. For instance from point C & E. in Figure 4, because the points are not adjacent to each other, it is not possible for one to travel directly from C to E. In the real world, it would be impossible for the user to penetrate through the wall to reach point E from point C, thus the user will need to go to point D before getting to point E. A user cannot travel to a new point unless it is an adjacent point. This rule enables the travel path to be more complete when obstacles such as objects, furniture and walls come into the picture in the real world. By joining all the tags with its adjacent tags, a complete state space and a search tree will be formed. This search tree is used by the shortest travel path search algorithm to perform calculations. The result of the calculation is the virtual path (consists of a string of waypoint tags) which indicates the shortest travel path to be taken.

The stair tag property indicates access to different floor levels. This parameter is important when the user is travelling between floors. If the users request a destination that is not on the current floor the stair tag property comes into play. The search algorithm will guide the user to the nearest stair tag which provides access to different floor levels. In other words, the stair tag property provides access between levels.

The virtually constructed search tree is used by the shortest travel path search algorithm to perform calculations while the virtual path will indicate the travel path to be taken. With a complete and detail tag mapping implemented via the database the performance and results of the search algorithm for navigation is guaranteed.

Search Algorithm

The search algorithm is performed after the RFID tags are properly mapped. The backbone of the search algorithm is the A* (pronounced A star) search algorithm. In the current scenario, A* is optimal (cost to the destination tag is never overestimated) and complete (all the tags and its positions are known) making it the best choice

Copyright © 2011, IGI Global. Copying or distributing in print or electronic forms without written permission of IGI Global is prohibited.

which minimizes the total estimated solution cost. The algorithm is enhanced further so that it will be able to perform search in a 3D environment as typical buildings consists of multiple floors.

The A* is a form of informed search utilizing the known position and distance between tags to obtain the cheapest path from the current stage to the goal. The A* search algorithm is a type of best-first search in which a node is selected for expansion based on an evaluation function f(n). The node with the lowest evaluation function is selected for expansion as the value of the evaluation function is the measured distance to the goal.

A* search algorithm evaluates nodes by combining $g(n)$, which is the cost to reach the node, and $h(n)$, the cost to get from that node to the goal: $f(n) = g(n) + h(n)$. Since $g(n)$ gives the path cost from the start node to node n and $h(n)$ is the estimated cost of the cheapest path from n to the goal, $f(n)$ is defined as the estimated cost of the cheapest solution through n (Russell & Novig, 2002).

A* is optimal in this case as the $f(n)$ is an admissible heuristic. The heuristic function h(n) never overestimates the cost as it is basically the straight line distance (h_{SLD}) from tag n to the goal (shortest distance from one point to another). On the other hand, $g(n)$ is the exact cost to reach n (total distance travelled). Thus it is an immediate consequence that $f(n)$ never overestimates the true cost of a solution through n. A* search algorithm is also complete in the sense that it will always find the solution when there is one (Wikipedia, 2008b). The search is always complete in this case as the solution is the user requested destination that is always available.

Referring to Figure 4, if a user request to travel from the main door (point A) to the telephone (point F), the shortest travel path using the A* algorithm would be A -> D -> F. The search algorithm will check on the current tag (point A) and all its adjacent tags (in this case the adjacent tags will be B, C and D). Utilizing the tag coordinates stored in the MySql database, the algorithm will then apply the evaluation function calculation and expand the nearest path as the one with the smallest heuristic distance (in this case it will be D with the smallest f(n)). Similarly, the algorithm will repeat itself by exploring all the adjacent tags of the subsequent state, in this case point D, and perform the heuristic calculation to decide which tag to expand until it reaches the goal state F. All the expanded tags will form the shortest path to the destination tag requested.

The 3D A* search comes into action when the destination requested is not on the same floor as the current position of the user. The algorithm will perform a search to locate the nearest gateway that provides access to different floors, in this case, stairs, escalators or elevator. The system will then provide the user navigation either up or down to the appropriate floor. The search will then continue to guide the user from the particular exit point of the gateway till the final destination which is now on the same floor.

Copyright © 2011, IGI Global. Copying or distributing in print or electronic forms without written permission of IGI Global is prohibited.

USER INTERFACE BY SPEECH

The speech layer is responsible to perform speech recognition and speech synthesis. A microphone acts as the main human interface of the SmartGuide system but inputting speech commands for them user (recognition) while a speaker/headphone is used to output instructions to provide navigation assistance (synthesis). The speech processor is the VR Stamp RSC-4X RPM microcontroller and software development supported by Phython Project-SE (Wikipedia, 2009a) IDE (Integrated Development Environment) which supports C language. Sensory Loader 4 is then used to burn the software into the VR Stamp via a development board.

The VR Stamp RSC-464 speech processor is a 8 bit programmable microcontroller with built-in ADC, DAC, RAM and a basic interpreter (PBASIC) built into the ROM. Utilizing the new Fluent-Chip technology and optimized audio processing blocks, the VR Stamp is capable of providing high performance I/O speech features to cost sensitive embedded and consumer products with improved noise control. The VR Stamp supports the capability of creating speaker independent recognition sets by simple typing in the desired recognition vocabulary. For development, the speech processor provides an unprecedented level of cost effective system-on-chip (SOC) integration, enabling many applications that require DSP or audio processing which be used as a general-purpose mixed signal processor platform for custom applications. Speech recognition is done via a hybrid Hidden Markov Model and Neural Net methods.

The VR Stamp supports and recommends fast rapid deployment by using Quick T2SI speech recognition software to construct words and phrase that make up the speech and command library. The command library is built on predefined user response various user responses maps to various actions that will be carried out by the speech recognition application. The speech library is responsible for speech synthesizing, outputting predefined navigation instructions by voice.

There are two types of speech interfacing methodologies, prompted recognition and continuous listening recognition. Command phrases are examples of prompted recognition where the application prompts for the user for further input to perform the required actions (initiative on application side). On the other hand, triggering phrases is an example of continuous listening recognition, and where the application reacts immediately once a speech input is received (initiative on user side). For either method, end-point detection is required to mark an end to the user's response. End point detection can be done via timeout (time elapsed with no input) and word spotting (predefined vocabulary).

Copyright © 2011, IGI Global. Copying or distributing in print or electronic forms without written permission of IGI Global is prohibited.

Figure 5. IntelNavWeb 3.0 main page

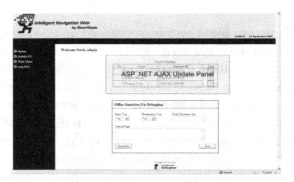

WEB-BASED INTELLIGENT APPLICATION SOFTWARE

The web-based software, "IntelNav Web 3.0" is built using ASP. NET. The web application utilizes ASP.NET AJAX framework extensively for bandwidth and speed enhancing. The web application performs partial page updates that refresh only the parts of the web page that have changed. Thus, improving the efficiency of the web application as part of the processing is performed by the browser. Figure 5 is a screen shot of the web application software.

CAMERA SENSOR NETWORK

To enhanced real time monitoring by the caregivers and system administrators, a camera sensor network is implemented on top of the SmartGuide system. The caregiver monitoring system automatically switches to the camera nearest to the user for live user tracking. The camera system network operated wirelessly consists of two basic elements, the visual camera node and the visual base node.

OmniVision OV9650 CMOS Camera

The visual camera node is made up of by the OmniVision OV9650 CMOS cameras connected to a Xilinx Spartan-3 FPGA. The Xilinx Spartan-3 FPGA used is part of a Celoxica RC10 development unit to process the captured images and control the ZigBee radio module. The information is sent wirelessly from the RC10 unit using the Telegesis ETRX2-PA ZigBee module to the data receiving end which is the visual base node on the PC/server side. For the vision nodes, the Telegesis

Copyright © 2011, IGI Global. Copying or distributing in print or electronic forms without written permission of IGI Global is prohibited.

Figure 6. Camera sensor network block diagram

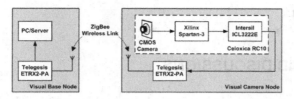

ETRX2-PA module is configured as a ZigBee router while the base node is configured as a coordinator.

By capturing and sending the images at a substantial rate, the camera sensor network can be used as a CCTV replacement and at the same time provide an extra layer of security to the SmartGuide system. Figure 6 illustrates the system block diagram for the camera sensor network.

Celoxica RC10 Development Board

The main function of the Spartan-3 FPGA Celoxica RC10 development board is to: (1) process incoming data from the camera, (2) control the camera via the SCCB interface, (3) store the captured image in a frame buffer, (4) structure the data in the frame buffer to be transmitted over the serial link and (5) control the Telegesis ZigBee module using byte sized AT commands.

The data from the camera is received in chunks of 16-bits (1 word), with 5-bits representing the Red and Blue channels and 6-bits representing the Green channel. The additional 1-bit allocated for the green channel is to provide more levels in this channel as the human vision is more sensitive to green than any other colour.

The RAW data sent from the camera is first converted to gray-scale by taking only the green channel and stored into the FPGA internal block RAM (i.e. the frame buffer). However, upon start up, the FPGA will most likely start receiving data from the camera that does not correspond to the beginning of a frame, i.e. the data the camera is sending is from halfway through a frame raster scan. This causes problems with data alignment at the receiving end. We have to ensure that the frame buffer is filled with exactly one complete frame. To overcome this, we have to ensure that what is stored in the frame buffer is a complete frame by detecting the x and y starting coordinates which should correspond to 0,0 at the beginning of a frame.

Once stored in the frame buffer, the data is restructured into 8-byte chunks. Before transmission over the wireless link can begin, the Telegesis module is setup to match the serial port parameters of the RC10. The transmission data packet is shown in Figure 3. The first packet to be sent tells the receiving end that it is a start

Copyright © 2011, IGI Global. Copying or distributing in print or electronic forms without written permission of IGI Global is prohibited.

of a new frame and similarly an end frame packet is sent to denote the end of the frame being sent.

RESULTS AND DISCUSSIONS

There are two experiments being carried out in this section. The accuracy of the dead reckoning device is tested thoroughly in the first experiment. Dead reckoning is a way of predicting the user's location while navigation assistance is temporarily lost when the user is travelling between tags. Section 7.1 provides the detail experiment done on the dead reckoning functionality of the system. In the second experiment the camera sensor nodes are tested. Important parameters such as data delay time and signal coverage ranges are obtained in order to determine the camera node network setup.

Dead-Reckoning Experiment Results

There are two experiment of dead reckoning method: continuous dead reckoning and zero dead reckoning method. Continuous dead reckoning is the continuous data collection from the start till the end of the navigation. Zero dead reckoning is the dead reckoning data from one point to another, meaning that the dead reckoning calculations is zeroed each time the user reaches a check point tag. The two sets of results collected are an average from three users. The users are blind folded, travelling from point A to point E shown in Figure 4. It took 10 steps to travel from the start to the destination calculated at an average stride length of 400mm. There are two sets of data collected the azimuth shows the heading of the user in degrees while the northing and easting shows how far the user has travelled from north and east of the starting position in meters.

For the continuous dead reckoning method, estimation error tends to grow with time and distance. Position estimation grows to a total of 1 meter till the end of the navigation in this case. Thus this method is not suitable to apply on the current system. On the other hand, the zero dead reckoning method upon arrival on each tag yields better results and the travel path is closer to the actual path travelled. Estimation error from the actual x and y axis is controlled at around 400 mm on average. In terms of real time performance, the estimation error is acceptable. In order to make use of the dead reckoning data and ensure the reliability of the user position tracking, the RFID tags can be enlarge to a minimum size 400mm by 400mm to contain the estimation error. Further calibration such as stride length, gyro default position, magnetic field and user body offset can be done to reduce the

Copyright © 2011, IGI Global. Copying or distributing in print or electronic forms without written permission of IGI Global is prohibited.

Figure 7. Continuous Dead Reckoning Coordinates vs. Actual Tag Coordinates

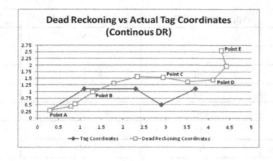

Figure 8. Zero Dead Reckoning Coordinates at each tag vs. Actual Tag Coordinates

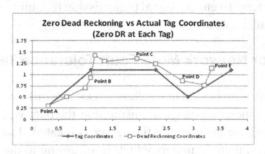

error estimation. Figure 7 and Figure 8 illustrates the dead reckoning performance of both methods in detail.

Wireless Sensor Network Range Tests

The range test is to determine the real maximum communication distance between two nodes during real time operation especially when the nodes are not in the line of sight. The testing is important as it determines the setup of the wireless sensor network to have maximum coverage area and sufficient fault tolerance. The experiment is being setup in the Faculty of Engineering where walls will acts as barricades and obstacles that affect RF signal transmissions which mimic real time operations in indoor buildings. The measurements of the range are an approximation which is referred to the floor plan. The results of the range test are shown in Table 2.

The measured maximum transmission range in real time shows discrepancy of 1 to 5 meters from the specification (30m in line of sight). As the motes are not in the line of sight from the base mote, signal is degraded when it penetrated through walls and floors. The measured results show that maximum node-node range is

Copyright © 2011, IGI Global. Copying or distributing in print or electronic forms without written permission of IGI Global is prohibited.

Table 2. Results of Transmission Range Test

Mote	Approximated Range	Line of sight	RF Signal
B	10m	No	Stable
C	21m	No	Unstable
D	5m	No	Stable
E	8m	No	Stable
F	14m	No	Stable
G	28m	No	No Signal
H	7m	No	Unstable

between 20 – 23 meters. To ensure signal transmission reliability each node is being setup within 20 meters apart.

Wireless Sensor Network Mote Fault Tolerance Test

The fault tolerance feature is vital in wireless sensor network communications. The nodes are setup in a mesh topology to ensure that the data will have at least two paths to relay to the base node where the server is located. The distance between each node is not more than 20 meters which is according to the range experiment carried out in Section 7.2. The system is being tested and results indicate that as long as a node is within the range of another node (20 m) data will be relayed safely to the base node regardless of the placement and the complexity of the node setup. The only flaw of the system is the base node where it is being positioned at the server side. It is the end point where all the data will pass through. If the base node fails, there will be no data flow to the server. This however can be solved by implementing two base nodes on two separate servers. The data is tested to be the same on both the server and base nodes.

Real Time System Test

The full system real time test is performed to benchmark the performance of the system. Figure 9 shows the SmartGuide System performing in real time via the observation from the software layer. The dynamically generated floor plan image displays the travel path calculated from the shortest path algorithm and an icon that estimates the user's current location. The search algorithm is performed and they dynamic travel path image is re-generated whenever the user reaches a way point tag. This is to ensure that the user can be guided to the right path in case of a path deflection.

Copyright © 2011, IGI Global. Copying or distributing in print or electronic forms without written permission of IGI Global is prohibited.

Figure 9. Real Time System Test shown in software layer

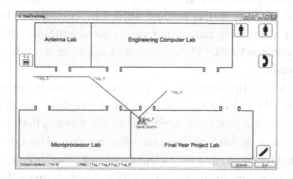

User position estimation and real time tracking is the core functionality of the system. The user icon with the user's name shown in Figure 9 is an estimation of the user's position. Real time user tracking is performed by using information provided by the SmartGuide hardware layer such as, easting, northing readings, heading angle. The user tracking algorithm utilizes these data to triangulate the current position of the user. The entire operation is performed at every pre defined interval (10 seconds).

FUTURE RESEARCH DIRECTIONS

Design Miniaturization

The author proposes PCB fabrication to achieve design miniaturization. The hardware components can be replaced by smaller SMD (Surface Mount Devices) or TSSOP (Thin Slim Small Outline Package) packages to minimize the physical size and weight or the system. On the other hand PCB hardware will have lower power consumption and better routing connections than physical wires. By fitting the entire hardware into a PCB, the overall size of the software will be 2 to 3 times smaller than the current design, offering fewer burdens and on the user side on the other hand improves usability.

Software Threading

Operating systems use processes to separate the different applications that they are executing. Threads are the basic unit to which an operating system allocates processor time, and more than one thread can be executing code inside that process. Each

Copyright © 2011, IGI Global. Copying or distributing in print or electronic forms without written permission of IGI Global is prohibited.

thread maintains exception handlers, a scheduling priority, and a set of structures the system uses to save the thread context until it is scheduled. The thread context includes all the information the thread needs to seamlessly resume execution, including the thread's set of CPU registers and stack, in the address space of the thread's host process.

An operating system that supports preemptive multitasking creates the effect of simultaneous execution of multiple threads from multiple processes. It does this by dividing the available processor time among the threads that need it, allocating a processor time slice to each thread one after another. The currently executing thread is suspended when its time slice elapses, and another thread resumes running. When the system switches from one thread to another, it saves the thread context of the preempted thread and reloads the saved thread context of the next thread in the thread queue (Wikipedia, 2009b).

The length of the time slice depends on the operating system and the processor. Because each time slice is small, multiple threads appear to be executing at the same time, even if there is only one processor. This is actually the case on multiprocessor systems, where the executable threads are distributed among the available processors.

Using more than one thread, however, is the most powerful technique available to increase responsiveness to the user and process the data necessary to get the job done at almost the same time. On a computer with one processor, multiple threads can create this effect, taking advantage of the small periods of time in between user events to process the data in the background. For example, a user can edit a spreadsheet while another thread is recalculating other parts of the spreadsheet within the same application (Microsoft, 2009).

By implementing threading on the current application software on windows and web version, communication to the database can be further enhanced. The user interface can remain responsive while allocating time to perform back ground processing tasks. Threading can dramatically increase user satisfaction especially running on a computer with more than one processor.

CONCLUSION

We have presented an intelligent assistive navigation management system. RFID tags planned in the infrastructure monitors the location of the users. Data is relayed to and fro via the tags in the wireless sensor network to software layer. The wireless sensor network is designed to be very low-power and fault tolerant by using a mesh network topology. The user friendly GUI enables the caregiver or the system administrator to access and manage the system with ease.

Copyright © 2011, IGI Global. Copying or distributing in print or electronic forms without written permission of IGI Global is prohibited.

The camera sensor network provides extra layer of security to the visually impaired uses. The caregivers were able to provide immediate attention during emergencies by able to monitor the user visually in real time.

Experiments carried out indicate that the wireless sensor network has minimal delay in data relaying even with walls and obstacles, thus it is concluded the system would work reliably in indoor environments.

REFERENCES

BrailleNote. (2009). *Braillenotes product information*. Retrieved April 29, 2009, from http://www.humanware.com/en-asia/products/blindness/braillenotes

Cardin, S., Thalmann, D., & Vexo, F. (2007). Wearable system for mobility improvement of visually impaired people. *The Visual Computer: International Journal of Computer Graphics, 23*(2), 109–118. doi:10.1007/s00371-006-0032-4

Chang, T. S., Ho, C. J., Hsu, D. C., Lee, Y. H., Tsai, M. S., Wang, M. C., & Hsu, J. (2005). *iCane-a partner for the visually impaired*. (pp. 393-402).

Crossbow Technology Inc. (2007a). *XServe user manual*. Retrieved January 2, 2009, from http://www.xbow.com/Support/Support_pdf_files/XMesh_Users_Manual.pdf

Crossbow Technology Inc. (2007b). *XMesh user manual*. Retrieved January 2, 2009, from http://www.xbow.com/Support/Support_pdf_files/XMesh_Users_Manual.pdf

D'Atri, E., Medaglia, C. M., Serbanati, A., Ceipidor, U. B., Panizzi, E., & D'Atri, A. (2007). *A system to aid blind people in the mobility: A usability test and its results*. Paper presented at the Second International Conference on Systems, Sainte-Luce, Martinique.

Microsoft. (2009). *Threads and threading*. Retrieved May 15, 2009, from http://msdn.microsoft.com/en-us/library/6kac2kdh(VS.71).aspx

Pun, T., Roth, P., Bologna, G., Moustakas, K., & Tzovaras, D. (2007). Image and video processing for visually handicapped people. *EURASIP Journal on Image and Video Processing*, 1–12. doi:10.1155/2007/25214

Ran, L., Helal, S., & Moore, S. (2004). *Drishti: An integrated indoor/outdoor blind navigation system and service*. Paper presented at the Second IEEE Annual Conference on Pervasive Computing and Communications.

Russell, S., & Novig, P. (2002). *Artificial intelligence: A modern approach* (2nd ed.). Prentice Hall.

Copyright © 2011, IGI Global. Copying or distributing in print or electronic forms without written permission of IGI Global is prohibited.

Wikipedia. (2008a). *Visual field*. Retrieved November 12, 2008, from http://en.wikipedia.org/wiki/Visual_field

Wikipedia. (2008b). *A* search algorithm*. Retrieved August, 2008, from http://en.wikipedia.org/wiki/A*_search_algorithm

Wikipedia. (2009). *Project-SE-integrated development toolset for sensory RSC4x microcontrollers*. Retrieved March 13, 2009, from http://www.phyton.com/htdocs/tools_se/PICE-SE.pdf

Wikipedia. (2009b) *Thread (computer science)*. Retrieved May 15, 2009, from http://en.wikipedia.org/wiki/Thread_(computer_science)

World Health Organization[WHO]. (2009). *Visual impairment and blindness*. Retrieved June 7, 2008, from http://www.who.int/mediacentre/factsheets/fs282/en/

KEY TERMS AND DEFINITIONS

Visually Impaired: Partial or Fully vision loss of a person to a degree as to qualify as a handicap

SmartGuide: The name of the proposed system.

Wireless Sensor Network: The transportation backbone of the system that utilizes sensor nodes which operated wirelessly.

Camera Sensor Network: A network of camera nodes operating wirelessly with the functionality similar to a CCTV.

Intelligent Navigation: The system computes the shortest path to the requested destination, at the same time, providing speech guidance.

Caregiver Monitoring: The system is being constantly monitored by caregivers such as security guards.

Fault Tolerant: The characteristic the data transmissions architecture of the system where data has more than one path to travel to the centralize server.

Copyright © 2011, IGI Global. Copying or distributing in print or electronic forms without written permission of IGI Global is prohibited.

Chapter 5

Collaborative Virtual Learning for Assisting Children with Cerebral Palsy

Nia Valeria
Swinburne University of Technology, Malaysia

Marlene Valerie Lu
Swinburne University of Technology, Malaysia

Lau Bee Theng
Swinburne University of Technology, Malaysia

ABSTRACT

Communication through speech is a vital skill, an innate ability in most human beings intended to convey thoughts, needs, and it is the very foundation of literacy. However, some people find it as one of the challenges in their lives, particularly children with Cerebral Palsy. Children with such disability suffer from brain injuries before, during, and after birth that evidently affect their motor, cognitive, and linguistic skills. Some of the additional complexities may also cause hearing, visual, and speech impairments that further decrease their learning abilities. Their development milestones in learning is slower than a typical child, thus they require intensive personal drilling. It is believed that the cognitive skills in these children can be improved to enable them to lead a more productive life. That was an antecedent that strongly motivated us to develop the proposed Virtual Collaborative Learning Tool. It aims to assist the learning ability of the targeted children through a

DOI: 10.4018/978-1-60960-541-4.ch005

Copyright ©2011, IGI Global. Copying or distributing in print or electronic forms without written permission of IGI Global is prohibited.

responsive avatar of their parents, teachers, or caretakers. A preliminary study was conducted on voluntary participants to evaluate the effectiveness of the proposed learning model. The results showed 80% of the participants were able to answer questions provided within the program.

INTRODUCTION

Children with Cerebral Palsy (CP) often have difficulties in developing speech, language, and gestural communication. Cerebral Palsy, which is known as CP, is an injury caused during prenatal, perinatal or postnatal where the brain is partly damaged, especially around the areas that control movements. It is a disorder that affects muscle tone, movement and motor skills, and it is a non-progressive disorders. Children who suffer from CP usually lack of control of their muscles. A group of studies have shown that speech disorders are associated with all types of Cerebral Palsy (Bax, Cockerill, & Carroll-Few, 2001).

Disabilities of one child with another child are different (Original of Cerebral Palsy, 2009; Peeters Verhoeven, Moor, & Balkom, 2009). The "disabilities" in this context includes the physical movement, speech impairment, hearing impairment, intellectual ability, seizures and other associated complications caused by the brain injury (Majumdar, Laisram, & Chowdhary, 2006).

A study shows that CP children have lower intelligence as compared to normal children (Valente, 1983). Children with CP suffer from a group of syndromes which does not only affect their intelligence but they also experience a range of disabilities as mentioned above. This can further affect their learning ability (Valente, 1983). Communication is essential and it encapsulates the very core of our existence and our civilisation. Without speech, people cannot express their needs, intentions or feelings. This is one of the major problems faced by CP children. These children suffer from motor speech disorder; a disturbance in the coordination of the muscles around the mouth and face. This speech impediment will greatly hamper them from producing intelligible speech, thus the inability to express oneself. Our objective is to introduce a conducive learning environment to aid in the learning process of these children.

When it comes to education, a two-way communication between the educators and child is vital, and should be established so that the educator is aware whether the child is able to catch or understand the materials that have been delivered. For some CP children who suffer from speech problems, they have non-verbal ways to communicate, either through gesture or gaze. However, sometimes the educa-

Copyright © 2011, IGI Global. Copying or distributing in print or electronic forms without written permission of IGI Global is prohibited.

tors do not understand the sign or gestures made by the child which cause further misunderstanding.

Therefore, in order to help those children to establish a proper communication flow between the educators and other people around them, many researchers have developed products (hardware and software) to assist those children in communicating with others. Those products are called Alternative and Augmentative Communication (AAC). Besides focusing on communication and interaction, it also provides a learning system to teach these children so that they can know and learn the things that they cannot learn effectively in the physical classroom. Most of them provide multimedia presentation, such as audio, image, text, video, etc, to assist the children in order to meet their daily needs (Lee, 2007).

'How was school today?' is one of the AAC products that allows disabled children such as cerebral palsy to communicate in a faster and more interactive way. It tracks the child's movement, responses to the questions and records his or her activities. The product is placed on the wheelchair (Meadows, 2009).Other AAC products such as Broadmaker (Mayer-Johnson, 2009), STANDUP (Waller et al., 2009), and other learning programs are introduced to teach the CP children in improving their learning skills. However, these AAC products require educators to teach and train the children.

Experienced special educational needs (SEN) teachers/educators are scarcely available. It is a profession shunned by many as it demands a greater level of commitment, motivation, passion and empathy towards children than a conventional job. Repetition is required in teaching those children; therefore an educator must be extra patient in handling the children. Such expertise and services are still unattainable in most countries.

As we immerse into an e-knowledge society, various ways are being explored with the available technology. Thus, a large variety of assistive tools or products for special educational needs children have been developed. However, most of these products require educator, parents or caregiver's supervision and guidance to operate. As knowledge increases with the growing research and the proliferation of technology, different ways are developed to evolve the approach used to produce a more adaptable and effective method. Hence, this research aims at crossing multidisciplinary boundaries by connecting several components through the application of IT ie. assistive, communicative and interactive components to produce an educational tool, wrapped within a learning environment and independent of any form of supervision. Collaborative Virtual Learning (CVL) provides a learning environment, where a user is accompanied by an avatar equipped with the function to teach and give responses to the user. This CVL is designed to be an assistive and educational technology.

Copyright © 2011, IGI Global. Copying or distributing in print or electronic forms without written permission of IGI Global is prohibited.

Transfer of Skills from Virtual Learning to Real World

Numerous applications have been developed using virtual reality (VR) like virtual offices (Weinstein, 2005), virtual kitchens (Safework, 2009b), virtual hotels (Safework, 2009a) and virtual pets (Vince, 2004). VR provides many alternatives for the users to choose, for instance immersive and non-immersive (desktop-based) VR. Desktop VR could be a useful approach for the children with CP where interaction between users and VR's objects can be mediated by interaction with another person sitting alongside the users (Parsons et al., 2000).

Virtual Reality has been known as a key communication and learning technology for the 21st century (Ausburn & Ausburn, 2004). Essentially, Virtual Reality, or known as VR, is defined as an interactive computer application where all of the objects are created in 3D models with real time performance. Real time performance is where the computer performs its ability to identify user's input and make changes based on the input, where the input can be made by having a gesture and verbal command (Burdea & Coiffet, 2003; Vince, 2004).

Concept of the VR development has been brought into the military industry and medical industry (Desbonnet, Rahman, & Cox, 1997). It can be used as a training, therapy or rehabilitation tools. Moreover, it has been brought as an entertainment tools and education tools (Burdea & Coiffet, 2003; Rizzo & Kim, 2005). Nowadays, the use of VR in medical industry has gained recognition in therapy and rehabilitation (Rizzo & Kim, 2005). Improvement in IT will provide a major means in improving health care in the next century (Gourlay, Lun, Lee, & Tay, 2000). Based on the studies that have been done by Gourlay et al. (2000), consideration to allow the users to transfer skills from virtual environment to their daily living tasks have led to the development of virtual reality as well.

VR was not merely effective in facilitating the acquisition of living skills but it aids in the transfer of skills from the virtual to the real environment. This is supported by McComas, Pivik, and Laflamme (1998b) in their research, where children were asked to find puzzle pieces hidden in a classroom. Result showed that children who have practiced in a VE performed as well as children who had done the same number of practice trial in a real environment. From the study, McComas, Pivik, and Laflamme (1998a) suggest that "VR has a role in providing children with opportunities to practise spatial skills and also that the learned skills can be transferred to a real-world spatial task".

Gourlay et al. (2000) in their study which involved an amnesia patient who was trained in route finding around a hospital rehabilitation unit by using a VE where the environment has been set based on the real unit. After 3 weeks of the practice, patient showed an improvement in recognizing 2 routes. She successfully performed the route based on the memory that she has during the practice within

Copyright © 2011, IGI Global. Copying or distributing in print or electronic forms without written permission of IGI Global is prohibited.

the VE. Result of this study indicates that training in VE may prove an effective method of teaching new information to the patients with severe memory impairments (Gourlay et al., 2000).

It has also been proven in the study conducted by Standen, Cromby, and Brown in 1998 cited by Standen and Brown (2006) on children with severe intellectual disabilities. Nineteen children participated in this study and they were brought to a supermarket to find four items from the shelves. All the children managed to find the items and brought them to the checkout counter. After that, these students were they divided into two groups. One group of children conducted similar task in a virtual supermarket twice a week and the remaining children did the same task in other virtual environment for the same duration of time. After training through the virtual environment, they were brought back to the real supermarket. The children who have been trained in the virtual supermarket performed significantly faster and more accurate in collecting the items than those who had not.

Avatar in Assisting Disabled Children's Virtual Learning

Fabri (2006) suggested that collaborative virtual environment has a good potential in addressing practical collaborative needs especially in gathering people virtually and engaging them in social interaction for learning, meetings, training, education, simulation, entertainment and therapy.

People gather and meet to gain knowledge through collaborative virtual environment. It allows multi-users communication between instructors and trainees with simulation and training applications being supported. Users can move about freely within the collaborative virtual environment, interacting with each other and sharing information of similar interested.

In collaborative virtual environment, users are represented by their avatars (Oliveira, Shen, & Georganas, 2000). Existence of the participant is visually represented by avatar and through this medium users can see other users (Fabri, 2006). The use of avatar coupled with an interactive chat environment allows the user to undergo an experimental learning without any repercussions. This serves as a pedagogical tool for learners to "learn by doing" in a rich and controlled environment which may lead to a better conceptual understanding eventually.

The avatar or user representation is useful in learning and providing response or feedback. Students may get frustrated in virtual world if there is no response from the virtual learning (Baig, n.d.). Moreover by implementing the user representation, students are able to access and get the instructions from the instructor anytime. This will alleviate boredom as the avatar will constantly be there during the learning process (Massaro, 2004). A companion in virtual learning helps the children achieve better performance instead of learning alone.

Copyright © 2011, IGI Global. Copying or distributing in print or electronic forms without written permission of IGI Global is prohibited.

Vygotsky (1978) found that "the zone of proximal development is the distance between the actual developmental level as determined by independent problem solving and the level of potential development as determined through problem solving under adult guidance or in collaboration with more capable peers". Based on this theory, they stated that a child achieves a higher developmental level of abstraction and performance with a knowledgeable and skilled partner than she achieves independently.

Theng and Paye (2009) found that children love avatars because they found enjoyment when they play or learn together with the virtual characters. Animated avatar offers an effective interaction for children to be more engaging and managing the overall learning context in the learning systems. For children, avatars are seen as virtual teachers, virtual instructors or virtual co-learners in their learning. In the domain of education and learning, avatars are widely deployed and essentially targeted for children to improve children's learning experiences. Theng and Paye (2009) reinforces that the main purpose in using the avatars is to attract children's attention and make them more engaged and motivated in their learning. As for children with autism, avatars help them to build their self-awareness because it engages them with facial expressions (Cheng, Moore, McGrath, & Fan, 2005).

Collaborative Virtual Learning for Disabled Children

Standen, Brown, and Cromby (2001) found that "students with intellectual disabilities find stimulation through *enjoyable repetition* and a gradual increase in level of challenge, words like '*handicapped*' and '*disabled*' imply dependence and powerlessness. With computers, disabled learners can be less dependent and more capable."

Brown, Standen, and Cobb (1998) also described why special needs children should learn from collaborative virtual environment. First, CVL permits self-directed activity. Self-directed is important in shaping and building the children' characters. In CVL, children with learning difficulties are able to do and explore some activities that they cannot do in real world. They feel empowered as they have control over their actions in the virtual learning. It offers a rich and varied set of opportunities to initiate self-directed activity in a safe arena.

Secondly, it provides motivation in learning for the disabled children who are able to control their own actions in the collaborative virtual learning. It inspires and motivates them to learn more as long as the contents are attractive and informative. It allows the children to work at their own pace; they are able to make as many mistakes as they want without getting de-motivated. A software neither feel tired of the children attempting in doing the same activity repetitively nor feel impatient even if they are slow in completing the task (Standen et al., 2001).

Copyright © 2011, IGI Global. Copying or distributing in print or electronic forms without written permission of IGI Global is prohibited.

Third, the role of play is given high importance in developmental theories of education. Due to the physical limitations of the disabled children, parents or care-takers tend to be over-protective. Hence, the disabled child does not have much real experience in life. Brown et al. (1998) commented that children are encouraged to explore and feel their environments. Since physical world does not permit, collaborative virtual learning grants them the chance to play as much as they wish with the instructor (avatar) in place to guide them whenever it is necessary.

Fourth, Brown et al. (1998) stated that "Collaborative virtual learning has their own natural semantics, the qualities of objects that can be discovered by direct interaction with them, compare to computer learning systems which rely on abstracted symbol systems, such as English or Mathematics". Thus, it can be used to facilitate concept achievement through practical activity (Standen et al., 2001). Practical learning experience is the best learning for the disabled children with learning difficulties since they are grouped as concrete thinker.

Fifth, collaborative virtual learning provides a safe space for the children to learn and practise the skills that they cannot do in real world, for instance some dangerous activities that are not suitable for their conditions. It is a training place, since it is not harmful for them and they are able to gain some experience about the activities that they have never done before. Lastly, collaborative virtual learning can be a great equalizer of physical abilities because it can be adapted to the children's condition since disabled children have many barriers in doing some activities in the real world due to the disabilities that they have. Children can operate or navigate the system. They can explore the virtual environment freely via touch screen, joystick, retina triggered mouse or switch and gain some experiences from it.

Cerebral Palsy and Collaborative Virtual Learning

Our targeted community is the children with spastic Cerebral Palsy between the ages of 9 to 15 years old. At this age, children have started to know how to communicate with and through computers. CP is an injury caused during birth or after birth where the brain is partly damaged, mainly the parts that control the movements, and causes them to acquire immature brain in their early lives (Werner, 1987; Miller, 2005). Due to their under-developed brains, it affects their muscle tone, movement and motor skills. United Cerebral Palsy Research and Educational Foundation in United States (United Cerebral Palsy, 2009) predicted that the number of children and adults with CP have reached between 1.5 – 2.0 million, where 1,200 to 1,500 children are recognized to have CP at their preschool age every year, and 10,000 occurred in infants.

The degrees of disabilities from one child to another child are different. One child may have a different type of CP from another child (Original of Cerebral

Copyright © 2011, IGI Global. Copying or distributing in print or electronic forms without written permission of IGI Global is prohibited.

Palsy, 2009; Peeters et al., 2009). If there are two children with Cerebral Palsy, the severity of their impairments, in terms of motor abilities and linguistics, will differ from each other. Some disabilities are curable while some of them are not curable. The classification of the CP is based on the movement disorders (Werner, 1987) clustered into three types which are (1) spastic CP or muscle stiffness, where the children have the difficulty in moving their position due to stiffness of their muscles, (2) athetoid CP, where the children are unable to control their movements of their feet, arms, hands or face muscles, where some muscles are too high and others are too low, (3) ataxic CP or poor balance, where the children find themselves with difficulty in controlling their arms, hands and legs, and lastly (4) mixed CP, where it is the combination of the above types of disordered movement. From those categorizations, the highest rate of children is found to have spastic CP which accounts for nearly 80% of CP children (Resource4 Cerebral Palsy, 2007; Werner, 1987).

Some of the disorders suffered by CP children include difficulty in fine motor skills, maintaining balance and walking, or involuntary movements such as uncontrollable writhing of the hands or drooling (Rajab et al., 2006). Moreover, some children may suffer from mental retardation which is one of results caused by the brain injury. Other than that, children may have one or two additional impairments, such as flawed vision, hearing, and intellectual ability, 25% may suffer from epilepsy and others from speech impairment (Falkman, 2005). The inability to produce incomprehensive speech can be caused by the muscles problem in moving the jaws and tongue to produce a word.

Children with Cerebral Palsy require special educators who are trained to teach them. In addition, educators have to be patient in drilling them repetitively due to their cognitive impairments. It is more effective to have a personal (one-to-one) teaching between the educator and the child as some of the children do not get proper attention from the educator in a classroom teaching style. Their inability to communicate creates a greater barrier with the educators. Children with CP require extra time in processing and absorbing the information compared to the normal children due to their low level of intelligence (Valente, 1983).

Virtual environment provides safety guarantee, repetition opportunities in learning and immersive feelings for the children with CP (Desbonnet et al., 1997; Chuah, Chen, & Teh, 2009; Chen, Toh, & Wan 2004; Reid, 2002). Collaborative virtual environment (CVE) offers collaboration during the learning through interaction with a virtual character that teaches and responses to them. The use of expressive emotional avatar integrated within the virtual environment makes the learning more interactive (Massaro, 2004). A collaborative virtual environment has the potential to provide some benefits to the children with CP as an assistive and educational technology. In terms of the lack of man power during/after the classroom learning session, CVE learning can be used as assistive tool to assist the educator in teach-

Copyright © 2011, IGI Global. Copying or distributing in print or electronic forms without written permission of IGI Global is prohibited.

ing the children. In terms of educational technology, the learning in CVE allows revisions to be done repetitively to drill and help the children to grasp the concepts taught. This research focuses on how the virtual collaborative learning environment can be integrated in the teaching and learning processes of the children with CP.

PROTOTYPING

Collaborative virtual learning has been proven to be effective for children with disability. Thus, we proposed collaborative virtual learning model to assist children with Cerebral Palsy in their daily learning.

Learning Environment

Collaborative Learning refers to having more than a person attempting to gain knowledge together in a physical environment in the form of a discussion, teaching, or meeting (Smith & MacGregor, 1992). In virtual world, *Collaborative Learning* refers to an electronic or web-based learning portal where each user has his own identity and interacts with other people through the avatar (Shih & Yang, 2008; McArdle, Monahan, Bertolotto, & Mangina, 2004).

Hence, our *Collaborative Learning* model has an avatar, representing the teacher who is able to deliver learning materials, give response or feedback to the user, sense and react to student's emotions throughout the learning. This is not a typical web based learning system where the avatar is displayed in a form of image or customizable object; instead a video is used where a teacher or trainer is able to record his learning materials and responses for the dedicated user.

As shown in Figure 1, collaborative learning is achieved through the interaction between the user and teacher in the virtual learning. It is analogous to a private classroom where there is only a teacher teaching a student. Emotions shown on a student's face are obtained through the facial expression system recognition while the attempts to the questions are collected from mouse input.

User Response

Inputs from the user with Cerebral Palsy are through mouse-clicks and facial expression recognition. Through mouse-clicking, the children are trained in fine motor skill coordination (Donker & Reitsma, 2007). This helps the children to have better coordination between their hands and eyes.

Some of the Cerebral Palsy children have speech disabilities which cause them to produce an incomprehensible speech. They are unable to voice out their opinions or

Copyright © 2011, IGI Global. Copying or distributing in print or electronic forms without written permission of IGI Global is prohibited.

Figure 1.Flowchart of the collaborative learning module and scenario

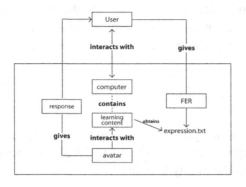

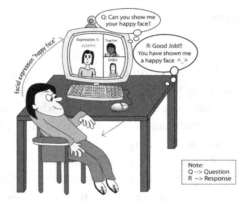

to give feedbacks as to whether they understand or are confused about the learning materials delivered by the teacher. However, responses from these children can be obtained from nonverbal communication through the expression reflected on their faces. Thus, with careful observation on these attributes, the teacher might be able to interpret their transitory mood or emotion. This is known as human intensive teaching and learning process. In order to identify the expressions shown by the user, our collaborative virtual learning model has incorporated a Facial Expression Recognition (FER) module to capture the user's emotion based on specific expression shown during the learning process.

For the Facial Expression Recognition to succeed, it has to be trained by feeding it with a dataset of each child's expression. This is to ensure that the module has the intelligence to recognize the user's expression. Each expression from the child is categorized under individual profiles.

As shown in Figure 2, FER module detects a face through the camera attached, then retrieves the facial expression, extracts the features, then matches the captured

Copyright © 2011, IGI Global. Copying or distributing in print or electronic forms without written permission of IGI Global is prohibited.

Figure 2.Flowchart of the FER application connect to the learning module

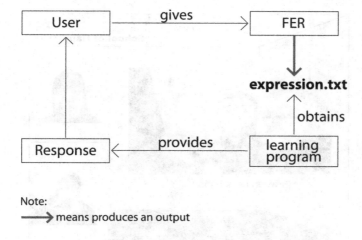

Note:
———> means produces an output

expression with the template images within the user's profile. If a match has been found, the emotional state of the user will be displayed on the screen. Therefore, the learning module is able to assess the response of the user and react accordingly to guide his learning.

Learning Contents

Animations are added in the learning materials in order to boost their learning spirit. The learning contents cover real world objects and scenes to create familiarity, otherwise it will not be effective. The contents have to be kept simple and ordinary (Figure 3).

System Architecture

Figure 4 shows the architecture of the virtual learning model. It consists of four layers which are the presentation layer, control layer, service layer and data layer. Those layers have its own components with different responsibilities in running the program. ApplicationUI (Presentation Layer) has the responsibility to introduce the learning model to the user. This component collaborates with the StoryBoard-Manager, which is resided within the control layer. Control layer provides all the functions that the system is supposed to have. In this layer, user is given the options to choose the learning content that they want to learn.

While in the service layer, each of the components collaborates with its respective component in the data layer. Service layer will process the function from the

Copyright © 2011, IGI Global. Copying or distributing in print or electronic forms without written permission of IGI Global is prohibited.

Figure 3. Sample of 3D content

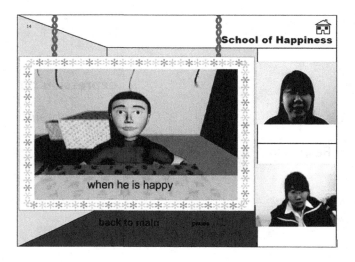

control layer and the data is obtained from the data layer. There are 3 components resided within the service layer. LearningContentGenerator has the responsibility to display the particular learning content to the screen. This component collaborates with LearningVideoAccessInterface in gaining the related video. AssessmentGenerator has the responsibility to provide and display the assessment content to the user. It collaborates with AssessmentVideoAccessInterface in obtaining the video file. And the last component is the AvatarGenerator. This component is responsible for displaying and generating the response from the avatar and displays it on the screen. It collaborates with ResponseVideoAccessInterface to provide the response.

Development Tools

This model is created by using Adobe Flash CS. This tool is suitable to develop interactive multimedia program. While, Autodesk 3Ds max 9 software is used to develop the 3D environment for learning contents. For the Facial Expression Recognition, it is developed using C++ programming language. As for the avatars, it is captured through video recorder in .avi format and converted into .flv format by using Adobe Flash CS3 Video Encoder in order to allow the program to read the file.

Preliminary Evaluation

The study aims to evaluate the effectiveness of collaborative virtual learning model for children with CP by conducting experimental study on different groups of par-

Copyright © 2011, IGI Global. Copying or distributing in print or electronic forms without written permission of IGI Global is prohibited.

Figure 4. UML component diagram

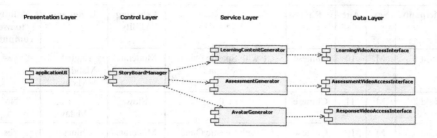

ticipants with different classification of CP. The results will be analysed, synthesized and a probable conclusion is derived.

Participant

Participants were chosen from one of the local schools for disabled children in Kuching. Prior to the beginning of the study, consents were obtained from the parents or guardian of the selected children.

Before testing was conducted, there were several criteria considered in selecting the participants:

1.   Must understand simple or brief verbal instructions in English, Bahasa Malaysia or Chinese.
2.   Must be able to focus their attention on a task or object for at least 5 seconds
3.   Has communication problem or produce incomprehensible speech
4.   Child can understand verbal English
5.   Participant can control their facial muscles to express some emotions

Based on the requirement given, a small sample which consists of 4 children (Table 1) has been selected to take part in this preliminary study. In order to protect the children's identity, the children will remain anonymous and shall be identified as child 1, child 2, child 3 and child 4.

1.   *Child 1*
    This child has been diagnosed to have CP with spastic quadriplegia, where the muscle stiffness affects both arms and legs. He has mild drooling and speech problem. He is unable to produce intelligible speech due to the damage on the area of the brain that is associated with speech. However, there is no problem in terms of his intelligence. He is able to understand

Copyright © 2011, IGI Global. Copying or distributing in print or electronic forms without written permission of IGI Global is prohibited.

Table 1. Participants' details

Participants	Sex	Age	Race	Diagnosis	Learning Ability	Language	Ability to use computer
Child 1	M	10	Chinese	CP with Spastic Quadriplegia	Moderate	English, Mandarin, Malay	Yes
Child 2	M	11	Chinese	CP	Slow	English, Malay	No
Child 3	M	10	Chinese	CP with Spastic Quadriplegia and asphyxia	Moderate	Chinese, Malay, English	Yes
Child 4	M	12	Dayak	CP with Spastic Quadriplegia	Good	English, Malay	Yes

what other people say, and he is able to communicate through gesture and gaze.

2. Child 2

    This child suffers from moderate Cerebral Palsy. He has problem with his leg movement. He needs to use wheelchair to support his body. He is able to move his hands even though it is very slow. He has made some improvement after he joined the school. However, his condition has deteriorated after suffering from high fever 2 years ago. He is able to understand simple instructions, and able to communicate with each other through body gesture.

3. Child 3

    This child suffers from CP with spastic quadriplegia and asphyxia. He has problem walking due to the muscle stiffness. He has a good sensory in seeing and listening. However, he only can make a simple speech like "koko (a call for elder brother)". He has a good coordination between his eyes and hands.

4. Child 4

    This child has been diagnosed to have CP with spastic quadriplegia. He has a movement problem with his leg and coordination problem with his arms. He is unable to control his arms while he is writing and eating. He has good intelligence in learning. However, he is able to communicate orally even though it is not very fluent. Another way for him to communicate is through his gaze and gesture.

Copyright © 2011, IGI Global. Copying or distributing in print or electronic forms without written permission of IGI Global is prohibited.

Scope

The prototype was used to teach the children with cerebral palsy on essential emotions. Children learnt 3 basic expressions which were happy, sad and surprised. It involved 2 stages: learning and assessment. In the learning stage, a child was given a simple situation where a particular facial expression is induced. Teaching content was animated and a video avatar of the teacher was played to accompany the child in learning.

Attention of the children in listening and watching the video was important since the questions in assessment stage were based on the learning stage. The questions were read out by the video avatar and was displayed in text form as well. The reason to display in those two modes was to train their reading and listening skill. The child could click on the "*play*" button under the video avatar if he wished the avatar to repeat reading the question. Since this is the basic stage of learning, there were only 2 answers to choose for each question to prevent him from getting confused.

There were 3 different assessments provided for each emotion. These assessment contents were inspired by Moore, Cheng, McGrath, and Powell (2005) who used the CVE technology in assisting people with autism.

The first assessment (Figure 5) required the child to select the situation to match a particular emotion. The rationale of this content was to teach them appropriate expression for various situations.

In the second assessment (Figure 6), the system required the child to match a particular expression given in the list of images provided based on what the question asked. The rationale reason behind this assessment was to help the children recognize basic emotions.

In the third assessment (Figure 7), the child was required to show his/her facial expression based on a particular emotion triggered by the system. The system then captured the expression reflected on the child's face. Thereafter it determined

Figure 5. 1ˢᵗ question in the assessment stage for each emotion

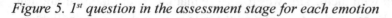

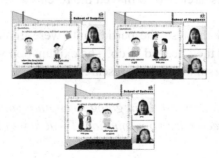

Copyright © 2011, IGI Global. Copying or distributing in print or electronic forms without written permission of IGI Global is prohibited.

Figure 6. 2nd question in the assessment stage for each emotion

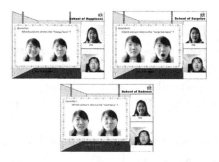

Figure 7. 3rd question in the assessment stage

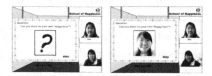

whether the child has shown the correct facial responses. This was to train the child to express his emotion on his face, so that other people will know how he feels. If the child was able to give the correct answer, his face will be displayed in the middle of the screen.

Setup

All of the tests were conducted in a quiet room within the child's school. This was to avoid any distractions to the participant or disruption to the class. The tests were given without a time limit and were presented to each child in the same order. Prior to the preliminary study, the researcher spent some time with the children in that school to bond with them. This was to ensure that they were familiar and felt comfortable with the researcher who played the role as a teacher in the collaborative virtual learning.

At the beginning of the test, the participants were given a short explanation regarding the tasks that they needed to do. The explanation was read aloud slowly so that they could understand what the researcher said.

"(Train the FER application) So, I am going to capture your facial expression so that the program can recognize your emotion. I will key in the text indicating an

Copyright © 2011, IGI Global. Copying or distributing in print or electronic forms without written permission of IGI Global is prohibited.

emotion, and you need to respond to it in front of the webcam. You need to express 4 emotions, which are happy, sad, surprised and neutral.

So, first, show me your neutral face. Next, show me your happy face. Next show me your sad face. And lastly, show me your surprised face.

(After training the system)

Next, I will run the learning program. Learning is started from school of happiness, followed by school of surprised and lastly the school of sadness. Video animation learning will be shown first, followed by a song and finally the assessment part. You need to understand the video in order to answer the assessment. In the assessment part, questions are given by the teacher. So, you have to listen carefully to what the teacher says.

(Start the learning program)"

When it came to the assessment, the participant was required to answer by clicking on the options given. The participant was required to answer 3 questions for each emotion tested. The researcher sat next to the participant to monitor the process of the testing, and to record the participant's progress. There were a few factors that must be observed during the testing.

1. *During the training session*
   For the training session, it was important to set the right lightings and distance between the user and the camera to ensure that the photo captured is clear. The child must be able to hold his/her facial expression for at least 10 seconds to obtain an accurate detection.
2. *During the learning session*
   During this session, their level of understanding was measured through the assessments given and the number of correct attempts.

Hardware and Software

In order to recognize each child's facial expression correctly, the Face Expression Recognition module was trained prior to commencing the evaluation. There were 3

Copyright © 2011, IGI Global. Copying or distributing in print or electronic forms without written permission of IGI Global is prohibited.

Figure 8. Sample of face expressions

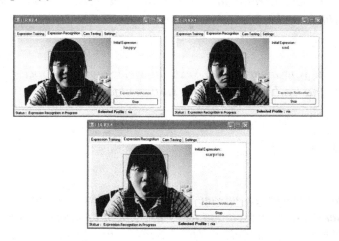

Figure 9. Needs of having 2 cameras

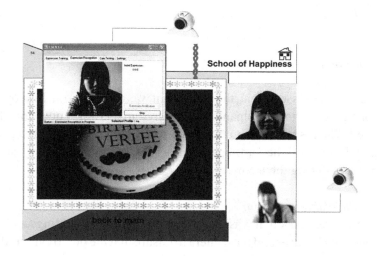

facial expressions that had to be captured from the child in this preliminary study. They were happy, sad, and surprised faces (Figure 8). This learning required 2 USB webcams installed on a laptop (Figure 9). One of the cameras was used to reflect the child's face on the monitor during the learning process and the other camera was used to capture the facial expression of the child. The reason for displaying the child's face on the monitor was to allow the child to see his expression and to train him to produce a consistent facial expression based on a specific emotional state.

Copyright © 2011, IGI Global. Copying or distributing in print or electronic forms without written permission of IGI Global is prohibited.

Training Session

The purpose of conducting the training session before the preliminary study was to train the program to recognize the participants' facial expression to enable the program to respond effectively. Several attempts were made to capture their facial expressions correctly but to no avail. The training could not be conducted as planned as it was hindered by several factors.

The first underlying factor was because the children were not able to hold their facial expression for approximately 10 seconds. They kept changing their expressions which affected the accuracy and consistency of the process involved in matching the emotion against the image captured. For instance, if the child showed a happy face, the system might detect it as a sad expression.

The other factor was their involuntary movements of their limbs and body. They kept jerking to the front and back, which disrupted the facial detection process. During the training, some of the children were just too excited to view their faces on the screen and they kept playing with it.

Lastly the participants did not know how to express a particular expression when asked. Some common expressions, like neutral, happy and sad were easy for them to express because they are familiar with it. However, they found it hard to express an angry, surprised, scared, and disgusted face. Therefore, the first training session was a failure.

At a latter time, another method was brought forward to resolve the obstacle mentioned above. Graphical items such as videos, pictures or sound were presented to the child and it successfully triggered the intended facial expressions. However, due to time constraint and lack of human resources, the training was not completed. Thus the testing process was conducted without any automated facial expression recognition.

Table 2. Participants' attempts in order to get the correct answer in 1st session

Participants	1st session					
	Correct (1st attempt)	Correct (2nd attempt)	Correct (3rd attempt)	Total Correct Answers	Total Wrong Answers	Don't know
Child 1	2	4	0	6	0	0
Child 2	4	1	0	5	1	0
Child 3	3	2	0	5	0	1
Child 4	5	1	0	6	0	0

Copyright © 2011, IGI Global. Copying or distributing in print or electronic forms without written permission of IGI Global is prohibited.

RESULT AND FINDINGS

Due to the failure in training the facial recognition system as explained in the training session, the third assessment was omitted. The results and findings below were collected from two assessments for each emotion.

Based on the observation done, all of the children were not able to answer the questions correctly in the first attempt of the first session (*Table 2*). As it has been explained before, the child is given 3 attempts to answer a question. A total of 6 questions were presented to the children.

After the first wrong attempts, some of the children were able to get the right answer when it came to the second attempt. However, some children still made the same mistake and some of them were not be able to answer some questions (*Table 2*). From the 3 attempts given to the participants, 2 children were not able to answer any question at all. They did not choose the question within the time frame given.

For each question, there were 2 options for the child to choose. If the first attempt to the question was incorrect, the child should be able to rule out that option and choose the next available option. (Figure 10). So, the probability for not being able to answer one question is very small, which is 0.125 (12.5%).

However, there was a child who made similar mistakes 3 times when answering a question (*Table 2*).

When the test was conducted for the second session, the result showed that most of the children performed worse than the first session. Based on general observation, the children did not pay much attention to the learning content during the second session. The duration of the learning part required a longer span of attention before the assessment took place. This may cause the child to lose focus even before the

Figure 10. Sample of wrong answer

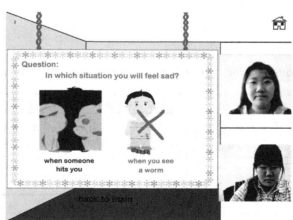

Copyright © 2011, IGI Global. Copying or distributing in print or electronic forms without written permission of IGI Global is prohibited.

Table 3. Total result for 1st and 2nd session (1st attempt)

Participants	1st Session		2nd Session	
	Correct	Wrong	Correct	Wrong
Child 1	2	4	0	6
Child 2	4	2	3	2
Child 3	3	2	4	1
Child 4	5	1	6	0

assessment was delivered. Another remark made from the observation was that the child was distracted by the video taking session. Thus their attention was strayed from its intended purpose. Only 1 child could score 6 out of 6 questions without making any mistakes (*Table 3*). Child 1 and child 2 obtained lower result compared to the first session. At the same time, child 3 was able to get better result in the first attempt of the second session, when compared to the first session. However, the percentage of not answering the questions was higher in the second round (*Table 4*).

From both types of questions given, almost all the children made similar mistakes in answering the question especially when answering question 2, where they were asked to choose the correct facial expression from the image given based on the question asked. Some possible factors may affect the results of the tests. It may be caused by the inappropriate usage of pictures which was not effective in portraying the intended expressions. The other reason may be the children did fully comprehend the question asked or they have difficulties in interpreting information.

From the graph below (Figure 11), child 1 made more mistakes in second session as compared to the first session. While child 3 and 4 made some improvements in the second session compared to others. Improvement is made because they paid more attention to the learning process than child 1.

The prime study of this research is to investigate the effectiveness of the collaborative learning model in assisting disabled children in their daily learning.

Table 4. Percentage of questions which were not answered by participants within the time frame given

Participants	Percentage for Don't Know (1st Session)	Percentage for Don't Know (2nd Session)
Child 1	0.00%	0.00%
Child 2	0.00%	**16.67%**
Child 3	16.67%	**16.67%**
Child 4	0.00%	0.00%

Copyright © 2011, IGI Global. Copying or distributing in print or electronic forms without written permission of IGI Global is prohibited.

Figure 11. False mistakes made by participants in all schools

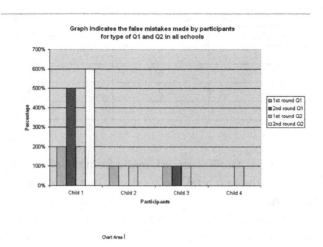

Moreover, we need to investigate whether this learning is able to attract their attention or not. Therefore, to assess the effectiveness of the learning, multiple choice questions have been devised with two options for each question. Three attempts were allowed for each question.

Learning Session

From the results elaborated above, some of the participants did not perform well in the learning stage. From the *Table 4* above, some of the children were not able to answer some of the questions at all within the time frame given, even though they have gone through the learning twice. From Figure 11, we can see that child 1 made more mistakes in the second session compared to the first session, so did child 2. While child 3 and child 4 made some improvements. They performed better in the second session than the first session. However, this result should not be used as evidence to conclude that this collaborative learning is not effective and not suitable to be used by Cerebral Palsy children. To set an unbiased point of view, there may be factors that caused the children to choose the right answer.

Based on the observation that has been done throughout the preliminary study, these children have problems controlling their limbs. Some children suffered from muscle stiffness, thus it was quite hard for them to control the mouse. They might accidentally click on the correct option, even though that was not their intention. The use of touch screen monitor can be an alternative way for them since it provides a wider surface area for them to make a selection.

Copyright © 2011, IGI Global. Copying or distributing in print or electronic forms without written permission of IGI Global is prohibited.

Other factors include poor command in English language and their inability to listen to, compute and focus on long instructions. Each of the learning content was developed using English language and took approximately 1 minute to complete. A child might not be able to fully understand the meaning conveyed due to their limited vocabulary scope. From the observation, when this happened, he started fidgeting and his attention strayed from the screen. To increase the interaction between the system and the child, the system was intended to monitor the child by capturing his facial expression while the video was playing and to respond accordingly. For instance, if the child looked confused, the system should be able to detect it through his facial expression and re-play the video. Due to the failure of the training session, the appropriate response could not be given to the child, and the video kept running until the end even though the child had lost his concentration. Therefore, to increase the effectiveness of the learning process, the system should be able to re-act to the child to ensure a successfully learning.

Some children did not have any problems with their language but they have lower ability to learn. For instance, child 1 is good in English. However, in his daily learning, he is categorized as a slow learner since he needs time to extract and understanding the contents. From *Table 3*, his performance dropped tremendously in the second session. Besides that, the child was easily distracted and had problems concentrating. He was too excited with the video taking session and was not able to focus on the learning content. As for child 4, his command in English language was moderate; however, he could answer all the questions correctly, even though he made a mistake in the first attempt. This was because he is more intelligent and is able to learn faster than the other children in the school.

From Figure 11, we can see that most of the participants could not answer question 2. Question 2 required the child to select the suitable expression from a list of images based on the question given. There was a possibility that the list of images given did not strongly reflect the intended emotion and were ambiguous. Another possibility is that children were not able to differentiate or identify the facial emotion. Therefore, the learning content has to be more real and natural.

FUTURE WORKS

The major aim of this research is to show the effectiveness of CVE in assisting CP children in learning. However, this learning module is not fully developed yet, therefore it did not meet the intended goal as a whole. There are some limitations to this learning module. It lacks user module implementation to maintain user's information, for instance to store their assessment records. This record will be useful in assisting the educators in keeping track of the user's learning progress. And

Copyright © 2011, IGI Global. Copying or distributing in print or electronic forms without written permission of IGI Global is prohibited.

it requires a more flexible control in the content management module to maintain the learning content. These limitations can be seen as the future works to provide an enhanced usability of the current model.

Another improvement that needs to be addressed is the lack of response from the avatar. As this program is about *"Collaborative"*, an intelligent response from the computer based on the user's input is required to establish a two-way communication. In addition to that, an enhancement on the learning content environment will be needed to make the learning more attractive, encouraging, and able to trigger their facial expression. This will eventually elevate the level of functionality and effectiveness of the program.

CONCLUSION

The introduction of the CVL (Collaborative Virtual Learning) in educational industry has been brought in to assist children with Cerebral Palsy in their learning. In this research, CVL program collaborates and integrates with the FER application (Face Expression Recognition) to produce an interactive system between the user and the program. This CVL program has been designed to assist, teach and assess the learning skills of children with Cerebral Palsy.

From the overall discussion, at this point, this program does not show the effectiveness in assisting the children in their learning. However, from the result presented above, some of the children are able to make some improvements from the learning process. This serves as a minor milestone for this research and it proves that the program is indeed able to teach the children to some degree. Although there are many errors and failure made by the participants, the results give grounds for optimism that CVL has the potential to be an assistive or learning tool in education field.

REFERENCES

Ausburn, L. J., & Ausburn, F. B. (2004). Desktop virtual reality: A powerful new technology for teaching and research in industrial teacher education. *Journal of Industrial Teacher Education, 41*(4). Retrieved October 05, 2009, from http://scholar. lib.vt.edu /ejournals/JITE/v41n4/ ausburn.html

Baig, M. A. (n.d.). Traditional v/s virtual learning environment. Retrieved October 26, 2009, from http://sites.google.com/ site/virtualearningorg/ Home/virtual-learning-environment /next

Copyright © 2011, IGI Global. Copying or distributing in print or electronic forms without written permission of IGI Global is prohibited.

Bax, M., Cockerill, H., & Carroll-Few, L. (2001). Who needs augmentative communication, and when? In Cockerill, H., & Carroll-Few, L. (Eds.), *Communication without speech: Practical augmentative & alternative communication* (pp. 65–71). London, UK: Mac Keith Press.

Brown, D. J., Standen, P. J., & Cobb, S. V. (1998). Virtual environments: Special needs and evaluative methods. In Riva, G., Wiederhold, B. K., & Molinari, E. (Eds.), *Virtual environments in clinical psychology and neuroscience* (pp. 91–102). Amsterdam, The Netherlands: Ios Press.

Burdea, G. C., & Coiffet, P. (2003). *Virtual reality technology* (2nd ed.). Hoboken, NJ: John Wiley & Sons.

Chen, C. J., Toh, S. C., & Wan, M. F. (2004). The theoretical framework for designing desktop virtual reality based learning environments. *Journal of Interactive Learning Research, 15*(2), 147–167.

Cheng, Y. F., Moore, D., McGrath, P., & Fan, Y. L. (2005). Collaborative virtual environment technology for people with autism. *Proceedings of the Fifth IEEE International Conference on Advanced Learning Technologies (ICALT'05),* (pp. 1-3).

Chuah, K. M., Chen, C. J., & Teh, C. S. (2009). ViSTREET: An educational virtual environment for the teaching of road safety skills to school students. In Zaman, H. B. (Eds.), *Visual informatics: Bridging research and practice* (pp. 392–403). Berlin/Heidelberg, Germany: Springer-Verlag. doi:10.1007/978-3-642-05036-7_37

Desbonnet, M., Rahman, A., & Cox, S. L. (1997). A virtual reality based training system for disabled children. In Anogianakis, G. (Eds.), *Advancement of assistive technology* (pp. 139–147). Amsterdam, The Netherlands: IOS Press.

Donker, A., & Reitsma, P. (2007). Young children's ability to use a computer mouse. *Computers & Education, 48*, 602–617. doi:10.1016/j.compedu.2005.05.001

Fabri, M. (2006). *Emotionally expressive avatars for collaborative virtual environments*. Unpublished doctoral thesis, Leeds Metropolitan University, United Kingdom.

Falkman, K. W. (2005). *Communicating your way to a theory of mind. The Development of mentalizing skills in children with atypical language development*. Sweden: Göteborg University.

Gourlay, D., Lun, K. C., Lee, Y. N., & Tay, J. (2000). Virtual reality for relearning daily living skills. *International Journal of Medical Informatics, 60*, 255–261. doi:10.1016/S1386-5056(00)00100-3

Copyright © 2011, IGI Global. Copying or distributing in print or electronic forms without written permission of IGI Global is prohibited.

Lee, L. W. (2007). Development of multimedia learning resources for children with learning disabilities in an undergraduate special education technology course. *MEDC, 1*. Retrieved October 12, 2009, from http://www.usm.my/education/MEDC/Vol1/4-%20DEVELOPMENT%20OF%20MULTIMEDIA%20LEARNING%20RESOURCES.pdf

Majumdar, R., Laisram, N., & Chowdhary, S. (2006). Associated handicaps in cerebral palsy. *IJPMR, 17*(1), 11–13.

Massaro, D. W. (2004). Symbiotic value of an embodied agent in language learning. In R.H. Sprague Jr. (Ed.), *IEEE Proceedings of the 37th Annual Hawaii International Conference on System Sciences* (10 pages). Washington, DC: IEEE Computer Society.

Mayer-Johnson. (2009). *Boardmaker plus! Adapt your curriculum to the needs of your students*. DynaVox Mayer-Johnson. Retrieved October 29, 2009, from http://www.mayer-johnson.com /products/boardmaker-plus /default.aspx

McArdle, G., Monahan, T., Bertolotto, M., & Mangina, E. (2004). *A Web-based multimedia virtual reality environment for e-learning*. Proceedings Eurographics 2004. Grenoble, France.

McComas, J., Pivik, J., & Laflamme, M. (1998a). Current uses of virtual reality for children with disabilities. In Riva, G., Wiederhold, B. K., & Molinari, E. (Eds.), *Virtual environments in clinical psychology and neuroscience*. Amsterdam, The Netherlands: Ios Press.

McComas, J., Pivik, J., & Laflamme, M. (1998b). Children's transfer of spatial learning from virtual reality to real environments. *Cyberpsychology & Behavior, 1*(2), 121–129. doi:10.1089/cpb.1998.1.121

Meadows, S. (2009). How was school today? Software helps Scottish children overcome communication difficulties. *Optimist News*. Retrieved October 19, 2009, from http://optimistworld.com/ Articles.aspx?id=9668562c- f119-4c92-8080-c39101198362 &style=news

Miller, F. (2005). *Cerebral palsy*. New York, NY: Springer.

Moore, D., Cheng, Y. F., McGrath, P., & Powell, N. J. (2005). Collaborative virtual environment technology for people with autism. *Focus on Autism and Other Developmental Disabilities, 20*(4), 231–243. doi:10.1177/10883576050200040501

Copyright © 2011, IGI Global. Copying or distributing in print or electronic forms without written permission of IGI Global is prohibited.

Oliveira, J. C., Shen, X., & Georganas, N. D. (2000). *Collaborative virtual environment for industrial training and e-commerce*. Workshop on Application of Virtual Reality Technologies for Future Telecommunication Systems, IEEE Globecom 2000 Conference, Nov-Dec. 2000, San Fransisco, CA.

Origins of Cerebral Palsy. (2009). Forms of cerebral palsy. *Origins of Cerebral Palsy*. Retrieved August 27, 2009, from http://www.originsofcerebralpalsy.com/ index.php

Parsons, S., Beardon, L., Neale, H. R., Reynard, G., Eastgate, R., Wilson, J. R., et al. Hopkins, E. (2000). Development of social skills amongst adults with Asperger's syndrome using virtual environments: The AS interactive project. *Proceedings of the 3rd International Conference on Disability, Virtual Reality & Associated Technologies* (pp. 163-170). Italy: Alghero.

Peeters, M., Verhoeven, L., Moor, J., & Balkom, H. V. (2009). Importance of speech production for phonological awareness and word decoding: The case of children with cerebral palsy. *Research in Developmental Disabilities*, *30*(4), 712–726. doi:10.1016/j.ridd.2008.10.002

Rajab, A., Yoo, S. Y., Abdulgalil, A., Kathiri, S., Ahmed, R., & Mochida, G. H. (2006). An autosomal recesive form of spastic cerebral palsy (CP) with microcephaly and mental retardation. *American Journal of Medical Genetics. Part A*, *140*(14), 1504–1510. doi:10.1002/ajmg.a.31288

Reid, D. T. (2002). Benefits of a virtual play rehabilitation environment for children with cerebral palsy on perceptions of self-efficacy: A pilot study. *Pediatric Rehabilitation*, *5*(3), 141–148.

Resource4 Cerebral Palsy. (2007). Cerebral palsy types. *Resource4 Cerebral Palsy*. Retrieved October 01, 2009, from http://www.resource4cerebralpalsy.com/ topics/ typesofcerebralpalsy.html

Rizzo, A., & Kim, G. (2005). A SWOT analysis of the field of virtual reality rehabilitation and therapy. *Presence (Cambridge, Mass.)*, *14*(2), 119–146. doi:10.1162/1054746053967094

Ryokia, K., Vaucelle, C., & Cassell, J. (2003). Virtual peers as partners in storytelling and literacy learning. *Journal of Computer Assisted Learning*, *19*, 195–208. doi:10.1046/j.0266-4909.2003.00020.x

Safework. (2009a). Virtual hotel. *Safework SA*. Retrieved June 05, 2010, from http://www.safework.sa.gov.au/ contentPages/Industry/Hospitality/ Resources/ VirtualHotel.htm

Copyright © 2011, IGI Global. Copying or distributing in print or electronic forms without written permission of IGI Global is prohibited.

Safework (2009b). Virtual kitchen. *Safework SA.* Retrieved June 02, 2010, from http://www.safework.sa.gov.au/ contentPages/Industry/Hospitality /Resources/ VirtualKitchen.htm

Shih, Y.-C., & Yang, M.-T. (2008). A collaborative virtual environment for situated language using VEC3D. *Journal of Educational Technology & Society, 11*(1), 56–68.

Smith, B. L., & MacGregor, J. T. (1992). What is collaborative learning? In Goodsell, A., Mahler, M., Tinto, V., Smith, B. L., & MacGregor, J. (Eds.), *Collaborative learning: A sourcebook for higher education* (pp. 9–22). University Park, PA: National Center on Postsecondary Teaching, Learning, and Assessment.

Standen, P. J., & Brown, D. J. (2006). Virtual reality and its role in removing the barriers that turn cognitive impairments into intellectual disability. *Virtual Reality (Waltham Cross), 10,* 241–252. doi:10.1007/s10055-006-0042-6

Standen, P. J., Brown, D. J., & Cromby, J. J. (2001). The effective use of virtual environments in the education and rehabilitation of students with intellectual disabilities. *British Journal of Educational Technology, 32*(3), 289–299. doi:10.1111/1467-8535.00199

Standen, P. J., Cromby, J. J., & Brown, D. J. (1998). Playing for real. *Mental Health Care, 1,* 412–415.

Theng, Y., & Paye, A. (2009). Effects of avatars on children's emotion and motivation in learning. In G. Siemens & C. Fulford (Eds.), *Proceedings of World Conference on Educational Multimedia, Hypermedia and Telecommunications 2009* (pp. 927-936). Chesapeake, VA: AACE.

United Cerebral Palsy. (2009). Cerebral palsy fact sheet. *United Cerebral Palsy.* Retrieved September 04, 2009, from http://www.ucp.org/uploads /cp_fact_sheet.pdf

Valente, J. A. (1983). *Creating a computer-based learning environment for physically handicapped children.* Unpublished doctoral dissertation, Massachusetts Institute of Technology, United States.

Vince, J. (2004). *Introduction to virtual reality.* London, UK: Springer-Verlag.

Vygotsky, L. (1978). Interaction between learning and development. In *Mind in Society.* (Trans. M. Cole, pp. 79-91). Cambridge, MA: Harvard University Press.

Waller, A., Black, R., O'Mara, D. A., Pain, H., Ritchie, G., & Manurung, R. (2009). Evaluating the STANDUP Pun generating software with children with cerebral palsy. *ACM Transactions on Accessible Computing, 1*(3), 1–27. doi:10.1145/1497302.1497306

Copyright © 2011, IGI Global. Copying or distributing in print or electronic forms without written permission of IGI Global is prohibited.

Weinstein, I. M. (2005). The arrival of the virtual office: Immediate access to colleagues and customers through an always-on virtual work environment. *Wainhouse Research.* Retrieved January 12, 2010, from http://www.wrplatinum.com /downloads/4256.aspx?relo=1

Werner, D. (1987). *Disabled village children: A guide for health workers, rehabilitation workers and families: Cerebral Palsy* (pp. 87–108). The Hesperian Foundation.

ADDITIONAL READING

Anolli, L., Mantovani, F., Balestra, M., Agliati, A., Realdon, O., & Zurloni, V. ... Confalonieri, L. (2005). The potential of affective computing in e-learning: MYSELF project experience. *International Conference on Human-Computer Interaction (Interact 2005).*

Arango, F., Aziz, E., Esche, S. K., & Chassapis, C. (2008, October). *A review of applications of computer games in education and training.* Paper presented at 38th ASEE/IEEE Frontiers in Education Conference, Saratoga Springs, NY.

Barrett, B. G. (n.d.). Using e-learning as a strategic tool for students with disabilities. Retrieved March 28, 2010, from http://wikieducator.org /images/9/98/PID_209.pdf

Blackstone, S. W. (2007). AAC research and development: Having an impact. *Augmentative Communication News,* 19(3), 1-8. Retrieved January 12, 2010, from http://www.augcominc.com/ newsletters/index.cfm/ newsletter_4.pdf

Bouras, Ch., Giannaka, E., & Tsiatsos, Th. (2008). Exploiting virtual environments to support collaborative e-learning communities. *Int. J. of Web-Based Learning and Technology,* 3(2), 1–22. doi:10.4018/jwltt.2008040101

Chase, C., Chin, D. B., Oppezzo, M., & Schwartz, D. L. (in press). Teachable agents and the protégé effect: Increasing the effort towards learning. *Journal of Science Education and Technology.*

Chen, C. J. (2006). The design, development and evaluation of a virtual reality based learning environment. *Australasian Journal of Educational Technology, 22*(1), 39–63.

Chung, D., deBuys, B. D., & Nam, C. S. (2007). Influence of avatar creation on attitude, empathy, presence, and para-social interaction. In Jacko, J. (Ed.), *Human-Computer Interaction, Part 1* (pp. 711–720). Springer-Verlag Berlin Heidelberg.

Copyright © 2011, IGI Global. Copying or distributing in print or electronic forms without written permission of IGI Global is prohibited.

Fabri, M., Elzouki, S., & Moore, D. (2007). Emotionally expressive avatars for chatting, learning and therapeutic intervention. In Jacko, J. (Ed.), *Human-Computer Interaction, Part III* (pp. 275–285). Springer-Verlag Berlin Heidelberg.

Fabri, M., & Moore, D. J. (2005, April). The use of emotionally expressive avatars in collaborative virtual environments. *Proceeding of Symposium on Emphatic Interaction with Synthetic Characters.* Paper presented at Artificial Intelligence and Social Behavior Convention 2005 (AISB 2005), UK: University of Hertfordshire.

Gombash, L. (1998). Cerebral palsy with hemiplegia. *Therapy Skill Builders: a division of The Psychological Corporation,* 1-2. Retrieved October 30, 2009, from http://www.pearsonassessments.com/ hai/Images/resource/techrpts/ TheraNotes/ TN_Ped_OT_pdf/ CP_W_Hemiplegia.pdf

Gonzales, C., Leroy, G., & De Leo, G. (2009). augmentative and alternative communication technologies. In M. M. Cunha, A. Tavares & R. Simoes (Eds.), *Handbook of research on developments in e-health and telemedicine: Technological and social perspectives.* Accepted for Publication.

Grynszpan, O., Martin, J.-C., & Nadel, J. (2008). multimedia interfaces for users with high functioning autism: An empirical investigation. *International Journal of Human-Computer Studies, 66,* 628–639. doi:10.1016/j.ijhcs.2008.04.001

Hadden, K. L., & von Baeyer, C. L. (2002). Pain in children with cerebral palsy: Common triggers and expressive behaviors. *International Association for the Study of Pain, 99,* 281–288.

Koubek, A., & Müller, K. (2002). Collaborative virtual environments for learning. *ACM SIG Proceedings* (pp. 16-20). United States: Louisiana.

Lányi, C. S., Basca, E., Mátrai, R., Kosztyán, Z., & Pataky, I. (2004). Interactive rehabilitation software for treating patients with aphasia. *Proc.5ᵗʰ Intl Conf. Disability, Virtual Reality & Assoc. Tech.* (pp. 233-238), UK: Oxford.

Lányi, C. S., Geiszt, Z., Károlyi, P., Tilinger, A., & Magyar, V. (2006). Virtual reality in special needs early education. *The International Journal of Virtual Reality, 5*(4), 55–68.

Lányi, C. S., Geiszt, Z., & Magyar, V. (2006). Using IT to inform and rehabilitate aphasic patients. *Informing Science Journal, 9,* 163–179.

Copyright © 2011, IGI Global. Copying or distributing in print or electronic forms without written permission of IGI Global is prohibited.

Lee, E. A. L., Wong, K. W., & Fung, C. C. (2009). Learning effectiveness in a desktop virtual reality-based learning environment. In S.C. Kong, H. Ogata, H.C. Arnseth, C.K.K. Chan, T. Hirashima, F. Klett, J.H.M. Lee, C.C. Liu, C.K. Looi, M. Milrad, A. Mitrovic, K. Nakabayashi, S.L. Wong, & S.J.H. Yang (Eds.), *Proceedings of the 17th International Conference on Computers in Education* (pp. 832-839). Hong Kong: Asia-Pasific Society for Computers in Education.

Li, K.-Y. R., Sofra, J., & Power, M. (2007). 3D avatars and collaborative virtual environments. *IGI Global*, 1-6.

Maguire, M., Elton, E., Osman, Z., & Nicolle, C. (2006). Design of a virtual learning environment for students with special needs. *An Interdisciplinary Journal on Humans in ICT Environments, 2*(1), 119–153.

Mantovani, F. (2001). VR learning: Potential and challenges for the use of 3d environments in education and training. In Riva, G., & Calimberti, C. (Eds.), *Towards CyberPsychology: Mind, Cognitions and Society in the Internet Age* (pp. 207–226). Amsterdam, Netherlands: Ios Press.

McIlhagga, M., & George, P. (1999). Communicating meaningful emotional information in a virtual world. *Proceedings of International Workshop on Affect in Interactions,* Italy, Siena.

Millar, D. C., Light, J. C., & Schlosser, R. W. (2006). The impact of augmentative and alternative communication intervention on the speech production of individuals with developmental disabilities: A research review. *Journal of Speech, Language, and Hearing Research: JSLHR, 49*, 248–264. doi:10.1044/1092-4388(2006/021)

Preston, D., & Carter, M. (2009). A review of the efficacy of the picture exchange communication system intervention. *Journal of Autism and Developmental Disorders, 39*(10), 1471–1486. doi:10.1007/s10803-009-0763-y

Stott, D. A. (2008). *Recognition emotion in facial expressions by children with language impairment.* Master Dissertation, Brigham Young University, United States.

Valk, J. E., & Ed, M. (2003). *Teaching imitation skills to preschool children with severe disabilities: The effects of embedding constant time delay within a small group activity.* PhD Dissertation, The Ohio State University, United States.

Zhao, Y., & Wang, W. (2008). Attributions of human-avatar relationship closeness in a virtual community. In Lytras, M. D., Carroll, J. M., Damiani, E., & Tennyson, R. D. (Eds.), *Emerging technologies and information systems for the knowledge society* (pp. 61–69). Springer-Verlag Berlin Heidelberg. doi:10.1007/978-3-540-87781-3_7

Copyright © 2011, IGI Global. Copying or distributing in print or electronic forms without written permission of IGI Global is prohibited.

KEY TERMS AND DEFINITIONS

Stands for Augmentative and Assistive Communication (AAC): An assistive or supplementation or replacement of natural speech and/or writing using aided and/or unaided symbols.

Asphyxia: A condition where the need of oxygen in the body is decreased cause the individual to not be able to breathe normally. Asphyxia can be induced by choking, drowning, electric shock, injury, or the inhalation of toxic gases.

Cerebral Palsy: A term used for a group of non-progressive disorder caused by an injury during or after birth that affects the motor control centres of the brain.

Cognitive Impairment: A term used for an impairment that affect their intellectual ability. Typically, individual with cognitive impairment have delayed intellectual development, inefficiency in learning, failure expectancy and social competency deficiencies.

Fine Motor Skill: Ability required in order to control the coordination of hand (fingers) movement with eyes.

Mental Retardation: A disability which is characterized with important limitations in intellectual functioning and in adaptive behaviour, where it is happen during the developmental period.

Non-Progressive Disorder: A disorder that will not get worst over the time.

Copyright © 2011, IGI Global. Copying or distributing in print or electronic forms without written permission of IGI Global is prohibited.

Chapter 6
Enabling Context Aware Services in the Area of AAC

Lau Sian Lun
University of Kassel, Germany

Klaus David
University of Kassel, Germany

ABSTRACT

Technology can be used to assist people with disabilities in their daily activities. Especially when the users have communication deficiencies, suitable technology and tools can assuage such needs. We envision that context awareness is a potential method suitable to provide services and solutions in the area of Assistive and Augmentative Communication (AAC). In this chapter, the authors give an introduction to context awareness and the state of the art. This is followed with the elaboration on how context awareness can be used in AAC. The Context Aware Remote Monitoring Assistant (CARMA) is presented as an application designed for a care assistant and his patient. A demonstration of a context aware component implemented in the CARMA application is shown in this chapter. An experiment that investigates movement recognition using an accelerometer in a smartphone and the obtained results are presented. This chapter ends with a discussion on challenges, future work and the conclusion.

DOI: 10.4018/978-1-60960-541-4.ch006

Copyright ©2011, IGI Global. Copying or distributing in print or electronic forms without written permission of IGI Global is prohibited.

INTRODUCTION

In our daily lives, we communicate with different parties as a matter of course. In human to human communication, languages and gestures help to convey one's thought to the other. We have the ability to interpret implicit information. This helps to reflect certain situations that take place around us. Our senses help us to accomplish this rather complicated task. Without this ability, communication can be challenging. When it comes to situations where communication cannot be carried out normally and naturally, we need appropriate applications and methods to fill the gap. Machines and systems can be designed to emulate human communication and comprehension capabilities. These capabilities can help those who need this assistance to fulfil communication needs.

People with certain disabilities or illnesses may have some communication deficiencies. For example, some children with cerebral palsy have difficulties to talk. People with Parkinson's disease may have motor deficits and communication difficulties, which cause them to face problems in carrying out daily activities and in interacting with others. Most of these people can be helped by using Assistive and Augmentative Communication (AAC) technology. Tools ranging from simple low-tech methods such as drawing and writing tools, to high-tech devices such as multi-purpose computer-based communication aids are being researched, designed and developed. When we look at the high-tech devices of the AAC technology, computing devices play an essential role in assisting both AAC users and people who need to communicate with them. These devices fulfil more complicated tasks including text-to-speech generation and eye-movement tracking techniques, especially for those who have speech and movement impairments.

In cases where an AAC user needs care and monitoring from a care assistant, the communication needs do not stop at face to face communication. The care assistant also potentially needs to have the means to keep track of the person he is taking care of, particularly if the AAC user has memory, motor or speech deficits. Instead of requiring the care assistant to manually perform these tasks, suitable devices and techniques can be used. For example, sensors can be installed to monitor different information regarding the AAC user. Implicit information can be captured and recorded. Based on this information, the care assistant can review and evaluate decisions suitable for the AAC user. Applications can also adapt to the captured information in order to serve the AAC user's needs.

One of the research areas that apply techniques similar to the above example is context awareness. The word context refers to the implicit information interpreted from different sensors. A context aware system utilizes context information to perform service behaviour adaptation. Depending on the contexts, the system may offer location or situation specific functions to the user. It can also automate processes when the

Copyright © 2011, IGI Global. Copying or distributing in print or electronic forms without written permission of IGI Global is prohibited.

obtained contexts fulfil pre-defined conditions. In other words, context awareness aims to "understand" and to satisfy the needs of a user by providing intelligent adaptation.

The following scenario is selected in order to demonstrate how context aware technology can be used in the area of AAC:

James is the care assistant for an AAC user, Bob. Bob has Alzheimer's disease. He can no longer independently carry out the various activities of daily living (ADLs). His condition requires constant supervision and monitoring in order to assist him and to ensure his safety. With the help of sensors and a context aware system, his activities and situations are constantly being measured and observed. He carries a smartphone, which is placed in a waist pouch. The rooms in his house are equipped with different types of sensors such as Bluetooth beacons, temperature sensors and humidity sensors. Bob stays alone in his home and he only gets occasional visits from his children.

James is responsible to take care of Bob and uses the system to keep track of Bob's activity. The system takes note of places Bob has visited throughout the day. James can check the location log to see which room Bob is currently in, and which rooms has Bob previously been to. If a certain home appliances had been left unattended, James gets a notification and it is also possible for James to remotely turn off the appliance.

On one particular day, Bob had an accident - he fell down at the corridor as he came out from the washroom. James almost immediately received a warning notification on his mobile phone that an accident had possibly taken place and Bob requires immediate assistance. While on his way to Bob's home, James enquired for status update from the system and was informed that all rooms were unoccupied and Bob was located in the corridor. This confirmed further that Bob was perhaps unconscious. James called paramedics immediately and arrived at Bob's home. He was able to locate Bob and attended to him in time, even before the paramedics arrived 5 minutes later. Bob was given first aid help immediately and then sent to the nearby hospital for further treatment.

In the scenario, the different sensors provide snapshots of information to the context aware system. There are sensors that collect information to obtain and describe context changes in the environment. Some of the example contexts are temperature changes, room occupancy and types of activity taking place in a given room. There are also sensors solely responsible to collect information of a given user. It can be a sensor that measures a person's current heart rate or his current position and acceleration force.

Copyright © 2011, IGI Global. Copying or distributing in print or electronic forms without written permission of IGI Global is prohibited.

By combining the available sensor information, a context aware system aims to provide contexts for the following purposes. Firstly, the contexts are used to explain implicit information. For instance, the activity and situation information of Bob are not directly measurable. However, the available information from sensors on and near Bob can be processed to give accurate recognition of his current activity. Secondly, based on the interpreted contexts and their changes, the context aware system can also trigger designated services to provide appropriate adaptations that serve Bob's needs. As presented in the scenario, the contexts obtained triggered an action that sends an emergency warning to James, when Bob is found to be in danger. Thirdly, context logs can be a useful tool for the monitoring of AAC users. The interpreted contexts are comprehensible information for the care assistants and family members. It reduces the sensor data dimensionality and simplifies the effort for human users to understand the recorded information. In situations where AAC users are no longer capable to communicate with other people, these context logs can be crucial in telling others, such as the paramedics, the information that will assist them to make correct decisions.

We envisioned that context awareness can be one of the applicable technologies to assist different tasks and needs in the area of AAC. We propose the use of non-obtrusive devices as part of a context aware enabled system. The users are not expected to explicitly wear multiple specialized hardware or systems in order to allow the system to monitor and observe context changes. A good example can be an off-the-shelf smartphone. The current smartphones available in the market have multiple sensor interfaces and can provide information such as time, radio signal or user acceleration. There are also a number of commercially available sensors that can be installed in rooms of a building for environmental sensor information. By carefully selecting the appropriate information, the sensor information can be processed and analysed to produce usable context information.

In the next sub chapter, at first a general introduction to context awareness is presented. This is followed by a discussion on how context awareness can be applied in the area of AAC. The sub chapter includes a brief overview on the design issues and requirements. The proposed vision is then explained by using the selected scenario with a concrete example implementation using acceleration data from a smartphone. The chapter concludes with lessons learnt and potential next steps.

Copyright © 2011, IGI Global. Copying or distributing in print or electronic forms without written permission of IGI Global is prohibited.

CONTEXT AND CONTEXT AWARENESS

History of Context and Context awareness

In the early 90s, Mark Weiser proposed the vision of ubiquitous computing (Weiser, 1991). He envisioned that in the future computers will eventually disappear and users are no longer required to interact with computers in the same way they use desktop computers. This vision challenges researchers to look into newer and more innovative approaches in different aspects, such as communications, human-computer interaction, applications and systems. An area that explores approaches that enable devices and systems to understand information in ubiquitous computing is context awareness.

The term context aware computing was first mentioned by Schilit and Theimer (1994). They defined context aware as "the ability of a mobile user's applications to discover and react to changes in the environment they are situated in". Context, according to Schilit, Adams, and Want (1994), is defined as location, identities, nearby people and objects, and changes to those objects. This was followed by subsequent work that further investigated the definition of context, context awareness and its potential applications. Another project at the University of Kent referred to context as information like the user's location, environment, identity of people around the user, time and temperature (Brown, 1996; Ryan, Pascoe, & Morse, 1998). Hull, Neaves, and Bedford-Roberts (1997) viewed context as different aspects of the current situation of the user.

Many of these definitions were made by example, i.e. they were defined either as synonyms for context or as aspects of information needed for their prototypes or applications. Dey and Abowd (2000b) argued that the definitions are too specific, and hence presented a more general definition as follows:

"Context is any information that can be used to characterize the situation of an entity. An entity is a person, place, or object that is considered relevant to the interaction between a user and an application, including the user and applications themselves."

The definition is widely accepted and used in various context aware related studies. However, some authors find this definition too general and abstract. For example, Crowley, Coutaz, Rey, and Reignier (2002) proposed that a clear semi-formal definition with an operational theory needs to be completed to apply context in the composition of perceptual processes. They made a distinction between the user's context and the system's context. Mäntyjärvi (2003) argued in his PhD thesis that the abstraction according to Dey is shifted from the definition of context to the definition of information and of knowledge. He pointed out that the definition does

Copyright © 2011, IGI Global. Copying or distributing in print or electronic forms without written permission of IGI Global is prohibited.

not indicate how context can be processed or how the relevancy of context can be acquired. Henricksen (2003) refined the definition of context as a set of information surrounding a given task that is needed for the completion of the task.

Throughout the development of context awareness, we have yet to identify a final and conclusive definition. The above definitions were made from individual perspectives. The earlier definitions were more intended for respective prototyping of initial context awareness ideas. This explains why these definitions are specific to the different pioneer context aware applications. The definition from Dey and its derivatives provide a general basis for all potential context aware applications, though it was not intended to specify how context should be modelled in an implementation. The definitions after Dey's were focused on context aware system designs. Therefore, in order to fully utilize the advantages of having contexts in the context aware system, it is necessary to have a more concrete definition for different parts of a system.

What is context?

The definition of context from Dey can be used as a basis. The evolution of context in the work after Dey has given a clearer picture how context can be applied in an implementation. As mentioned by Henricksen (2003), Dey did not clarify what he meant by "the situation of an entity". However, the concept of situation is not just a simple word. It is a complex yet definable concept.

In some of the earlier research, contexts were mainly used to reveal further information that is comprehensible by both application and the users. For example, the Active Badge system (Want, Hopper, Falcão, & Gibbons, 1992) allowed the receptionists to see a user's possible last detected location. Schilit et al. (1994) demonstrated in their PARCTAB work a context aware application that is able to present information to users based on proximity to services. Devices can be turned on or reconfigured according to the location of the users and adapted services can be executed automatically. In these examples, users can see which contexts have been recognized by the application (e.g. location of a user). At the same time, devices and services were started and executed based on the obtained contexts.

Sigg (2008) argued that context should be defined in a general yet clear manner. By adapting the definition from Dey, he further refined the concept of contexts with a more detailed categorization called aspects. Independent from applications or tasks, the different aspects of context can provide a structured and extended distinction of context types. A depiction of the aspects of context is shown in Figure 1.

Context can have different levels of abstraction. According to the above definitions from different researchers, the information measured and provided by a sensor is a context, while the interpreted information based on this sensor measurement is

Copyright © 2011, IGI Global. Copying or distributing in print or electronic forms without written permission of IGI Global is prohibited.

Figure 1. Aspects of context (© 2008, Stephan Sigg. Used with permission.)

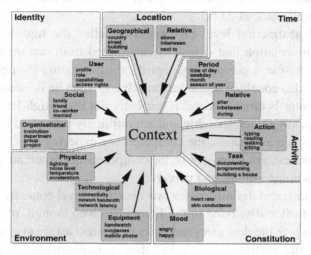

also considered as a context. The abstraction levels can be seen as a way to view context from a computational point of view (Sigg, 2008). The first hand information obtained from a sensor device can be referred to as raw data. The processing of this raw data produces low level context. The low level context can be further processed to obtain high-level context. The process is illustrated in Figure 2. Note that a high-level context can be processed to produce another high-level context.

The low-level context is normally a direct interpretation of the information obtained from a context source, i.e. a sensor. It gives a semantic meaning to the obtained value in order to allow further usage of this context. For example, the temperature sensor gives a reading of the voltage potential differences that represents the current temperature of the object or environment it measures. By giving the

Figure 2. Relationship between different levels of abstraction for contexts

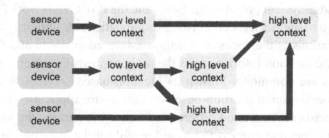

Copyright © 2011, IGI Global. Copying or distributing in print or electronic forms without written permission of IGI Global is prohibited.

corresponding calculation to this value, one can then obtain the current temperature with a desired unit, such as 23 °C.

The second abstraction level of context is called the high-level context. It expresses the information that is usually interpreted from one or more low-level contexts. For example, a person may regard the surrounding temperature 23°C as warm. One can also conclude that a person is busy, when he is located in his office while his computer is turned on and is currently not idle. High-level contexts are usually semantically understandable and are implicitly perceived by human automatically. In context awareness, the computers are expected to be able to produce and use these contexts. In other words, the computers can potentially "understand" what and how a human thinks and perceives.

The distinctions and definitions for raw data, low-level contexts and high-level contexts are not often discussed in the literature. Even though, these distinctions are necessary to provide designers and users of context aware systems a better understanding for the required contexts in a desired implementation and usage. The abstraction levels are useful to allow human users to understand what a system has processed and interpreted. For a computing device, the different abstractions are basically still strings, where these strings are results from the processing of the sensor data (Sigg, 2008).

The process to obtain low- and high-level contexts from sensor data is commonly known as context modelling. A context model defines context data that is understandable by machines and sometimes users. Strang and Popien (2004) presented a summary on most relevant context modelling approaches. They are Key-Value, Markup scheme, Graphical, Object oriented, Logic based and Ontology based models. The authors concluded that ontology based models are most expressive and suitable approach for their requirements. In our opinion, one needs to analyse his own application and requirement in order to identify the most suitable modelling approach. There are cases where an ontology is required for its expressiveness, but there are also cases where simple key-value implementations will suffice.

Context aware applications and systems

The Active Badge system (Want et al., 1992) and the PARCTAB work (Schilit et al., 1994) were two of the earliest context aware applications. A similarity among these earliest applications is the focus on location-aware adaptations and functions. In other words, the location information is the main contexts considered and applied. These systems are commonly known as location-based services today. Another common demonstration of location-based context aware application is a tour guide system. As tourists move around different attractions in a town, the tour guide can make use of the location context to present useful tourist information of different

Copyright © 2011, IGI Global. Copying or distributing in print or electronic forms without written permission of IGI Global is prohibited.

nearby highlights. Some examples are the work of Abowd et al. (1997) and Cheverst, Davies, Mitchell, Friday, and Efstratiou (2000).

As mentioned by Schmidt, Beigl, and Gellersen (1999), there are more contexts than location. This can be observed in later work after the end of the 1990s. For example, the CybreMinder system (Dey & Abowd, 2000a) is a context aware application that sends out reminders based on time, location and situational contexts. Several other domains that have adopted the context aware approaches are smart home (Roy, Roy, & Das, 2006), personalization (Sutterer, Droegehorn, & David, 2008) and health care (Bardram & Nørskov, 2008; Matic, Mehta, Rehg, Osmani, & Mayora, 2010).

There are also different context aware frameworks proposed in the past years. These frameworks include the Context Toolkit (Dey, Abowd, & Salber, 2001), the Context Management Framework (CMF) (Korpipää, Mäntyjärvi, Kela, Keränen, & Malm, 2003), the Context Broker Architecture (CoBrA) (Chen, Finin, & Joshi, 2003), the Context aware Sub-Structure (CASS) middleware (Fahy & Clarke, 2004) and the Service-Oriented Context aware Middleware (SOCAM) (Gu, Pung, & Zhang, 2005). As we analyse and observe these different context aware frameworks, there are a number of similarities between them. These systems may use different names or categorizations of their functions, but it is possible to summarize them in a generalized layer framework for understanding purposes. This framework, as depicted in Figure 3, gives an overview of the core functions of the different roles and components found in a context aware system.

The first layer is where the sensors are found. The sensors are responsible for the sensing of information that can be used to derive usable contexts. The processes that derive contexts are found in the second layer. Context processing includes a number of functions, such as filtering, context learning, context interpretation, context reasoning and prediction. Many context awareness related research projects

Figure 3. A generalized context aware layer framework

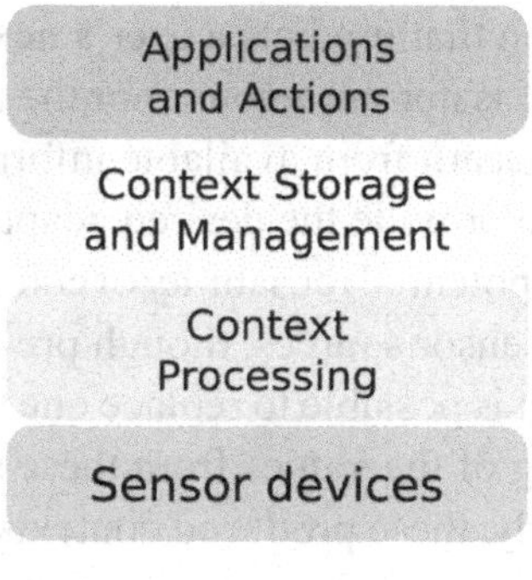

Copyright © 2011, IGI Global. Copying or distributing in print or electronic forms without written permission of IGI Global is prohibited.

focus in this layer. On top of context processing is the context storage and management layer. It deals with the issues on how the derived and produced contexts are stored and managed. Components such as context repository and context broker are found here. The final layer utilizes components from the second and third layers for potential applications and actions. The available contexts for a specific application domain may be used by respective applications for display and adaptation purposes. It is also possible that a context aware application automatically invokes desired actions that are triggered by context-changes.

Differences between Context Awareness and Current Systems

To date there are already many consumer products that perform smart adaptations and controls for various applications. These products can be seen as smart systems. For instance, modern Heating, Ventilating, and Air Conditioning (HVAC) systems installed in homes can be programmed to automatically adjust different settings of controls according to the users' preferences. Heaters can be turned on and adjusted to the optimum temperature throughout the day, adapting to the indoor and outdoor temperature of a given day. There are electrical toothbrushes that give instruction to their users on how one should brush his teeth correctly. According to the definitions and concepts mentioned above, these products are not context aware.

These smart systems are commonly designed in such a way that they react and response based on pre-defined thresholds. The threshold values are usually set according to the sensor measured data. For example, a HVAC system configured to provide optimum heating needs information such as the indoor and outdoor temperature, time and also day of week. Once the system is programmed with the desired room temperature for specific days of a week, heating process takes place as long as the pre-defined conditions are satisfied. The system neither initiates the heating because it knows that someone is going to use the room in the next hour, nor it turn off the heater when the user leaves the room or feels it is too warm. A context aware version of such a system uses context information as triggering conditions. Therefore, a context aware HVAC system will be able to adapt its heating period by receiving context information that predicts a user's next location and arrival time. Note that the distinction here is not the amount nor the types of conditions used for triggering. It is the ability to learn from available information to obtain the needed contexts and subsequently to provide the desired adaptations.

Another distinction is the potential reusability of context information. In a context aware system, the different sensor sources, though pre-defined and known, are not necessary closed and fixed. It is possible to replace one with the other, as long as the interpretation and processing of the values from these sensor sources can produce the desired contexts. Similarly, these produced contexts are also not limited to only

Copyright © 2011, IGI Global. Copying or distributing in print or electronic forms without written permission of IGI Global is prohibited.

one application. If there are several applications available simultaneously, they can all use the same contexts for different adaptation and tasks. One has to consider the issue of trust and privacy, particularly if the contexts reveal private information that are not meant for other people except for the user.

The above comparison and distinction are presented to help us understanding how we can differentiate context aware systems from current smart systems. We also see context aware systems as potential extensions for current systems. In other words, the use of contexts can be integrated in some existing systems to compliment the available functions.

Applying Context Awareness in the Area of AAC

There have been a number of investigations in the past that applied context aware techniques in AAC to help users who are disabled or ill. Davis, Moore, and Storey (2003) presented a context aware framework that provides conversation prediction for a disabled user. The proposed framework focuses on using context aware user profiles to analyze contextually relevant information from the interaction between the user and his visitor. The stored contextual information is then used for future conversations. Betz et al. (2007) proposed a general architecture of Context aware Adaptable System (CAAS) that aims to use context aware ubiquitous devices to help people with disabilities by automatically detecting changes in the surrounding.

Catarinucci, Colella, Esposito, Tarricone, and Zappatore (2009) proposed a context aware system based on RFID sensor-tags that can be applied in the health-care domain. The hardware and software issues were investigated in order to achieve a system that is cost-effective, easy to use and reconfigurable. Paganelli and Giuli (2007) proposed a context-management system for a home-based continuous care system. Adaptive and automated services are enabled in their proposed system using an ontology-based context management middleware. The UCare (Vales-Alonso et al., 2008) is a context aware architecture that provides rich environment adaptation services to disabled users. The system supports interactive and non-interactive operation modes with the use of service and user profiles. Similar to our vision, they proposed the use of commercially available devices such as smartphones and PDAs in the systems.

The combination of context awareness in assistive technology and systems is seen as a challenging task (Nehmer, Becker, Karshmer, & Lamm, 2006; Varshney, 2007; Vales-Alonso et al., 2008). Such a system must fulfil requirements such as availability, adaptability, human-computer interaction and security. The existing work, described above, shows the potential for creating innovative context aware applications and systems for the area of AAC. In the next section, a discussion on design issues and requirements is presented. This is followed by a brief overview

Copyright © 2011, IGI Global. Copying or distributing in print or electronic forms without written permission of IGI Global is prohibited.

on hardware and software infrastructures that are commonly found in a context aware system.

Design Issues and Requirements

There exist different tasks and needs for the AAC users. Therefore, we can use a top down approach to analyse the tasks. By identifying what is needed to help and to solve the tasks, it will lead us to the required contexts. Once context types are determined, it is necessary to investigate how the system can obtain these contexts. This includes the analysis of possible abstraction levels of contexts and the techniques needed to evaluate and produce them. Only then, one can consider which type of sensors is required to produce the desired low-level and high-level contexts.

During the process of identifying the different tasks, contexts and sensors, one should also consider the target users of the context aware applications. It is crucial to know whether the selected sensors are available for a real implementation. The sensors should also be as non-obtrusive as possible, in order not to discourage or bring discomfort to the potential users. Especially for the AAC users, this consideration is necessary since they may have different preferences and needs as compared to normal users.

One should also consider the issue of trust and privacy. If the users are going to be monitored, whether periodically or on-demand, the measured information should only be made accessible for authorized people. The availability and validity of sensor data and contexts information must be well managed and checked. This also affects the decision on how and where the data and contexts are stored.

The automatic adaptation of services and tasks in a context aware system will potentially reduce the need for direct user instructions and actions. Consequently, the interaction between human users and the system will also be different as compared to conventional computing devices. It is recommended to consider the user requirements for a good design of context aware systems. The users need to have control over the adaptation and functions of the system. It should be possible for users to know, at a comprehensible level, what the context aware system is doing or going to do. The designed system should allow interventions and changes from the users. An ideal situation is where a balance can be achieved between user control and the system adaptation.

A context aware application is not restricted to only a device. In many examples it is usually a combination of different hardware and software components. Depending on the target environment, this decision can vary according to the tasks and needs. In the next sub section we look into this area.

Copyright © 2011, IGI Global. Copying or distributing in print or electronic forms without written permission of IGI Global is prohibited.

Hardware Infrastructures

For a context aware application there is generally no given guideline in deciding which type of hardware infrastructure one should use. However, from previous work and results, we can generally categorize them into the following categories:

Sensor Devices

Sensors play an essential role in a context aware system. They provide information to derive the context needed in the system. Some examples are listed in the literature such as (Schmidt & Laerhoven, 2001). We would like to categorize the sensors into three large groups:

1. **Environmental sensors:** In places where the application is implemented, sensors can be installed to provide information regarding the surrounding of the users. Typical examples are environmental information such as temperature, humidity, brightness and noise level. In some cases one can also use RFID tags to provide customized information related to the place a user is currently located. This type of sensor is usually fixed and is location specific. The communication between sensors and the application can be performed either via wired or wireless medium.
2. **Body-worn sensors:** It is also possible to put sensors on a user to provide information about and around him. Body-worn sensors should be small and robust. They should also be non-obtrusive for the user. Due to this factor, often such sensors connect to a device carried by the user using wireless communication. These sensors should also have reasonable battery time to measure the desired information. The sensors remain with the user wherever he goes and to measure respective information whatever he does.
3. **Virtual sensors:** The above two categories of sensors are physical sensors. It is however possible to have software that provides specific type of information that can be useful. Such type of information source can be called virtual sensors. For example, by getting the information from a calendar system, a virtual sensor can provide the availability or a location of a person. The information provided by virtual sensors may not be only raw data. It is also possible to obtain directly low- or high-level contexts from a virtual sensor.

The above categorization of sensors intends to help context aware designers to select and decide suitable sensor sources. In a case where the application should react according to contexts related to a user's movement and situation, it may be sufficient to only use selected body-worn and virtual sensors. If the application

Copyright © 2011, IGI Global. Copying or distributing in print or electronic forms without written permission of IGI Global is prohibited.

aims to provide a context aware HVAC control for a building, it may need all three groups of sensors.

Communication Devices

Quite a number of the previous context aware systems were implemented using multiple devices. Often the different components, found in different layers of the generalized layer framework, are deployed on these devices in a distributed manner. These components require different types of communication channel to enable the exchange of data. For example, the wireless sensors connect to the context processing components via ZigBee while the latter communicates with the storage server via an Ethernet connection. The different connection possibilities require a careful selection for the designated scenario.

The availability and economic factors of the communication channel are another two consideration factors. Some connections are not always on or are distance dependant. For example, communications using Bluetooth or IR are bound to a limited radius of operation. Cost of communication may give a certain amount of restrictions, such as the choice between fixed broadband and mobile Internet. Besides costs, other factors that affect the decision of communication devices also include speed, performance and reliability of the selected communication channel.

User Interaction Devices

Users need suitable interaction devices to use context aware systems. They cannot be excluded from the systems. In previous work we see large choices of possibilities - from simple buttons to touch screens, tablets, personal digital assistant and smartphones. Most of the applications use a software graphical user interface (GUI) to allow users to view information, and to interact with the system. The decision of user interaction devices is particularly crucial for the AAC users. The selected user interaction devices have to be simple and direct. With context awareness, the application attempts to learn and understand the user's needs and service usage behaviours. Adaptation and automation reduce the need for the user to instruct or interact with the application. Consequently, it also reduces the frequency of direct user involvement and the possible inconvenience caused. We foresee the use of contexts can lessen tedious and repetitive interactions with the system, and hence can improve user experience and comfort.

Copyright © 2011, IGI Global. Copying or distributing in print or electronic forms without written permission of IGI Global is prohibited.

Computing Devices

Different functions in the second layer to forth layer of the generalized layer framework are provided by software running on computing devices. Apart from the required computing power and time, there is usually no restriction or specific requirement on the computing devices. One can use a full-scale computer server with multiple processors or just an embedded system packed in a small case.

The decision of where a component should be deployed is a necessary consideration, especially in a more complex implementation where redundant components are available. Such implementations usually use distributed approaches like client-server or peer-to-peer (P2P). The context aware system is responsible to manage and distribute tasks and information from and to the designated computing devices.

Software Infrastructures

A context aware application consists of a collection of software components. These components perform specific functions such as sensor data collection, context processing and context management. From the previous and existing context aware systems, there is also no so-called standard software infrastructure. However, it is observed that many systems were implemented using concepts and techniques based on service oriented architecture (SOA) (MacKenzie, Laskey, McCabe, Brown & Metz, 2006). A middleware is used in an implementation to provide deployment, management and execution of the designated context aware related functions. Some examples can be observed in the Context aware Sub-Structure (CASS) middleware (Fahy & Clarke, 2004) and Service-Oriented Context aware Middleware (SOCAM) (Gu, Pung, & Zhang, 2005). Dey, Abowd, and Salber (2001) implemented the Context Toolkit using a widget based design.

CARMA - THE CONTEXT AWARE REMOTE MONITORING ASSISTANT

In this sub chapter we present a context aware application that demonstrates a part of the scenario mentioned in the introduction. We name this application CARMA (Context aware Remote Monitoring Assistant). It is an application designed to help care assistants to remotely monitor the progress and well-being of their patients. CARMA aims to provide the following functions:

1. Monitoring of the patient's movement
2. Monitoring of the patient's location

Copyright © 2011, IGI Global. Copying or distributing in print or electronic forms without written permission of IGI Global is prohibited.

3.   Automated notification based on contexts
4.   Reminder system for the patient of his past activity and location

As mentioned in the scenario, the patient stays in his own apartment. The care assistant visits his patient according to fixed schedules. During his absence, the CARMA application is responsible to keep him informed. To simplify the implementation, we limit the needed computing devices to three main devices. The mobile devices are carried by the users and function as interaction interfaces and also sensor devices (for the patient). The context server (CS) is responsible to store the sensor and context data of the patient. Core functions such as context processing, learning and reasoning take place at the CS. It also serves as the central communication point for both care assistant and patient. We assume there is constant connectivity for the CS and both mobile devices.

The patient is equipped with a smartphone as a body-worn device. Besides being a communication device, it is also used to detect the movement of the patient with the built-in accelerometer. The smartphone detects also nearby radio signals for localization purposes. Usable radio information can be wireless LAN (WLAN) access point addresses and Bluetooth addresses. Additional sensor information can be obtained using current smartphones. Within the scope of this chapter we describe the use of accelerometer and radio signal information in the example implementation.

The care assistant also uses a mobile device such as a smartphone to use the CARMA application. He can view the movement and the location history of his patient using the smartphone. It is also possible to select desired notifications to be sent to the care assistant's smartphone. In this way, he does not need to perform manual monitoring and constant checks on the patient, especially when everything is fine. Since the device is a smartphone, he should be reachable most of the time via different possible communication channels, such as voice call, Internet and short messaging system (SMS).

The CARMA application is built on top of a Java service execution environment (SEE). The SEE provides basic features such as service deployment, service life cycle management, service repository and eventing. It supports the execution of the context aware components.

Functional Components in CARMA

The functional view on CARMA can be described in three types of functional components: context acquisition, context processing and service action. The following sections elaborate on each component:

Copyright © 2011, IGI Global. Copying or distributing in print or electronic forms without written permission of IGI Global is prohibited.

Context Acquisition Components

The context acquisition components collect the sensor information from selected sensor sources. For the CARMA application, this collection process takes place on the context server and the smartphones. The momentary sensor values are measured and sent over to the context server. In our scenario, the smartphone on the patient collects the needed sensor data. We name this component on the mobile device a context acquisition (CA) component.

CA components run on the smartphone as a background process, and measure the values from the select sensors at pre-defined rates. Depending on the requirements for context processing and reasoning, the sampling rate and method of data transmission may vary. For example, for real time recognition each instance of sensor data should be sent to the CS immediately. For simply logging purposes, it may be sufficient to have the collected data sent at a longer interval, such as once every hour.

Context Processing Components

The context processing (CP) processes takes place usually at a device with sufficient computing power and storage space. In our implementation, the CP components are found at the CS. We divide context processing into two categories. The first category is responsible to derive contexts from the available collected data. We name this component the context interpreter. A context interpreter evaluates the collected data and provides contexts as results. In some literature this interpretation process is also known as context reasoning or context inference. The output contexts are usually known as low and high level contexts. Low level contexts are derived from the sensor data using simple techniques such as matching of key-value pairs. Context interpretation can also be performed by using more complicated approaches such as classification, clustering or ontology modelling. Classification and clustering based approaches require usually pre-processing techniques like filtering or feature extraction. For an ontology based approach, an ontology is defined by system designers to obtain the desired context-model. Regardless of the approach, a context interpreter produces new contexts that can be used for other components or further context interpretation.

The second category of context processing is known as context prediction. Context prediction is used in context awareness to provide proactive adaptation. It is used to predict future contexts that can help the context aware application to react timely. As an example, a context aware application uses context prediction to obtain next location and activity of a user. The adaptation takes place as soon as he enters a new location, when the application predicts this location correctly. There are situations where adaptation needs to start before a user enters the premises, such

Copyright © 2011, IGI Global. Copying or distributing in print or electronic forms without written permission of IGI Global is prohibited.

as to pre-heat a room or a car automatically and timely. Context prediction is seen as an important but relatively new field in context awareness.

We group these two categories in context processing because they process the given data based on available past knowledge to produce new contexts. Whether it is context interpretation or context prediction, the produced contexts are essential in context awareness for the intended adaptations.

Service Action Components

The third component in CARMA is the service action components. They are components designed to carry out tasks. For example, the care assistant wishes to receive a notification when the patient stays in a place without movement for an unusual longer period of time. He can instruct CARMA to observe a number of contexts, such as the patient's movement, location and duration of the same movements. At runtime, the designated context interpreters interpret these contexts at desired interval. As soon as the contexts obtained satisfy the above situation, the notification service action component is invoked.

A system can have different types of service action components. It can be seen as a break down of functions for the required and defined tasks. The concept of these service action components is similar to the enabler concept defined by the Open Mobile Alliance (OMA, 2010).

Movement Recognition using a Smartphone

Based on the above overview of CARMA, we present an implementation of a context interpreter component in this sub chapter. This component provides the movement recognition function. By measuring the acceleration of the patient's smartphone, the component uses a classification algorithm to tell what the patient is possibly doing at a given time. This elaboration of the context interpreter implementation intends to give an idea how one can investigate suitable techniques that produce the desired contexts.

The input data required by the context interpreter for movement recognition is obtained from the built-in accelerometer in a smartphone. The choice of using this sensor device instead of a dedicated standalone accelerometer has the following reasons. Firstly, we would like to utilize non-obtrusive devices for our applications. A smartphone with built-in sensors is an ideal choice, because users do not need to explicitly put on additional dedicated sensors in order to use the CARMA application. Secondly, a smartphone also has ready computing and communication capabilities. The collected data can be either locally processed or sent to a remote computing

Copyright © 2011, IGI Global. Copying or distributing in print or electronic forms without written permission of IGI Global is prohibited.

device for processing. Thirdly, it is also expected that more phones, if not all, will be equipped with accelerometers in the future (iSuppli, 2010).

The accelerometer found in smartphones is usually a micro-electro-mechanical system (MEMS). An acceleration deflects the proof mass (the body of the sensor), and this creates a differential capacitance between the proof mass and the fixed sets of fingers. The capacitance differences are converted into values that represent the acceleration in the respective axes. This method provides two types of acceleration sensing - dynamic acceleration that shows shock or vibration, and static acceleration that shows the tilt or gravity. The usages of accelerometer in smartphones include automatic screen orientation change, gesture-based application control and stabilization function for image capture.

The idea to use or include an accelerometer for movement recognition is observed in past work and is still an ongoing research area. There were a number of investigations on movement recognition using different sensors, including the use of accelerometers. Some earlier investigation such as Bao and Intille (2004), Kern, Schiele, and Schmidt (2007), Laerhoven and Cakmakci (2000), Mantyjarvi, Himberg, and Seppanen (2001) and Ravi, Dandekar, Mysore, and Littman (2005) demonstrated that the usage of dedicated accelerometers can provide good results in the area of activity recognition. The first three investigations used multiple accelerometers placed on different parts of the body, either wired or wireless, and users were required to perform designated movements. The work of (Mäntyjärvi, 2003) and (Ravi et al., 2005) used a combination of sensor board with accelerometer combined with a mobile device (a mobile phone or a personal digital assistant) for movement recognition. The ideas were expanded with the inclusion of additional sensor information. For example, in (Tapia et al., 2007) a heart rate monitor was coupled with data taken from five accelerometers to detect physical activities. The team at Intel Research in Seattle and University of Washington used the multi-modal sensor board (MSB) that had accelerometer, audio, temperature, IR/visible/high-frequency light, humidity, barometric pressure and digital compass (Lester, Choudhury, & Borriello, 2006). They investigated activity recognition classification of physical activities with multiple MSBs. The group in (Cho, Nam, Choi, & Cho, 2008) used a tri-axial accelerometer together with a wearable camera to recognize human activity.

The results obtained in the above investigations were between 83% and 99%. These investigations have shown that the accelerometer data can be use to provide movement and activity recognition. However, these set ups required multiple accelerometers to be worn and observed. For a typical real user, it can be rather obtrusive and troublesome to attach multiple sensors or sensor boards to specific parts of the body. This factor also partly motivated us to use a smartphone as a non-obtrusive

Copyright © 2011, IGI Global. Copying or distributing in print or electronic forms without written permission of IGI Global is prohibited.

sensor source. As shown in previous work, the inclusion of other sensors did give a slight improvement on accuracy rate.

Recently, the three-dimensional accelerometer integrated in smartphones was also investigated as a potential sensor for movement recognition. In (Mladenov & Mock, 2009), the accelerometer of a Nokia N95 was used as a step counter. The results showed that such smartphones can provide accurate step-counts comparable to some of the commercial, dedicated step counter products, provided the phone is firmly attached to the body. The DiaTrace project (Bieber, Voskamp, & Urban, 2009) uses a mobile phone with accelerometers for physical activity monitoring. The proof of concept prototype obtained a recognition accuracy of >95% for activity types of resting, walking, running, cycling and car driving. Brezmes, Gorricho, and Cotrina (2009) used also the accelerometer data collected with a Nokia N95 with K-nearest neighbour algorithm to detect common movements. They argued that the selected algorithm dynamically deletes previously saved records on the ongoing training. This removes possible conflicts and improves accuracy. Lau and David (2010) used a Nokia N95 8GB smartphone for daily movements such as walking, sitting, standing, walking upstairs and downstairs. They showed that even with a relatively low sampling rate (10-20Hz) and only two simple features (mean and standard deviation of the accelerometer data) it is possible to achieve recognition accuracy of >90%. These investigations show that movement recognition using accelerometer in smartphones can be an attractive and useful option as compared to dedicated accelerometer sensors.

Recognition can be achieved by building the needed model. One of the methods is to use classification algorithms to analyse and classify the obtained data. The built model can be used at run time to detect the user's movement. We present three core steps that enable a context interpretation component in the following sections.

Feature Extraction

The process of feature extraction aims to obtain useful features for a classification process. It is a pre-processing step to measure heuristic properties from a given data set. Feature extraction process can potentially reduce the dimensionality of the data. By carefully selecting the correct amount and types of features, it helps to improve classification results. Acceleration data is a time series data that describe changes in an object's acceleration and movements. As stated by Dorian (Pyle, 1999), this type of data is not suitable to be analysed and processed by classification algorithms. Therefore, feature extraction is used in CARMA to pre-process the accelerometer data.

Copyright © 2011, IGI Global. Copying or distributing in print or electronic forms without written permission of IGI Global is prohibited.

Context Modelling

The process of context modelling models a given situation or behaviour of an entity. In our implementation, the movements of the designated user are analysed and modelled using selected classification methods. The required training data for modelling is obtained by combining the features computed in the feature extraction and the corresponding movements. Therefore, the patient is requested to perform the movements and these movements should be labelled along with the sensor measurement. We used a graphical user interface on a Nokia N800 tablet to record the performed movements with time stamp. A script was used to combine the movement records and the features as training data.

The results of modelling evaluation give an overview of how well the selected features and classification algorithms perform. A common technique for this type of evaluation is the 10-fold cross-validation method. This provides an estimation how well the models will perform generally. We will present the modelling evaluation in the later section using an experiment.

Context Interpretation

For the CARMA application, we intend to have the context interpretation executed on the context server. By using the model built using the Weka Toolkit (Hall et al., 2009) and the selected classifier, the context interpretation component evaluates the incoming data to perform movement recognition. We call this context interpretation component the Movement Classifier (MC). The input data for MC is the computed features using the feature extraction component. This is similar to the context modelling process. In the implementation of MC for CARMA, we use the API provided by the Weka toolkit to integrate classification in MC. The generated model produced in context modelling is used to classify the given input data in the interpretation process.

Experiment for Context Modelling

In this section we use an experiment to demonstrate the context modelling process. It involves the above steps. The accelerometer data will be first collected with the corresponding movements recorded in a supervised manner. This provides the annotated accelerometer data. The features are then computed to produce the training data. The Weka toolkit is used to produce the desired models from the obtained training data. A model is a classifier built using Weka based on the training data. The classifier deduces patterns found in the training data and use these patterns to classify the movement with given test data. Selected classification algorithms use

Copyright © 2011, IGI Global. Copying or distributing in print or electronic forms without written permission of IGI Global is prohibited.

in the experiment are k-nearest neighbour (KNN), decision tree (DT), rule based learning (JRip) and Naive Bayes (NB). The models are evaluated using the 10-fold cross-validation method to compare the accuracy of the models built using each classification algorithm.

The previous work commonly used statistical methods for feature extraction. Most used features observed are mean, standard deviation, correlation and entropy of the Fast Fourier Transform (FFT) (Bao & Intille, 2004; Ravi et al., 2005; Lester et al., 2006). The goal of these selections is to be able to use these features to classify the given data. The sliding window technique is commonly used in many investigations. Most of them compute the features using sliding windows with 50% overlapping.

In our context interpretation component we use the same technique. The obtained data is divided into fixed window lengths with 50% overlapping. The features are then computed for each window of every available sensor data type. For our experiment, we use the data collected from all three axes of the accelerometer in a smartphone.

In our experiment, we want to answer the following questions:

1. Which algorithm provides best accuracy with our training data?
2. Which combination of features and parameters for the construction of the sliding windows are most suitable?

The answers to the questions are the criteria for the design of the context interpretation component. The first question helps us to decide on the choice of classifier, while the second question provides the parameters needed for suitable feature extraction.

We have used the accelerometer in a Nokia 5730 smartphone as our sensor device. A script was written using the m-Shell scripting environment to record the accelerometer data. Five common movements were chosen – sitting, standing, walking, going upstairs and downstairs. The accelerometer data was recorded at a higher sampling rate then converted to 10Hz, 25Hz and 50Hz to simulate the individual sampling rate. The produced training data is then processed with different window size combinations to compute the selected features. The sampling rate and window size combinations are 10Hz with 25, 50 samples, 25Hz with 50 and 100 samples, and 50Hz with 100 and 200 samples per window. In the experiment we examined three features combinations: combination C1 with only the mean and standard deviation values of all three accelerometer axes, combination C2 with only the mean and standard deviation values of the three axes' FFT coefficient values, and combination C3 with all four types of features. The evaluation results are summarized in Table 1.

It is observed that among the best results, NB and KNN gave the highest accuracies. DT's accuracies were good as well. The results also showed that it is possible to obtain accuracy > 94% with KNN and DT at lower sampling rate such

Copyright © 2011, IGI Global. Copying or distributing in print or electronic forms without written permission of IGI Global is prohibited.

Table 1. The result of the classifier evaluation

Combination	Algorithm	Sampling Rate (Hz)	Window Size (samples)	Accuracy (%)
C1	NB	50	200	97.51
C3	NB	50	200	96.41
C1	KNN	50	200	96.13
C1	KNN	10	25	95.51
C1	KNN	50	100	95.17
C3	KNN	10	25	95.07
C3	DT	50	200	95.03
C3	DT	10	25	94.96
C1	KNN	25	50	94.87
C1	DT	10	25	94.85

Table 2. The result of the classifier evaluation using combination C2 only

Combination	Algorithm	Sampling Rate (Hz)	Window Size (samples)	Accuracy (%)
C2	DT	20	50	84.93
C2	JRip	25	50	84.86
C2	DT	10	25	84.74
C2	JRip	25	50	83.86
C2	JRip	50	100	83.49
C2	JRip	10	25	83.17
C2	DT	25	50	83.08
C2	DT	10	25	82.69

as 10Hz and 25Hz. The combinations C1 and C3 were generally more accurate than the combination C2. The best results with combination C2 is shown in Table 2.

The combination C2 gave lower accuracies (>10% lower). It is also shown that both DT and JRip performed better than KNN and NB for the combination C2.

The accuracies of data with smaller sampling rate (10Hz and 25Hz) are shown in Table 3. The results indicated that a combination of 10Hz and window size of 25 samples can potentially be sufficient to provide accuracies of more than 90%. All the tested algorithms gave similar accuracies with differences within 1%.

We conclude that the mean and standard deviation values of all three accelerometer axes and the mean and standard deviation values of the three axes' FFT coefficient values are suitable to be used as features. In situations where less features

Copyright © 2011, IGI Global. Copying or distributing in print or electronic forms without written permission of IGI Global is prohibited.

are desired, we can take only the mean and standard deviation values of all three accelerometer axes. This is the same with the choices of sampling rate and windows size. Though the sampling rate 50Hz combined with window size 200 gave best results with NB and KNN, lower sampling rates such as 10Hz and 25Hz are still able to give comparatively good accuracies. This may be practical where the smartphone needs more resources and hence can only provide the accelerometer data at a lower sampling rate.

Based on the obtained result, we can select NB or KNN as the choice algorithm for the MC. It is observed that the sampling rates of 10Hz, 25Hz and 50Hz with a window size of > 2 seconds are suitable. For the case of the CARMA application, higher sampling rates can also be used because it performs context interpretation on the context server. There will be sufficient resources for data storage and context interpretation during runtime. In a situation where the context interpretation takes place on a smartphone, it may be necessary to use a lower sampling rate and a less computing intensive algorithm for this purpose.

Putting the Components Together

In order to enable context aware notification and movement recording, the application CARMA needs another component. We introduce a software agent called Business Rule Evaluator (BRE). The BRE runs as a manager and reacts based on defined policies. A policy is a set of rules that enables service action component triggering when certain conditions are met. The BRE works in two modes. Firstly, it reviews the defined policies periodically. This is suitable for non-time critical tasks. Secondly, it starts evaluating the policies as soon as a needed context changes. This mode is suitable for real-time monitoring or execution.

As the name suggests, the BRE policies are rules. We use if-then rule relations to define the needed context aware functions. For example, the care assistant can define the following rules:

if *(movement is walking)* and *(location is outside)*
then *SMS 0180-12345678*
if *(movement is not sitting)* and *(time is daytime)*
then *record (5, location, movement)*

With this approach, the care assistant can add, remove and review the list of rules according to his needs. The BRE subscribes to the defined context interpreters, i.e. movement, location and time in the above rules, and executes the defined service action component. For example, the first rule sends an SMS to the given destination number when the patient walks out from the home premises. The sec-

Copyright © 2011, IGI Global. Copying or distributing in print or electronic forms without written permission of IGI Global is prohibited.

Figure 4. The visual service editor

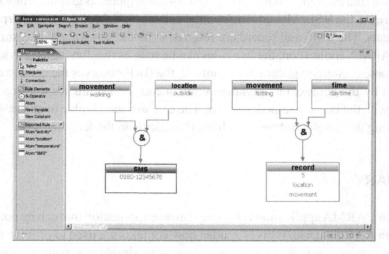

ond rule records the current location and movement of the patient every 5 minutes when the patient is not sitting during the day. The example rules demonstrate how the combination of context interpretation and service action components can build simple context aware services.

The definition of the policies we use the Visual Service Editor (VSE). It compliments the CARMA application by providing graphical service creation. The VSE lists the available components in the CARMA application and allows the users to connect the desired components with logical relations graphically. This "draw-a-service" concept is introduced in (Lau et al., 2008). It aims to provide an easy and effective way for end-users to create context aware services. A screenshot of the VSE with the defined rules is depicted in Figure 4:

The left palette of the VSE displays a list of available context interpretation and service action components found in the CARMA application (under "Imported Rules"). If the care assistant wishes to use additional components, he can use the component discovery feature in VSE to locate them. Alternatively, he can also create a new block in the VSE. He must define the block using suitable keywords that describe the functions of the component. At runtime, the BRE is responsible to locate the desired component using the underlying semantic service discovery feature. In our work we propose the use of technology agnostic service description (Lau et al., 2008). This approach enables the users of VSE to define service functions without the need of technical know-how regarding the available components. The semantic service discovery feature matches the terms given by the users to the designated components.

Copyright © 2011, IGI Global. Copying or distributing in print or electronic forms without written permission of IGI Global is prohibited.

The two rule examples shown in the Figure 4 are depicted as graphical blocks in the canvas area of the VSE. Movement, location and time are three context interpretation components. The SMS and record are referred to as the service action components. In the CARMA application, the two rules can be seen as two functions provided by a simple context aware application. At runtime, the BRE observes the context changes produced by the context interpretation components, and evaluates the two defined policies with the latest obtained contexts. The care assistant is able to add new "functions" using the drag-and-drop tools from the palette on the left hand side.

SUMMARY

The given CARMA application is a context aware application that can be potentially used in an AAC scenario. It gives an idea how contexts are used to provide context-triggered services. It is currently a prototype with simple components running on a Java service execution environment.

The prototype demonstrates the role of context in an implementation. The intended adaptation and tasks can only be performed when the system can produce usable contexts. A context aware application consists of components that carry out the context-related tasks, such as acquisition and processing. There are a large number of techniques, framework and algorithms proposed and investigated in previous work in this specific area. There is, however, no one-size-fits-all solution. One has to determine the designated environment and purpose of the context aware application. This provides a clearer idea on which contexts are available and can be obtained through context acquisition and processing techniques. Existing context aware systems can be evaluated, and one can adapt or extend a suitable existing system for the targeted tasks.

If a new context acquisition or processing component has to be created, it is necessary to identify the requirements for the context information. This is usually essential because the needed contexts are not available with existing components. In this case, one needs to investigate which sensor data is suitable and usable. The same goes for the decision on appropriate context interpretation techniques. The application designer needs analysis and experiments to find the most suitable modelling technique that produces the desired contexts accurately.

CHALLENGES AND FUTURE WORK

The previous sub chapters elaborated the vision and approaches of using context awareness to assist and simplify tasks and needs for AAC users. This sub chapter

Copyright © 2011, IGI Global. Copying or distributing in print or electronic forms without written permission of IGI Global is prohibited.

presents some challenges in research and development of context aware computing applications for the field of AAC.

CHALLENGES

The modelling of needed contexts is still an open question for researchers, especially if there is still no context modelling techniques investigated for a specific target environment. In some cases, even if substantial work has been performed, one still needs to test and evaluate the proposed approaches in order to ensure these approaches are suitable for the needed application. Though it is not realistic to have components that work everywhere and are suitable for every situation, reusable components can still be created for specific platform and sensor devices.

The usage of context awareness in the area of AAC is faced with the challenge of trust and privacy issues. In situations where personal sensor data and interpreted contexts are collected and stored, suitable solutions and approaches that ensure privacy protection are essential. The trustworthiness of context information, context and sensor sources, different components and the underlying software platform needs to be checked, especially when the context aware applications are supposed to run without constant human control and intervention.

The evaluation of context aware applications is also a topic of interest. It is not easy to put two context aware applications side-by-side and decide which is suitable. The word "suitable" is difficult to justify. Additionally, the evaluation of a context aware application needs to include user feedback. This put forth the challenge to identify suitable evaluation methods that can provide a good overview of the strength and weaknesses of a given context aware application. With the obtain evaluation results, context aware applications can be improved to provide the desired adaptation and services for the targeted users and environment.

FUTURE WORK

The CARMA application is a demonstration of how contexts are used for AAC scenarios. In the future we intend to extend the number of context interpretation components to provide additional contexts types. With the increase of context types, we also need to provide more service action components. This will give a wider scope of newer context aware services. It is also necessary to evaluate the CARMA application with real users. The evaluation will give insights on how suitable the selected idea and approach can really help the designated AAC users. The use cases can also be extended according to the feedback from the care assistant and the patient.

Copyright © 2011, IGI Global. Copying or distributing in print or electronic forms without written permission of IGI Global is prohibited.

The performed experiment has shown that the accelerometer in a smartphone can be used to provide movement recognition. The chosen algorithm and feature extraction parameters should be further tested and evaluated. Real test data can be used to evaluate the built model. We also wish to investigate other modelling techniques such as clustering or pattern matching. The idea of being able to recognize movement without the need of training data and manual labelling is advantageous and attractive, since it reduces the dependency of the training phase and relieves the targeted user from the modelling process.

CONCLUSION

This chapter introduced the basic concepts of context awareness. It gave an overview of the state of the art work in this area of research. Definitions of context aware related terms and discussions were made to provide a clear understanding of the core characteristics and techniques in context awareness. This is followed with a presentation of the proposal to apply context awareness in the area of AAC. The presented proposal included the design issues and requirements identified and an outline of the needed hardware and software infrastructure.

The chapter continued with the elaboration of the Context aware Remote Monitoring Assistant (CARMA) application. The functions and components found in the application were described with the intention to summarize the features of this application. The movement recognition component was highlighted in order to demonstrate how a concrete context interpretation component is designed and implemented. This is followed by introducing a graphical approach for context aware service creation.

We hope the researchers are motivated with this chapter to start exploring the potential of context aware based application and solutions for the area of AAC. The proposed idea and examples in the chapter are presented as pointers to provide a foundation for researchers to engage in this approach. It opens up newer application domains and helps to improve the available techniques and ideas.

ACKNOWLEDGMENT

The authors would like to acknowledge the German Federal Ministry of Education and Research (BMBF) for funding the project MATRIX (Förderkennzeichen 01BS0802). The authors are responsible for the content of the publication.

The authors are involved in the VENUS research project. VENUS is a research cluster at the interdisciplinary Research Center for Information System Design (ITeG)

Copyright © 2011, IGI Global. Copying or distributing in print or electronic forms without written permission of IGI Global is prohibited.

at Kassel University. We thank Hesse's Ministry of Higher Education, Research, and the Arts for funding the project as part of the research funding program "LOEWE - Landes-Offensive zur Entwicklung Wissenschaftlich-ökonomischer Exzellenz". For further information, please visit: http://www.iteg.uni-kassel.de/venus.

The authors would also like to thank Niklas Klein for his valuable discussion and suggestions.

REFERENCES

Abowd, G. D., Atkeson, C. G., Hong, J., Long, S., Kooper, R., & Pinkerton, M. (1997). Cyberguide: A mobile context aware tour guide. *Wireless Networks, 3*(5), 421–433. doi:10.1023/A:1019194325861

Bao, L., & Intille, S. S. (2004). *Activity recognition from user-annotated acceleration data*. Pervasive Conference 2004, (pp. 1–17).

Bardram, J. E., & Nørskov, N. (2008). A context aware patient safety system for the operating room. In *Ubicomp '08: Proceedings of the 10th international conference on ubiquitous computing* (pp. 272–281). New York, NY: ACM.

Betz, M., Huq, M., Pipek, V., Rohde, M., Stevens, G., & Englert, R. (2007). An architecture for adaptive and adaptable mobile applications for physically handicapped people. In Stephanidis, C. (Ed.), *Hci (5) (Vol. 4554*, pp. 335–344). Springer.

Bieber, G., Voskamp, J., & Urban, B. (2009). Activity recognition for everyday life on mobile phones. In Stephanidis, C. (Ed.), *Hci (6) (Vol. 5615*, pp. 289–296). Springer.

Brezmes, T., Gorricho, J., & Cotrina, J. (2009). Activity recognition from accelerometer data on a mobile phone. *In Proceedings of the 10th International Work-Conference on Artificial Neural Networks: Part II: Distributed Computing, Artificial Intelligence, Bioinformatics, Soft Computing, and Ambient Assisted Living,* (pp. 796-799). Salamanca, Spain: Springer-Verlag.

Brown, P. J. (1996). The stick-e document: A framework for creating context aware applications. In *Proceedings of EP '96, Palo Alto* (pp. 259–272).

Catarinucci, L., Colella, R., Esposito, A., Tarricone, L., & Zappatore, M. (2009). A context aware smart infrastructure based on RFID sensor-tags and its application to the healthcare domain. In *ETFA '09: Proceedings of the 14th IEEE International Conference on Emerging Technologies & Factory Automation* (pp. 1356–1363). Piscataway, NJ: IEEE Press.

Copyright © 2011, IGI Global. Copying or distributing in print or electronic forms without written permission of IGI Global is prohibited.

Chen, H., Finin, T., & Joshi, A. (2003, October). An intelligent broker for context aware systems. *Adjunct Proceedings of Ubicomp, 2003*, 183–184.

Cheverst, K., Davies, N., Mitchell, K., Friday, A., & Efstratiou, C. (2000). Developing a context aware electronic tourist guide: Some issues and experiences. In *Chi '00: Proceedings of the Sigchi Conference on Human Factors in Computing Systems* (pp. 17–24). New York, NY: ACM.

Cho, Y., Nam, Y., Choi, Y., & Cho, W. (2008). SmartBuckle: Human activity recognition using a 3-axis accelerometer and a wearable camera. In *Proceedings of the 2nd international Workshop on Systems and Networking Support for Healthcare and Assisted Living Environments* (pp. 1–3). Breckenridge, CO: ACM.

Crowley, J. L., Coutaz, J., Rey, G., & Reignier, P. (2002). *Perceptual components for context aware computing*. In Ubicomp 2002, International Conference on Ubiquitous Computing, Goteborg (pp. 117–134).

Davis, A. B., Moore, M. M., & Storey, V. C. (2003). Context aware communication for severely disabled users. In *CUU '03: Proceedings of the 2003 Conference on Universal Usability* (pp. 106–111). New York, NY: ACM.

Dey, A. K., & Abowd, G. D. (2000a). Cybreminder: A context aware system for supporting reminders. In *Huc '00: Proceedings of the 2nd International Symposium on Handheld and Ubiquitous Computing* (pp. 172–186). London, UK: Springer-Verlag.

Dey, A. K., & Abowd, G. D. (2000b). *Towards a better understanding of context and context awareness*. CHI 2000 Workshop on the What, Who, Where, When, and How of Context awareness.

Dey, A. K., Abowd, G. D., & Salber, D. (2001). A conceptual framework and a toolkit for supporting the rapid prototyping of context-aware applications. *Human-Computer Interaction, 16*(2-4), 97–166. doi:10.1207/S15327051HCI16234_02

Fahy, P., & Clarke, S. (2004). *CASS-a middleware for mobile context aware applications*. In Workshop on Context Awareness, Mobisys.

Gu, T., Pung, H. K., & Zhang, D. (2005). A service-oriented middleware for building context aware services. *Journal of Network and Computer Applications, 28*(1), 1–18. doi:10.1016/j.jnca.2004.06.002

Hall, M., Frank, E., Holmes, G., Pfahringer, B., Reutemann, P., & Witten, I. H. (2009). The weka data mining software: An update. *SIGKDD Explorations*, 11.

Copyright © 2011, IGI Global. Copying or distributing in print or electronic forms without written permission of IGI Global is prohibited.

Henricksen, K. (2003). *A framework for context aware pervasive computing applications*. Unpublished doctoral dissertation, School of Information Technology and Electrical Engineering, The University of Queensland.

Hull, R., Neaves, P., & Bedford-Roberts, J. (1997). Towards situated computing. In *Iswc '97: Proceedings of the 1st IEEE International Symposium on Wearable Computers* (p. 146). Washington, DC: IEEE Computer Society. iSuppli. (2010, March). *One-third of mobile phones to use accelerometers by 2010, spurred by iPhone and Palm Pre*. Retrieved March 25, 2010, from http://www.isuppli.com/News/Pages/One-Third-of-Mobile-Phones-to-Use-Accelerometers-by-2010-Spurred-by-iPhone-and-Palm-Pre.aspx

Kern, N., Schiele, B., & Schmidt, A. (2007). Recognizing context for annotating a live life recording. *Personal and Ubiquitous Computing, 11*(4), 251–263. doi:10.1007/s00779-006-0086-3

Korpipää, P., Mäntyjärvi, J., Kela, J., Keränen, H., & Malm, E. J. (2003). Managing context information in mobile devices. *IEEE Pervasive Computing / IEEE Computer Society [and] IEEE Communications Society, 2*, 42–51. doi:10.1109/MPRV.2003.1228526

Laerhoven, K. V., & Cakmakci, O. (2000). What shall we teach our pants? In *Iswc '00: Proceedings of the 4th IEEE International Symposium on Wearable Computers* (p. 77). Washington, DC: IEEE Computer Society.

Lau, S. L., & David, K. (2010). Movement recognition using the accelerometer in smartphones. *Proceedings of Future network & Mobilesummit 2010.*

Lau, S. L., Klein, N., Pirali, A., Koenig, I., Droegehorn, O., & David, K. (2008). *Making service creation for (almost) everyone*. Stockholm: In ICT-MobileSummit.

Lester, J., Choudhury, T., & Borriello, G. (2006). A practical approach to recognizing physical activities. In Fishkin, K. P., Schiele, B., Nixon, P., & Quigley, A. J. (Eds.), *Pervasive* (pp. 1–16). Springer. doi:10.1007/11748625_1

MacKenzie, C. M., Laskey, K., McCabe, F., Brown, P. F., & Metz, R. (2006). *Reference model for service oriented architecture 1.0*. Tech. rep., 2006. Retrieved March 25, 2010, from http://docs.oasis-open.org/soa-rm/v1.0/soa-rm.pdf

Mäntyjärvi, J. (2003). *Sensor-based context recognition for mobile applications*. Unpublished doctoral dissertation, University of Oulu.

Copyright © 2011, IGI Global. Copying or distributing in print or electronic forms without written permission of IGI Global is prohibited.

Mantyjarvi, J., Himberg, J., & Seppanen, T. (2001). Recognizing human motion with multiple acceleration sensors. In *Proceedings of 2001 IEEE International Conference on Systems, Man, and Cybernetics* (Vol. 2, pp. 747–752).

Matic, A., Mehta, P., Rehg, J. M., Osmani, V., & Mayora, O. (2010). *aid-me: Automatic identification of dressing failures through monitoring of patients and activity evaluation*. In 4th International Conference on pervasive computing technologies for healthcare 2010 (pervasive health 2010).

Mladenov, M., & Mock, M. (2009). A step counter service for Java-enabled devices using a built-in accelerometer. In *Cams '09: Proceedings of the 1st International Workshop on Context-Aware Middleware and Services* (pp. 1–5). New York, NY: ACM.

Nehmer, J., Becker, M., Karshmer, A., & Lamm, R. (2006). Living assistance systems: An ambient intelligence approach. In *Icse '06: Proceedings of the 28th International Conference on Software Engineering* (pp. 43–50). New York, NY: ACM.

Open Mobile Alliance. (2010). *Released enablers*. Retrieved March 25, 2010, from http://www.openmobilealliance.org/technical/released enablers.aspx

Paganelli, F., & Giuli, D. (2007). A context-aware service platform to support continuous care networks for home-based assistance. In *Uahci '07: Proceedings of the 4th International Conference on Universal access in Human-Computer Interaction* (pp. 168–177). Berlin/ Heidelberg, Germany: Springer-Verlag.

Pyle, D. (1999). *Data preparation for data mining*. San Francisco, CA: Morgan Kaufmann Publishers Inc.

Ravi, N., Dandekar, N., Mysore, P., & Littman, M. L. (2005). *Activity recognition from accelerometer data*. American Association for Artificial Intelligence.

Roy, N., Roy, A., & Das, S. K. (2006). Context-aware resource management in multi-inhabitant smart homes: A Nash h-learning based approach. In *Percom '06: Proceedings of the Fourth Annual IEEE International Conference on pervasive computing and communications* (pp. 148–158). Washington, DC: IEEE Computer Society.

Ryan, N. S., Pascoe, J., & Morse, D. R. (1998). Enhanced reality fieldwork: The context-aware archaeological assistant. In Gaffney, V., van Leusen, M., & Exxon, S. (Eds.), *Computer applications in archaeology 1997*. Oxford, UK: Tempus Reparatum.

Copyright © 2011, IGI Global. Copying or distributing in print or electronic forms without written permission of IGI Global is prohibited.

Schilit, B. N., Adams, N. I., & Want, R. (1994). Context-aware computing applications. In *Proceedings of the Workshop on Mobile computing systems and applications, 1994.* (p. 85-90).

Schilit, B. N., & Theimer, M. (1994). Disseminating active map information to mobile hosts. *Network, IEEE, 8*(5), 22–32. doi:10.1109/65.313011

Schmidt, A., Beigl, M., & Gellersen, H. W. (1999). There is more to context than location. *Computers & Graphics, 23*(6), 893–901. doi:10.1016/S0097-8493(99)00120-X

Schmidt, A., & Laerhoven, K. V. (2001). How to build smart appliances. *IEEE Personal Communications, 8*, 66–71. doi:10.1109/98.944006

Sigg, S. (2008). *Development of a novel context prediction algorithm and analysis of context prediction schemes.* Unpublished doctoral dissertation, University of Kassel.

Strang, T., & Linnhoff-Popien, C. (2004). *A context modeling survey.* In First International Workshop on advanced context modelling, reasoning and management, Nottingham, England.

Sutterer, M., Droegehorn, O., & David, K. (2008). Upos: User profile ontology with situation-dependent preferences support. In *Achi '08: Proceedings of the First International Conference on advances in computer-human interaction* (pp. 230–235). Washington, DC: IEEE Computer Society.

Tapia, E. M., Intille, S. S., Haskell, W., Larson, K., Wright, J., & King, A. (2007). *Real-time recognition of physical activities and their intensities using wireless accelerometers and a heart rate monitor.* In Wearable computers, 2007 11th IEEE international symposium (pp. 37–40).

Vales-Alonso, J., Egea-Lopez, E., Muoz-Gea, J. P., García-Haro, J., Belzunce-Arcos, F., Esparza-García, M. A., et al. (2008). Ucare: Context-aware services for disabled users in urban environments. In *Ubicomm '08: Proceedings of the 2008 the Second International Conference on mobile ubiquitous computing, systems, services and technologies* (pp. 197–205). Washington, DC: IEEE Computer Society.

Varshney, U. (2007). Pervasive healthcare and wireless health monitoring. *Mobile Networks and Applications, 12*(2), 113–127. doi:10.1007/s11036-007-0017-1

Want, R., Hopper, A., Falc, V., & Gibbons, J. (1992). The active badge location system. *ACM Transactions on Information Systems, 10*(1), 91–102. doi:10.1145/128756.128759

Weiser, M. (1991). The computer for the 21st century. *Scientific American, 265*(3), 66–75. doi:10.1038/scientificamerican0991-94

Copyright © 2011, IGI Global. Copying or distributing in print or electronic forms without written permission of IGI Global is prohibited.

KEY TERMS AND DEFINITIONS

Activity: Activity represents the contexts that can explain the situation or task a user is currently undertaking.

Activity Recognition: Activity recognition is the ability to detect and understand which activity a user is currently performing or has performed.

Context: Context is any information that can be used to characterize the situation of an entity. An entity is a person, place, or object that is considered relevant to the interaction between a user and an application, including the user and applications themselves. Context consists of various aspects such as time, location, identity, activity, environment and constitution.

Context Awareness: Context awareness is the ability of the applications to discover, understand and react to the contexts and the context changes of users and the environment they are situated in".

Patient Monitoring: Patient monitoring is a task or service that keeps track of a patient's condition, and activity and well-being.

Service: Service is an application that offers one or more functions to the users.

Service Adaptation: Service adaptation is the ability to change a service's function(s) or behaviour(s) according to the needs and contexts of the user(s) it is (currently) serving.

Smartphone: A mobile phone that offers advanced capabilities, which often can be compared to PC-like functionality and capabilities in terms of hardware and software.

Copyright © 2011, IGI Global. Copying or distributing in print or electronic forms without written permission of IGI Global is prohibited.

Chapter 7
Spatial Knowledge Communication to Visually Challenged People

Kanubhai K. Patel
Ahmedabad University, India

Sanjay Kumar Vij
Sardar Vallabhbhai Patel Institute of Technology, India

ABSTRACT

A computational model of non-visual spatial learning through virtual learning environment (VLE) is presented in this chapter. The inspiration has come from Landmark-Route-Survey (LRS) theory, the most accepted theory of spatial learning. An attempt has been made to combine the findings and methods from several disciplines including cognitive psychology, behavioral science and computer science (specifically virtual reality (VR) technology). The study of influencing factors on spatial learning and the potential of using cognitive maps in the modeling of spatial learning are described. Motivation to use VLE and its characteristics are also described briefly. Different types of locomotion interface to VLE with their constraints and benefits are discussed briefly. The authors believe that by incorporating perspectives from cognitive and experimental psychology to computer science, this chapter will appeal to a wide range of audience - particularly computer engineers concerned with assistive technologies, professionals interested in virtual environments, including computer engineers, architect, city-planner, cartographer, high-tech artists, and mobility trainers, and psychologists involved in the study of spatial cognition, cognitive behaviour, and human-computer interfaces.

DOI: 10.4018/978-1-60960-541-4.ch007

Copyright ©2011, IGI Global. Copying or distributing in print or electronic forms without written permission of IGI Global is prohibited.

INTRODUCTION

About 314 million people are visually challenged worldwide; 45 million of them are blind. One out of every three blind people in the world lives in India - that comes to approximately 15 million. The inability to travel independently around and interact with the wider world is one of the most significant handicaps that can be caused by visual impairment or blindness, second only to the inability to communicate through reading and writing. The difficulties in the mobility of visually challenged people in new or unfamiliar locations are caused by the fact that spatial information is not fully available to them as against it being available to sighted people. Visually challenged people are thus handicapped to gather this crucial information, which leads to great difficulties in generating efficient cognitive maps of spaces and, therefore, in navigating efficiently within new or unfamiliar spaces. Consequently, many blind people become passive, depending on others for assistance. More than 30% of the blind do not ambulate independently outdoors (Clark-Carter, Heyes & Howarth, 1986; Lahav & Mioduser, 2003).

This constraint can be overcome by communicating spatial knowledge of the surroundings and thereby providing some means to generate cognitive mapping of spaces and of the possible paths for navigating through these spaces virtually, which are essential for the development of efficient orientation and mobility skills. It is obvious that reasonable number of repeated visits to the new space leads to formation of its cognitive map subconsciously. Thus, a good number of researchers focused on using technology to simulate visits to a new space for building cognitive maps. It need not be emphasized that the strength and efficiency of cognitive map building process is directly proportional to the closeness between the simulated and real-life environments. However, most of the simulated environments reported by earlier researchers don't fully represent reality. The challenge, therefore, is to enhance and enrich simulated environment so as to create a near real-life experience.

The fundamental goal of developing virtual learning environment for visually challenged people is to complement or replace sight by another modality. The visual information therefore needs to be simplified and transformed so as to allow its rendition through alternate sensory channels, usually auditory, haptic, or auditory-haptic. One of the methods to enhance and enrich simulated environment is to use virtual reality along with advanced technologies such as computer haptics, brain-computer interface (BCI), speech processing and sonification. Such technologies can be used to provide learning environment to visually challenged people to create cognitive maps of unfamiliar areas. We aim to present various research studies including ours for communicating spatial knowledge to visually challenged people and evaluating it through virtual learning environment (VLE), and thereby enhancing spatial behaviour in real environment. This chapter proposes taxonomy of spatial

Copyright © 2011, IGI Global. Copying or distributing in print or electronic forms without written permission of IGI Global is prohibited.

learning and addresses the potential of virtual learning environment as a tool for studying spatial behaviour of visually challenged people and thereby enhancing their capabilities to interact in a spatial environment in real life. It would be useful to understand as to how they learn and acquire basic spatial knowledge in terms of landmarks and configuration of spatial layout and also how navigation tasks are improvised. Understanding the use of such knowledge to externalize and measure virtually perceived cognitive maps is also important.

Following questions are addressed in this chapter:

- Does virtual learning environment (VLE) contribute to communicate the spatial knowledge and thereby the formation of a cognitive map of a novel space?
- Which are the major factors that influence the spatial knowledge communication to visually challenged people through VLE?
- Which are the factors that mediate for enhancement of the navigation performance of visually challenged people?
- Is learning via VLE more effective, accurate, interesting, and enjoyable than learning via conventional methods?
- How is the effectiveness of cognitive maps measured?
- Can we consider trajectory of subjects as cognitive map?
- Does the type of locomotion interface impinge on accuracy of spatial learning?
- Is navigating through treadmill-style locomotion interface less disruptive than navigating via conventional devices?

A computational model of non-visual spatial learning through virtual learning environment (VLE) is presented in this chapter. The inspiration has come from Landmark-Route-Survey (LRS) theory (Siegel & White, 1975), the most accepted theory of spatial learning. This NSL model is created by undertaking thorough literature review of the material existing in the area of spatial cognition and computer science. An attempt has been made to combine the findings and methods from several disciplines including cognitive psychology, behavioral science and computer science (specifically virtual reality (VR) technology). The study of influencing factors on spatial learning and the potential of using cognitive maps in the modeling of spatial learning are described. Motivation to use VLE and its characteristics are also described briefly. Different types of locomotion interface to VLE with their constraints and benefits are discussed briefly. We believe that by incorporating perspectives from cognitive and experimental psychology to computer science, this chapter will appeal to a wide range of audience - particularly computer engineers concerned with assistive technologies; professionals interested in virtual

Copyright © 2011, IGI Global. Copying or distributing in print or electronic forms without written permission of IGI Global is prohibited.

environments, including computer engineers, architect, city-planner, cartographer, high-tech artists, and mobility trainer; and psychologists involved in the study of spatial cognition, cognitive behaviour, and human-computer interfaces.

Modeling Spatial Environment

The topological component of map consists of a set of N place nodes and a set of links that connects pairs of places. Various objects like places, paths, obstacles etc. can be represent in topological map of an environment. They are linked by the various relations among them like places are along the paths, place is on left or right side of other place or path, etc. Before we explore this modeling technique, we should understand basic concepts of space and spatial cognition.

Space

Space (and time) is very elementary and ubiquitous for almost all human behaviour and reasoning (Freksa, 1997). Yet, it is difficult (or impossible) to find a single definition that covers all aspects of space. For example, while in mathematics the term space is frequently used to describe the dimensionality of sets or vectors (Bronstein & Semendjajew, 1979); this has little to no relevance in the context of human behaviour. However, since computers heavily rely on mathematical concepts, oftentimes spatial knowledge is stored in cartesian coordinates (e. g. in geographical information systems (GIS)). This somewhat contradicts the naive perception most people have of space as being the physical environment, in which we live and act. In psychology and other disciplines such as architecture, (everyday) space is often seen as being structured and hence being perceived differently according to its scale (see, for example, (Lynch, 1960). After initial approaches which introduced a binary portioning (e. g. Ittelson, 1973; Downs & Stea, 1977), the distinction between small- and large-scale spaces has been further refined (Freundschuh & Egenhofer, 1997).

Montello (Montello, 1993), for example, distinguishes four main categories of space as,

- Figural space
- Vista space
- Environmental space
- Geographical space

Figural space encompasses the space within the direct reach of a person, which is smaller than the body of the observer. Another term that is frequently used to describe this kind of space is table-top space (Ittelson, 1973). Vista space is the

Copyright © 2011, IGI Global. Copying or distributing in print or electronic forms without written permission of IGI Global is prohibited.

space that can be perceived visually from a single location without locomotion falls in this category. For example, the room a person is located in lies in vista space. If a portion of space cannot be perceived from a single location without the observer moving around, it can be classified as belonging to environmental space. A city is an example for an entity existing in this type of space. Montello defines geographical spaces as spaces that cannot be apprehended even with extensive knowledge but have to be reduced to figural or vista space in order to do so. This is the space of countries or continents. These different types of spaces are closely related to how humans encode and memorize spatial information such as constellations or routes.

Spatial Knowledge

When humans explore space they not only perceive it but they build up a mental representation of it (Tversky, 1993). Generally, we can distinguish three classes of spatial knowledge: landmark knowledge, route knowledge and survey knowledge (Werner, Krieg-Bruckner, Mallot, Schweizer & Freksa, 1997). Landmarks are objects, which are embedded in the environment and which differ from other objects in their vicinity in one or more respects such as visual salience and/or conceptual salience (see, for example, Sorrows & Hirtle, 1999). Since they 'stand out' from their environment they are not only easy to remember but also easy to recognize. Therefore, they are highly relevant in a number of spatial processes such as object localization (Gapp, 1995) or wayfinding (Lynch, 1960; Raubal & Worboys, 1999). Landmark knowledge actually links specific landmarks to other knowledge. For example, by associating a turn instruction with a landmark at a decision point, a person can decide which path to follow in order to get to her target location. Route knowledge (also known as procedural knowledge) is most frequently gained from actively exploring the environment. (Alternatively, people can acquire route knowledge indirectly, e. g. by listening to route instructions.) Route knowledge consists of a series of spatial actions such as turning or following a road, which together form a route from one location to another. Survey knowledge encodes information about the topology and/or spatial constellations in an area. People mainly acquire survey knowledge by extensively exploring a region of space, which enables them to establish multiple relationships between various locations within that area. Maps also represent survey knowledge, and hence, support the acquisition of survey knowledge. The main difference between survey knowledge and the two other categories lies in the way in which knowledge is organized: survey knowledge abstracts from single experiences and observations to form an integrated model. The amalgamation of spatial knowledge that is encoded in different ways forms the basis for human spatial reasoning, and is often defined as a cognitive map (Tolman, 1948) or cognitive collage (Tversky, 1993). It is important to highlight that these cognitive maps

Copyright © 2011, IGI Global. Copying or distributing in print or electronic forms without written permission of IGI Global is prohibited.

do not result from a homomorphic mapping of the real world to a representation, but that they are a conglomeration of possibly contradicting pieces of information. Nevertheless, they enable humans to efficiently store spatial information and to interact with space in a meaningful way most of the time.

SPATIAL RELATION

Not only do humans act within space they also talk about it or refer to it verbally or by other means such as gestures. A frequent means to realize spatial references consists of spatial relations (Herrman & Grabowski, 1994). The region connection calculus (RCC) serves for qualitative spatial representation and reasoning. RCC abstractly describes regions (in Euclidian space or in a topological space) by their possible relations to each other. RCC8 consists of 8 basic relations (see Figure 1) that are possible between two regions:

- disconnected (DC)
- externally connected (EC)
- equal (EQ)
- partially overlapping (PO)
- tangential proper part (TPP)
- tangential proper part inverse (TPPi)
- non-tangential proper part (NTPP)
- non-tangential proper part inverse (NTPPi)

From these basic relations, combinations can be built. For example, proper part (PP) is the union of TPP and NTPP.

Figure 1. The RCC8 calculus can be used for reasoning about spatial configurations

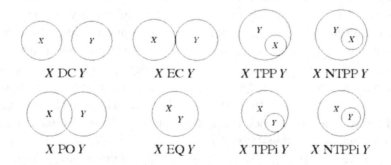

Copyright © 2011, IGI Global. Copying or distributing in print or electronic forms without written permission of IGI Global is prohibited.

Other versions of the region connection calculus include RCC5 (with only five basic relations - the distinction whether two regions touch each other are ignored) and RCC23 (which allows reasoning about convexity).

Spatial Layout Designer

The topographical layout, color-coded identifiers for objects, and force feedback correlation with objects can develop through man-machine interaction. The Spatial Layout Designer mainly helps to create layout of particular area or premises easily and without having any technical knowledge. It should provide a user friendly interface to quickly design and develop virtual environment of particular area or premises easily by placing objects (such as places and paths) of different sizes and shapes. Vector graphics technique of graphics drawing to draw objects is to be used. It has advantages compare to raster graphics technique.

Objects are provided in the toolbox under different categories viz. building, road, obstacle, gate, entrance, etc. Various attributes of objects such as size, location, direction and form of an object can be set or updated through property window. These objects may also have default attributes such as color, speech tag, label tag, movement, type and intensity of force feedback. Force feedback effect and audio label to these components can be set or updated. Different shapes of objects to be covered are square, rectangle, circle, line polygon, curve polygon, line, curve and oval etc. Different types of objects are mainly covering areas (places), passages/roads and boundaries. User can create templates for objects for future requirements also.

Following are the colors that may be used to encode some of the objects (see as an example Table 1).

Using Spatial Layout Designer, one can proportionately map the real world's objects to their size and their distance from other objects. Various properties like position, shape, orientation, height, and size of objects can be set or updated through drag and drop also. Simple to complex environments can be created trivially. There should be relation between Macro and Micro level objects. It means user can create

Table 1.Predefined color code for various segments

Objects	Color
Building	Red
Road, Path	Black
Garden	Green
Entrance/Door	Yellow
Parking Area	Grey

Copyright © 2011, IGI Global. Copying or distributing in print or electronic forms without written permission of IGI Global is prohibited.

hierarchy of the objects. One object can have multiple parents. Layout can be stored in either in XML format, EMF or in database.

Non-Visual Spatial Learning Research Background

In recent years, a plethora of assistive navigation technologies have been designed to enhance and maintain the independence of the community of blind and visually challenged. The available spatial learning aids for the visually challenged can be categorized into,

1. Passive aids
2. Active aids and
3. VR based aids

Passive aids are providing the user with information before his/her arrival to the environment. For example, verbal description, tactile maps, strip maps, Braille maps, and physical models (Ungar, Blades, & Spencer, 1996; Rieser, 1989).

Active aids are providing the user with information while navigating, for example, Sonicguide (Warren, & Strelow, 1985), Talking Signs or embedded sensors in the environment (Crandall, Bentzen, Myers & Mitchell, 1995), and Personal Guidance System, based on satellite communication (Golledge, Klatzky, & Loomis, 1996). The research results indicate a number of limitations in the use of passive and exclusive devices, for example, erroneous distance estimation, underestimation of spatial components and objects dimensions, low information density, or misunderstanding of symbolic codes used in the representations.

Virtual reality has been a popular paradigm in simulation-based training, game and entertainment industries (Burdea, & Coiffet, 2003). It has also been used for rehabilitation and learning environments for people with disabilities (e.g., physical, mental, and learning disabilities) (Standen, Brown, & Cromby, 2001; Schultheis, & Rizzo, 2001). Recent technological advances, particularly in haptic interface technology, enable blind individuals to expand their knowledge as a result of using artificially made reality through haptic and audio feedback. Research on the implementation of haptic technologies within virtual navigation environments has yielded reports on its potential for supporting rehabilitation training with sighted people (Giess, Evers, & Meinzer, 1998; Gorman, Lieser, Murray, Haluck & Krummel, 1998), as well as with people who are blind (Jansson, Fanger, Konig & Billberger, 1998; Colwell, Petrie, Kornbrot, Hardwick & Furner, 1998).

This research can also be classified into navigational assistance for

Copyright © 2011, IGI Global. Copying or distributing in print or electronic forms without written permission of IGI Global is prohibited.

1.   Indoor environments (e.g. Sabelman, et. al., 1994),
2.   Outdoor environments (e.g. Strothotte et. al., 1996; Dodson, Moore, & Moon, 1999), and
3.   A combination of both (e.g. Golledge, Klatzky, Loomis, Speigle & Tietz, 1998; Helal, Moore, & Ramachandran, 2001).

In relation to outdoor environments, Petrie (1995) distinguishes between 'micro-navigation' technologies, which provide assistance through immediate environment, and 'macro-navigation' technologies, which provide assistance through the distant environment. For instance, ETAs (Electronic Travel Aids) such as obstacle avoidance systems (e.g. Laser Cane (Kay, 1980) and ultrasonic obstacle avoiders (Bradyn, 1985) have been developed to assist visually challenged travelers for micro-navigation. Whereas, Global Positioning Systems (GPS) and Geographical Information System (GIS) have been used to assist visually challenged for macro-navigation. Examples include the MOBIC Travel Aid (Strothotte, et. al., 1996), Arkenstone system (Fruchterman, 1995) & Personal Guidance System (Golledge, et. al., 1998). Radio Frequency (RF) beacons have also been used to assist navigation for both micro and macro navigation (Kemmerling, & Schliepkorte, 1998).

Navigation through indoor environments, on the other hand, has been developed using similar systems. As GPS is ineffective inside buildings, most systems depend on relative positioning using sensors such as digital tags, active badge, accelerometers, temperature, photodiodes and beacons (Ertan, Lee, Willets, Tan & Pentland, 1998; Golding, & Lesh, 1999; Long, Aust, Abowd & Atkeson, 1996).

Human navigation and wayfinding consists of both sensing the immediate environment for obstacles and hazards, and navigating to remote destinations beyond the immediately perceptible environment (Loomis Golledge & Klatzky, 2001). Navigation therefore involves updating one's orientation and position; a process involving position-based navigation, velocity-based navigation, and acceleration-based navigation (all of which are described by Loomis et al. (2001). Visually challenged people are therefore at a huge disadvantage in unfamiliar routes, as they 'lack much of the information needed for planning detours around obstacles and hazards, and have little information about distant landmarks, heading and self-velocity'(Loomis et al., 2001).

Cognitive mapping research focuses on how individuals acquire, learn, develop, think about and store data relating to the everyday geographic environment (e.g. encoding locations, attributes and landmark orientations to navigate) (Downs, & Stea, 1997). Jonsson (2002) describes how maps can change for one particular area depending on the (i) time of day (i.e. day/night), (ii) season (e.g. summer vs. winter), and (iii) direction of travel (traveling the same route forward or back).

Copyright © 2011, IGI Global. Copying or distributing in print or electronic forms without written permission of IGI Global is prohibited.

A number of theories (e.g. landmark-based learning strategies and route-based strategies) and mechanisms (e.g. images, dual coding, genetic coding, etc.) have been advanced to account for how knowledge is learned, stored, and structured. However, the unique strategies and mechanisms used by visually challenged people have not been given sufficient investigation in current research (Kitchin, Blades, & Golledge, 1997). Kitchin and Jacobson (1997) argue that cognitive mapping research could reveal 'what spatial information should be given to visually challenged pedestrians, in what form and at which particular locations'.

Different forms of visual impairment might also impact on cognitive map development. Someone experiencing a loss of central vision would perhaps find reading text (e.g. road signs) extremely difficult, whereas someone with only one half of their field of vision would possibly be more dependent on information within the side that was lost. The use of VE technology helped people who are blind in exploring an unknown novel room (Lahav & Mioduser, 2003). Research on the use of haptic devices by people who are blind for construction of cognitive maps includes (Lahav & Mioduser, 2003; Semwal & Evans-Kamp, 2000).

Motivation for VR Based Assistance

Some of the many general factors underlying the idea that VE technology is likely to be useful for training spatial behavior in the real world are summarized (by Darken, Cockayne, & Carmein, 1997) in the following paragraphs.

- Training in the real space may be inappropriate or impossible because of inaccessibility, cost, excessive danger, security requirements, etc.
- A single VE installation can be used for training individuals in a wide variety of tasks in a wide variety of spaces because it is software reconfigurable.
- When a VE system is used for training, it is possible to automatically and reliably (a) provide immediate feedback to the trainee and (b) record the trainee's actions for later analysis.
- VE training systems can be used to assess basic spatial abilities and skills and to upgrade these abilities and skills, as well as to train individuals to perform specific tasks in specific spaces.
- VE training systems can be modified adaptively in real time to optimize the training of specific individuals at specific stages of learning under the guidance of specific instructors.
- VE training systems can be used for training team behavior not only by providing common, shared environments in which real team members can interact, but also by providing virtual team members with whom an individual trainee can interact.

Copyright © 2011, IGI Global. Copying or distributing in print or electronic forms without written permission of IGI Global is prohibited.

- VE training systems can be used to provide unreal situations especially designed to enhance training effectiveness.

An understanding of formation of cognitive maps by VIP for successful navigation and wayfinding through non-visual virtual environment is required for designing computer-simulated (virtual) environment.

A Computational Model of Non-Visual Spatial Learning (NSL)

Although isolated solutions have been attempted, no integrated solution of spatial learning to visually impaired people (VIP) is available to the best of our knowledge. Yet no researcher has given a computation model to cover all the aspects of the non-visual spatial learning process. Our non-visual spatial learning (NSL) model provides abstraction of non-visual spatial learning by VIP. Special emphasis is placed on internalizing and externalizing cognitive maps and online assessment of perceived cognitive maps by users. Understanding how spatial learning tasks are constructed is useful in determining how best to improve performance. We should decompose the various tasks of spatial learning in a generic way. So that we might be able to determine where assistance is needed, or where training can occur.

To describe the computational model of the spatial learning, we divided whole process into following four steps (see Figure 2).

Figure 2. Components of non-visual spatial learning (NSL) model

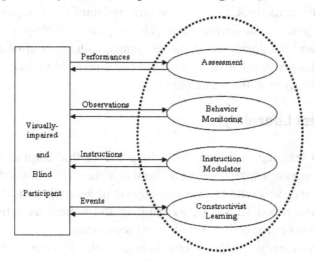

Copyright © 2011, IGI Global. Copying or distributing in print or electronic forms without written permission of IGI Global is prohibited.

1. Constructivist Learning
2. Instruction modulator
3. Behavior monitoring
4. Assessment

The model works like this. In first phase, a constructivist learning experience is to be provided that emphasizes the active participation of users in spatial learning through virtual environment exploration. This is kind of learning-by-exploring approach of learning. Virtual environment exploration should be as familiar and natural as actually walking through the regions. In second phase, simulated agent explores the area and creates the knowledgebase to provide guidance and directs user by generation of the various kinds of instructions. Instructor modulator conforms the instructions and conveys to the participant in various ways (speech, force feedback, and/or non-speech sound). Besides this assistance, the participant can get contextual cues that help them to structure cognitive maps. The participant can interact with the various objects of virtual environment and structure cognitive map of an environment. In third phase, partial cognitive map build till now, it is evaluated in terms of the participant's behavior, navigating style (i.e. normal walk or drunkard/random walk) and the participant's course with obstacles (where and when). Need based further instructions may be provided for any adjustment.

In the final phase, once the participant gets confident and memorizes the path and landmarks between source and destination, he is allowed to go for assessment. The participant's navigation performance, such as path traversed, time taken and number of steps taken to complete the task are recorded and evaluated. The participant's performance is evaluated in terms of statistical measures like bi-dimensional correlation coefficients (BCC), navigation time and number of steps taken to reach the destination place from source place. The sequence of objects falling on the traversed path and the positions where he seemed to have confusion (and hence took relatively longer time) are also recorded and conveyed to them. Performance feedback is to be given to the participant.

Constructivist Learning

A constructivist learning experience is to be provided that emphasizes the active participation of users in spatial learning through virtual environment exploration. The participant interacts with the various objects of an environment. Also virtual environment exploration should be as familiar and natural as actually walking through the regions portrayed on a traditional paper map.

A constructivist learning experience is to be provided that emphasizes the active participation of users in spatial learning through virtual environment exploration. This

Copyright © 2011, IGI Global. Copying or distributing in print or electronic forms without written permission of IGI Global is prohibited.

is kind of learning-by-exploring approach of learning. The participant interacts with the various objects of an environment. The participant can load layout of premise or area through interface easily and can get the brief description of the layout in the beginning through text-to-speech conversion. The participant can choose starting location and destination through speech recognition guided selection. The participant can start session by pressing a particular key (for say F5). Session start date-time (that is also start break date-time for first break) is to be stored by system. Now the participant can start navigation. The participant navigates or explores the virtual environment using a force feedback joystick, mouse or locomotion interface. Virtual environment exploration should be as familiar and natural as actually walking through the regions. Before starting training session, the participant can configure (a) foot step size, (b) height and (c) length of their foot. System maintains session starting and ending time. The participant can end the session by pressing a particular key.

In case of confusion or any difficulty, the participant can take assistance from system. The participant can get information regarding orientation, whenever needed, through help key (for say F3). The participant can also get information (help) regarding Near-by (, near to near-by, or far) objects from his current location (i.e. knowing orientation) by pressing key (for say F4). The participant also gets options and direction available to move by pressing key (for say F8), number of steps taken and distance covered from origin or from particular location and distance remains to travel to reach the destinations. When the participant takes these type of helps, system stores information regarding helps taken (i.e. When and Where – Current location). This information is used to find the confidence level of the participant. The System also generates audible and vibration alerts when the participant is approaching any obstacle.

Following are the some of the common operations need to be implemented that performed by the participant:

- Load layout (as prepared by sighted)
  void loadLayout(layout_name);
- Select source and destination locations
  void selectSourceLocation(location_name);
  void selectDestinationLocation(location_name);
- Starting and ending session
  int startSession();
  void endSession(sessionNumber);
- Take break
  int takeBreak(); return next break number.
- Get orientation help
  String[] getOrientationHelp();

Copyright © 2011, IGI Global. Copying or distributing in print or electronic forms without written permission of IGI Global is prohibited.

- Get present route help
  String getPresentRouteHelp();
- Taking assistance
  void askOptionToMove(presentPosition);

Following are the some of the common operations need to be implemented that performed by system:

- Transition / Acceleration
  void transition (stepNumber);
  void accelerate();

Instruction Modulator

This is kind of directed mode of navigation. The basic concept of directed mode of navigation is to augment the standard user interface in a virtual environment with a system that has knowledge about the content of the virtual world and lets users find objects and locations through assistance.

The simulated agent explores the area and creates the knowledgebase to provide guidance and directs user by generation of the various kinds of instructions. Instructor modulator conforms the instructions and conveys to the participant in various ways (speech, force feedback, and/or non-speech sound).

Following are the type of instructions generated by the Instruction modulator:

1. Directional Instructions
2. Obstacles avoidance Instructions
3. Orientation Instructions
4. Contextual Instructions
5. Temporal Instructions

In this mode of navigation, the Instruction modulator guides the blind participant through speech by describing surroundings, guiding directions, and giving early information of a turning, crossings, etc. Additionally, occurrences of various events (e.g. arrival of a junction, arrival of object(s) of interest, etc.) are signaled through vibration using consumer-grade devices. Current position in virtual environment is changed as user walks on the locomotion interface. They may use the force feedback joystick, mouse to control and move the current position indicator (referred to as cursor in this paper). System generates (non-speech) sound for each step taken by User. Whenever the cursor is moved onto or near an object, its sound and force feedback features are activated. Thus a particular sound, which may also be a pre-

Copyright © 2011, IGI Global. Copying or distributing in print or electronic forms without written permission of IGI Global is prohibited.

recorded message, will be heard by the participant. As long as the cursor is on the object, the participant will feel the force feedback effect associated with this object. The participant can get contextual information continuously during navigation according to session's time like Morning, Afternoon, Evening, or Night. Contextual information is also according to different events of the place. For example for Railway station, contextual information is different for different events like at train arrival time, departure time and normal waiting time period. When the participant is approaching or passing through class room (for school or college premises) he gets sound of teacher and students with Doppler Effect. When the participant is passing through fountain or river, they heard the sound of flowing of water. The participant gets information about path surface (i.e. Sandy, Muddy, Concrete, Slippery, or Grass-root/loan etc.) through tactile effects.

Optimal Path Finding

As mentioned earlier various objects like places, paths etc. in topological map of an environment are linked by the various relations among them like places are along the paths, place is on left or right side of other place or path, etc. An algorithm is formulated for finding optimal path between two places in topology map based on Boundary Relation Heuristic (BRH). According to the BRH, boundary relations supply sub goals for the wayfinding algorithm.

Here first Route-to-route relation matrix and Route-to-place relation matrix (see Table 2) are to be created based on boundary relation. We use two basic behavioral modes, wall following and object avoidance. In the wall following mode, the blind person tries to stay close to the wall, once it detected one. This is a more opportunistic strategy. As per this strategy, simulated agent finds the exact route with number of steps and directions to reach the destination. Object avoidance is implemented by turning away from objects upon contact, to avoid collision in the near future. Object avoidance is an exploratory strategy. Consider the following layout (Figure 3) which has eight places (P1, P2,..., P8) and three routes (R1, R2 and R3).

Table 2. Route-to-route connectivity matrices

Route-to-route connectivity matrix (reach-ability matrix)			
Route	R1	R2	R3
R1	-	1	∞
R2	1	-	1
R3	∞	1	-

Copyright © 2011, IGI Global. Copying or distributing in print or electronic forms without written permission of IGI Global is prohibited.

Figure 3. Optimal route by the simulated agent

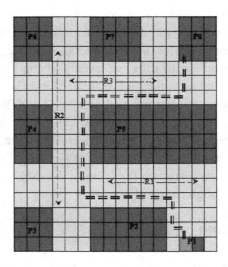

In our algorithm, search process to be guided by the BRH by providing sub goals and then the way in which sub goals can be further explored. This algorithm uses various wayfinding strategies of human being for these sub goals. As shown in Figure 3 to reach P8 (that is Computer lab) from P1 (that is entrance), system finds out the route R1-> R2->R3 from route-to-route connectivity matrix.

Here R2 is on left side of R1, so we get the route along the P2 building for R1->R2. The heuristic estimates the cost to reach the goal node from the current node; the heuristic estimate is usually referred to as the h(n) value. It also keeps track of

Table 3. Place-to-route connectivity matrices

Place-to-Route connectivity matrix			
Route	R1	R2	R3
Place			
P1	1	∞	∞
P2	∞	1	∞
P3	∞	1	∞
P4	∞	1	∞
P5	∞	1	∞
P6	∞	1	∞
P7	∞	∞	1
P8	∞	∞	1

Copyright © 2011, IGI Global. Copying or distributing in print or electronic forms without written permission of IGI Global is prohibited.

the cost needed to get to the current node from the start node, this cost is generally referred to as g(n). The total cost of a node, f(n), is the sum of the cost to reach the current node from the start node and the heuristic estimate.

The simulated agent moves to a successor node by choosing the most promising node (the one with the lowest f(n) value) from it's list of potential successor nodes (i.e. from the open list). An OpenList contains all the nodes that have been reached but haven't been visited and expanded yet and ClosedList contains all the nodes that have been visited and expanded, i.e. they have been removed from the open list and added to the closed list.

Behavior Monitoring

The system continuously monitors and records following type of the participant's behaviors:

- Navigating style (normal /random walk)
- Mental state (confusion/fear/lost/excited/confident)

During learning, the system continuously monitors and records the participant's navigating style (i.e. normal walk or drunkard/random walk) and the participant's course with obstacles (where and when). The participant can take break at any time during the session by pressing the Escape key. System stores break number, break start time and end time, and user's trajectories in the database. Once the system finds the participant confident and memorizes the path and landmarks between source and destination, it allows him to go for assessment. The system monitors the number of step taken and distance traveled by the participant for the each break and session. If these two values are reducing or coming near the expected values and if the participant's navigation style is proper then system finds that the participant is confident and ready for performance test.

Assessment

In the assessment phase, the participant navigates without system's help and trying to reach the destination. The participant gets only contextual information. The system records the participant's navigation performance, such as path traversed, time taken and number of steps taken to complete this task. It also records the sequence of objects falling on the traversed path and the positions where he seemed to have confusion (and hence took relatively longer time). The System evaluates the participant's performance in terms of statistical measures like bi-dimensional correlation coefficients (BCC), navigation time and number of steps taken by the

Copyright © 2011, IGI Global. Copying or distributing in print or electronic forms without written permission of IGI Global is prohibited.

Table 4. Algorithm

ALGORITHM	
1:	INPUT:: StartNode and GoalNode
2:	OpenList ← ⊘; ClosedList ← ⊘;
3:	Insert StartNode to OpenList;
4:	while OpenList is not empty
5:	Pick the node n which has the least f(n) value from OpenList; //make it the current node
6:	if isGoal(n) then
7:	Return (n);
8:	End if
9:	Find all successor nodes of n;
10:	For each successor node n' of n do
11:	g(n') = g(n) + the cost to get from n to n';
12:	find n' on OpenList;
13:	if (n' is on OpenList && has lower g(n')) then
14:	continue;
15:	End if
16:	If (n' is on ClosedList && has lower g(n')) then
17:	continue;
18:	End if
19:	Delete all occurrences of n' from OpenList and ClosedList;
20:	Parent(n') ← n;
21:	Find h(n'); //Use the heuristic to estimate the distance to the goal node
22:	Insert n' to OpenList;
23:	End for
24:	Insert n to ClosedList;
25:	End while

participant to reach the destination place from source place and gives performance feedback to the participant.

As mentioned earlier the simulated agent finds out the possible best path(s) between source place and destination using optimal path algorithm. The System compares optimal paths with the participant's earlier recorded navigation path (during un-guided VE navigation). Navigation paths of the participant are evaluated quantitatively using bi-dimensional regression analysis developed by Tobler (1976). Bi-dimensional regression is applied to calculate the bi-dimensional correlation coefficients. The value of BCC near to 1 indicates that the participant's performance

Copyright © 2011, IGI Global. Copying or distributing in print or electronic forms without written permission of IGI Global is prohibited.

is satisfactory and cognitive maps are satisfactorily formed. If its value is one then the cognitive map is almost precise. The trainer may ask the participant to give a verbal description of the area and then performs orientation and mobility tasks in the real target space.

Quality Factors for Spatial Learning Techniques

There are few categories of virtual environment applications that are currently in use for productive, consistent work, but the requirements of these applications for spatial learning techniques cover a wide range. Further, there are many new applications of VEs being researched, which also may require spatial learning techniques with different characteristics. It is therefore impractical to evaluate spatial learning techniques directly within each new application. Instead, we propose a more general methodology, involving a mapping from spatial learning techniques to a set of quality factors. Quality factors are measurable characteristics of the performance of a technique. With this indirect mapping, application designers can specify desired levels of various quality factors, and then choose a technique which best fits those requirements. Our current list of quality factors for VR-based spatial learning techniques includes:

1. Speed of learning (time taken to develop cognitive map)
2. Navigation Efficiency (Distance traveled, number of steps taken and time taken to complete the task)
3. Accuracy (proximity to the desired target)
4. Spatial Awareness (the user's knowledge of his position and orientation within the environment during and after exploration)
5. Ease of Learning (the ability of a novice user to use the technique)
6. Ease of Use (the complexity or cognitive load of the technique from the user's point of view)
7. Information Gathering (the user's ability to actively obtain information from the environment during exploration)
8. Presence (the user's sense of immersion or 'being within' the environment due to navigation)
9. User Comfort (lack of simulator sickness, dizziness, or nausea)

This list may not be complete, but it is a good starting point for quantifying the effectiveness and performance of virtual spatial learning techniques. Some of the quality factors, such as speed, navigation Efficiency and accuracy, are simple to measure quantitatively. Others, however, are difficult to measure due to their inherent subjective nature. To quantify these factors, standard questionnaires for factors such

Copyright © 2011, IGI Global. Copying or distributing in print or electronic forms without written permission of IGI Global is prohibited.

as ease of use (e.g. Chin, Diehl, & Norman, 1988), presence (e.g. Slater, Usoh, & Steed, 1995), and simulator sickness (e.g. Kennedy, Lane, Berbaum, & Lilienthal, 1993) should be part of the experimental method.

Measuring Cognitive Load

A person has a limited amount of cognitive resources which they must allocate amount all mental tasks being concurrently performed. Cognitive load refers to the total amount of mental activity on working memory at an instance in time (Cooper, 2004). Short term memory is limited in the number of elements it can contain simultaneously (Chandler, & Sweller, 1999). If a design requires the user to hold too many items in short term memory, it will fail (Balogh, Michael, & Giangola, 2004). When a user's working memory is available to concentrate on the details of to-be-used information, usability is increased (Cooper, 2004).

There are many different methods of measuring a user's cognitive load, ranging from direct measurement of neuro-physiological response to post-event questions. While techniques measuring physical responses such as EEG and pulse rates are very accurate, they are also expensive and require special equipment and training. Following are the three methods which are easily applied within a simple usability test.

NASA TLX

The NASA TLX test was developed to measure the overall work load of equipment operation. "It can be used to assess workload in various human-machine environments such as aircraft cockpits; command, control, and communication (C3) workstations; supervisory and process control environments; simulations and laboratory tests". To assess the workload experienced while completing multiple tasks, six rating scales have been established: mental demand, physical demand, temporal demand, performance, effort, frustration. The user rates each of these on a Likert scale and then has 15 questions that pair up two scales and ask the user to select the one which is the most important contributor to workload for the task.

The concept of the NASA-TLX is to allow the user time to access the workload situation once the testing is complete. The subscales provide detailed information, not just one-answer questions. We must consider that it measures workload as an afterthought. NASA-TLX does not test the user while they are in the process of completing the task. The user is forced to rely on what they remember and provide and opinion based on memory. NASA TLX is designed for work loads which often had a higher physical component than computer mouse operations. On the other

Copyright © 2011, IGI Global. Copying or distributing in print or electronic forms without written permission of IGI Global is prohibited.

hand, for the information seeking activities which are the norm on web sites, the cognitive load a person experiences tends to be directly related to the work load.

An electronic version of the test can be downloaded at http://www.nrl.navy.mil/aic/ide/NASATLX.php.

Sternberg Memory Test

As originally designed, the Sternberg Memory Test was designed to measure how quickly people can search for and retrieve information from short-term memory. People were give a small set of number (1-6) to memorize and were then give a sequence of probe numbers. The subjects had to respond yes/no to whether the probe number was one of the numbers they had memorized. For example, you memorize 3 and 6. The probe number is 8, you say "no." The probe number is 6, you say "yes." The part of the website or system using high cognitive resources can be determined because the yes/no response will take longer. According to Sternberg (Sternberg, 1969), several theories of short-term memory can be tested by altering the number of items on the list. Sternberg (Sternberg, 1969) found that as the theory set increased, reaction times increased, and whether the probe was or was not committed to memory, did not alter the reaction time (Cog Lab Wadsworth). While this test sounds very simple, the speed of response (saying yes/no) varies with the cognitive load. For high load situations, a user responds slower and if they are overloaded, there could be a substantial delay or out-right forgetting of some of the numbers which were memorized (Miyake, Yohei, & Ernst, 2004).

Tapping Test

Using tapping is a simple way of imposing a secondary load on the user. If the subject's concentration is focused at processing information other than tapping, it is hard for subjects to apply the concentration needed to execute the tapping task (Miyake, et al., 2004). While seemingly a trivial task, it does require cognitive resources to continue to rhythmically tap either a finger or foot. This imposes the additional load which helps push the user into cognitive overload.

Simulator Sickness

The Simulator Sickness Questionnaire (SSQ) introduced by Kennedy et al. (Kennedy, et al., 1993) can be used as a measure in the simulator sickness experiments. There is an ambiguity in the use of the term "simulator sickness". In informal usage, "simulator sickness" tends to refer to the generic experience of feeling sick as a result of exposure to computer-generated stimuli. However, it is frequently used in

Copyright © 2011, IGI Global. Copying or distributing in print or electronic forms without written permission of IGI Global is prohibited.

a more restricted sense, as including only the sickness caused by poor simulations. For instance, Pausch, Crea, and Conway (1992) mention that "The term simulator sickness is typically used to refer to sickness caused by the incorrect aspects of the simulation, not sickness caused by a correct simulation of a nauseating experience, such as a turbulent airplane flight." Else where in the same special issue on simulator sickness, one may find "simulator sickness" used in the more generic sense. For instance, in the preceding article Biocca (1992) states that "Simulator sickness is the term that has been attached to a host of symptoms associated with visual and vestibular disturbances that resemble motion sickness." The generic usage of "simulator sickness" is implicit in the title of the special issue, "Spotlight On: Simulator Sickness" (covering all sickness symptoms induced by simulators).

To take another example of the generic usage, Kennedy et al.'s widely-used "Simulator Sickness Questionnaire" (Kennedy, et al., 1993) records motion sickness symptoms. It appears that there are three ideas present for which only two terms are in wide-spread use. The best solution is to introduce a third term. The three ideas are:

1. The generic feeling of sickness resulting from exposure to a computer-generated space.
2. The component of "1" which is inherent to the stimulus itself, and which would be present even if the simulation were a perfect representation of the real world.
3. The component of "1" which results from an imperfect simulation, for instance due to lag, poor inter-ocular adjust, poor resolution, etc.

There is general agreement that "2" should be referred to as "motion sickness". The problem lies with "1" and "3". Both are important ideas, and the term "simulator sickness" tends to oscillate between them depending on the topic of discussion.

Locomotion in Virtual World

Virtual reality provides for creation of simulated objects and events with which people can interact. The definitions of virtual reality (VR), although wide and varied, include a common statement that VR creates the illusion of participation in a synthetic environment rather than going through external observation of such an environment (Earnshaw, Gigante, & Jones, 1993). Essentially, virtual reality allows users to interact with a computer-simulated environment. Users can interact with a virtual environment either through the use of standard input devices such as a keyboard and mouse, or through multimodal devices such as a wired glove, the Polhemus boom arm, or else omni-directional treadmill. The locomotion interface is used to simulate walking from one location to another location. The device is

Copyright © 2011, IGI Global. Copying or distributing in print or electronic forms without written permission of IGI Global is prohibited.

needed to be of a limited size, allow a user to walk on it and provide a sensation as if he is walking on an unconstrained plane.

Generally, a locomotion interface should cancel the user's self motion in a place to allow the user to go to anywhere in a large virtual space on foot. For example, a treadmill can cancel the user's motion by moving its belt in the opposite direction. Its main advantage is that it does not require a user to wear any kind of devices as required in some other locomotion devices. However, it is difficult to control the belt speed in order to keep the user from falling off. Some treadmills can adjust the belt speed based on the user's motion. There are mainly two challenges in using the treadmills. The first one is the user's stability problem while the second is to sense and change the direction of walking. The belt in a passive treadmill is driven by the backward push generated while walking. This process effectively balances the user and keeps him from falling off.

The problem of changing the walking direction is addressed by Brooks (1986) and Hirose & Yokoyama (1997), who employed a handle to change the walking direction. Iwata, and Yoshida, (1999) developed a 2D infinite plate that can be driven in any direction and Darken, et al. (1997) proposed an Omni directional treadmill using mechanical belt. Noma, and Miyasato (1998) used the treadmill which could turn on a platform to change the walking direction. Iwata and Fujji (1996) used a different approach by developing a series of sliding interfaces. The user was required to wear special shoes and a low friction film was put in the middle of shoes. Since the user was supported by a harness or rounded handrail, the foot motion was canceled passively when the user walked. The method using active footpad could simulate various terrains without requiring the user to wear any kind of devices.

Type of Locomotion in Virtual World

It has often been suggested that the best locomotion mechanism for virtual worlds would be walking, and it is well known that the sense of distance or orientation while walking is much better than while riding in a vehicle. However, the proprioceptive feedback of walking is not provided in most virtual environments. Good number of devices has been developed over the last two decades to integrate locomotion interfaces with VR environments. We have categorized the most common VR locomotion approaches as follow:

- Treadmills-style interface (Darken, et al., 1997; Hollerbach, Xu, Christensen, & Jacobsen, 2000; Iwata, & Yoshida, 1999; De Luca, Mattone, & Giordano, 2007),
- pedaling devices (such as bicycles or unicycles) (Iwata & Fuji, 1996),
- walking-in-place devices (Sibert, et al., 2004),

Copyright © 2011, IGI Global. Copying or distributing in print or electronic forms without written permission of IGI Global is prohibited.

- the motion foot pad (Iwata, Yano, Fukushima, & Noma, 2005),
- actuated shoes (Iwata, Yano, & Tomioka, 2006),
- the string walker (Iwata, Yano, & Tomiyoshi, 2007), and
- Finger walking-in-place devices.

CONCLUSION AND FUTURE DIRECTIVES

Knowledge based systems help to enhance capacity of machine or computer system to behave intelligently, similar to human being in some aspects at least. Machine based training simulators are equivalent or better than human trainers in terms of efficiency and effectiveness. Our Non-visual spatial navigation (NSL) model provides computational framework for spatial knowledge representation, acquisition and assessment of the acquired spatial knowledge. This model is effective to promote the development and online evaluation of cognitive maps of users. We are encouraged by preliminary results from our prototype implementation, which suggest that such spatial learning techniques would help visually challenged and blind people to get effectively learned for independent navigation. This is an ongoing study and we feel that our system based on our NSL model will be progressively enriched to become increasingly effective for spatial learning by them.

REFERENCES

Balogh, J., Michael, C., & Giangola, J. (2004). *Voice user interface design: Minimizing cognitive load.* Addison Wesley Professional.

Biocca, F. (1992). Will simulation sickness slow down the diffusion of virtual environment technology? *Presence (Cambridge, Mass.), 1*(3), 334–343.

Bradyn, J. A. (1985). A review of mobility aids and means of assessment. In Warren, D. H., & Strelow, E. R. (Eds.), *Electronic spatial sensing for the blind* (pp. 13–27). Martinus Nijhoff.

Bronstein, I. N., & Semendjajew, K. A. (1979). *Taschenbuch der mathematik.* Verlag Harri Deutsch, Thun and Frankfurt am Main, reprint of the 20th edition.

Brooks, F. P., Jr. (1986). Walk through- a dynamic graphics system for simulating virtual buildings. *Proceedings of 1986 Workshop on Interactive 3D Graphics*, (pp. 9-21).

Burdea, G., & Coiffet, P. (2003). *Virtual reality technology.* New York, NY: John Wiley & Sons.

Copyright © 2011, IGI Global. Copying or distributing in print or electronic forms without written permission of IGI Global is prohibited.

Chandler, P., & Sweller, J. (1999). *Cognitive load while learning to use a computer program. Applied Cognitive Psychology*. University of New South Wales.

Chin, J., Diehl, V., & Norman, K. (1988). Development of an instrument measuring user satisfaction of the human-computer interface. *Proceedings of CHI*, (pp. 213-218).

Clark-Carter, D., Heyes, A., & Howarth, C. (1986). The effect of non-visual preview upon the walking speed of visually impaired people. *Ergonomics*, *29*(12), 1575–1581. doi:10.1080/00140138608967270

Colwell, C., Petrie, H., Kornbrot, D., Hardwick, A., & Furner, S. (1998). Haptic virtual reality for blind computer users. In *Proceedings of the 3rd International ACM Conference on Assistive Technologies (ASSETS '98)*, (pp. 92–99). Marina del Rey, Calif, USA.

Cooper, G. (2004). *Research into cognitive load theory and instructional design at UNSW*. University of New South Wales. Retrieved from http://www.google.com/scholar?hl=en&lr=&q=cache:BP2uyE_8R1EJ:www.uog.edu/coe/ed451/tHEORY/LoadTheory1.pdf+research+into+cognitive+load+theory+and+instructional+design+at+unsw

Crandall, W., Bentzen, B., Myers, L., & Mitchell, P. (1995). *Transit accessibility improvement through talking signs remote infrared signage, a demonstration and evaluation*. San Francisco, Calif, USA: Tech. Rep., The Smith-Kettlewell Eye Research Institute, Rehabilitation Engineering Research Center.

Darken, R. P., Cockayne, W. R., & Carmein, D. (1997). The omni-directional treadmill: A locomotion device for virtual worlds. *Proceedings of UIST*, *97*, 213–221. doi:10.1145/263407.263550

De Luca, A., Mattone, R., & Giordano, P. R. (2007). *Acceleration-level control of the CyberCarpet*. 2007 IEEE International Conference on Robotics and Automation, Roma, I, (pp. 2330-2335).

Dodson, A. H., Moore, T., & Moon, G. V. (1999). *A navigation system for the blind pedestrian. GNSS 99* (pp. 513–518). Italy: Genoa.

Downs, R. M., & Stea, D. (1977). *Maps in minds: Reflections on cognitive mapping*. New York, NY: Harper and Row.

Downs, R. M., & Stea, D. (1997). Cognitive maps and spatial behaviour: Process and products. In R.M. Downs & D. Stea (Eds,), *Image and environment* (pp. 8-26). Chicago, IL: Aldine.

Earnshaw, R. A., Gigante, M. A., & Jones, H. (Eds.). (1993). *Virtual reality systems*. Academic Press.

Copyright © 2011, IGI Global. Copying or distributing in print or electronic forms without written permission of IGI Global is prohibited.

Ertan, S., Lee, C., Willets, A., Tan, H., & Pentland, A. (1998). *A wearable haptic navigation guidance system*. 2nd International Symposium on Wearable Computer, Pittsburgh, PA, (pp. 164-165).

Freksa, C. (1997). *Spatial and temporal structures in cognitive processes* (pp. 379–387). (LNCS 1337). Berlin/Heidelberg, Germany & New York, NY: Springer.

Freundschuh, S. M., & Egenhofer, M. J. (1997). Human conceptions of spaces: Implications for geographic information systems. *Transactions in GIS, 2*(4), 361–375.

Fruchterman, J. (1995). Archenstone's orientation tools: Atlas speaks and strider. In J. M. Gill, & H. Petrie (Eds.), *Orientation and navigation systems for blind persons*. Hatfield, UK. 1-2 February 1995. RNIB.

Gapp, K. P. (1995). An empirically validated model for computing spatial relations. In I. Wachsmuth, C. R. Rollinger, & W. Brauer (Eds.), *KI-95: Advances in Artificial Intelligence. 19th Annual German Conference on Artificial Intelligence*, (pp. 245–256). Berlin/Heidelberg, Germany & New York, NY: Springer.

Giess, C., Evers, H., & Meinzer, H. (1998). Haptic volume rendering in different scenarios of surgical planning. In *Proceedings of the 3rd Phantom Users Group Workshop (PUG '98)*, (pp. 19–22). Massachusetts Institute of Technology, Cambridge, MA, USA.

Golding, A. R., & Lesh, N. (1999). *Indoor navigation using a diverse set of cheap, wearable sensors*. Third International Symposium on Wearable computers, San Francisco, CA, (pp. 29-36).

Golledge, R., Klatzky, R., & Loomis, J. (1996). Cognitive mapping and wayfinding by adults without vision. In Portugali, J. (Ed.), *The construction of cognitive maps* (pp. 215–246). The Netherlands: Kluwer. doi:10.1007/978-0-585-33485-1_10

Golledge, R. G., Klatzky, R. L., Loomis, J. M., Speigle, J., & Tietz, J. (1998). A geographical information system for a GPS based personal guidance system. *International Journal of Geographical Information Science, 12*(7), 727–749. doi:10.1080/136588198241635

Gorman, P., Lieser, J., Murray, W., Haluck, R., & Krummel, T. (1998). Assessment and validation of force feedback virtual reality based surgical simulator. In *Proceedings of the 3rd Phantom Users Group Workshop (PUG '98)*. MIT, Cambridge, MA, USA.

Helal, A. S., Moore, S. E., & Ramachandran, B. (2001). *Drishti: An integrated navigation system for visually impaired and disabled*. 5th International Symposium on Wearable Computers, Zurich, Switzerland.

Copyright © 2011, IGI Global. Copying or distributing in print or electronic forms without written permission of IGI Global is prohibited.

Herrman, T., & Grabowski, J. (1994). *Sprechen–Psychologie der Sprachproduktion.* Berlin/Heidelberg, Germany: Spektrum Akademischer Verlag.

Hirose, M., & Yokoyama, K. (1997). Synthesis and transmission of realistic sensation using virtual reality technology. *Transactions of the Society of Instrument and Control Engineers, 33*(7), 716–722.

Hollerbach, J. M., Xu, Y., Christensen, R., & Jacobsen, S. C. (2000). Design specifications for the second generation Sarcos Treadport locomotion interface. *Haptics Symposium, Proc. ASME Dynamic Systems and Control Division, DSC-Vol. 69-2,* Orlando, Nov. 5-10, 2000, (pp. 1293-1298).

Ittelson, W. (1973). Environment and cognition. In *Environment perception and contemporary perceptual theory* (pp. 1–19). New York, NY: Seminar Press.

Iwata, H., & Fujji, T. (1996). Virtual preambulator: A novel interface device for locomotion in virtual environment. *Proceedings of IEEE VRAIS, 96,* 60–65.

Iwata, H., Yano, H., Fukushima, H., & Noma, H. (2005). CirculaFloor. *IEEE Computer Graphics and Applications, 25*(1), 64–67. doi:10.1109/MCG.2005.5

Iwata, H., Yano, H., & Tomioka, H. (2006). *Powered shoes.* SIGGRAPH 2006 Conference DVD.

Iwata, H., Yano, H., & Tomiyoshi, M. (2007). *String walker.* Paper presented at SIGGRAPH 2007.

Iwata, H., & Yoshida, Y. (1999). Path reproduction tests using a torus treadmill. *Presence (Cambridge, Mass.), 8*(6), 587–597. doi:10.1162/105474699566503

Jansson, G., Fanger, J., Konig, H., & Billberger, K. (1998). Visually impaired persons' use of the phantom for information about texture and 3D form of virtual objects. In *Proceedings of the 3rd Phantom Users Group Workshop,* MIT, Cambridge, MA, USA.

Jonsson, E. (2002). *Inner navigation: Why we get lost and how we find our way* (pp. 27–126). New York, NY: Scribner.

Kay, L. (1980). Air sonar with acoustical display of spatial information. In Busnel, R. G., & Fish, J. F. (Eds.), *Animal sonar system* (pp. 769–816). New York, NY: Plenum Press.

Kemmerling, M., & Schliepkorte, H. (1998). *An orientation and Information System for blind people based on RF-speech-beacons.* Helsinki: TIDE.

Copyright © 2011, IGI Global. Copying or distributing in print or electronic forms without written permission of IGI Global is prohibited.

Kennedy, R. S., Lane, N. E., Berbaum, K. S., & Lilienthal, M. G. (1993). Simulator sickness questionnaire: An enhanced method for quantifying simulator sickness. *The International Journal of Aviation Psychology, 3*(3), 203–220. doi:10.1207/s15327108ijap0303_3

Kitchin, R. M., Blades, M., & Golledge, R. G. (1997). Understanding spatial concepts at the geographic scale without the use of vision. *Progress in Human Geography, 21*(2), 225–242. doi:10.1191/030913297668904166

Kitchin, R. M., & Jacobson, R. D. (1997). GIS and people with visual impairments or blindness: Exploring the potential for education, orientation, and navigation. *Transactions in Geographic Information System, 2*(4), 315–332.

Lahav, O., & Mioduser, D. (2003). A blind person's cognitive mapping of new spaces using a haptic virtual environment. *Journal of Research in Special Educational Needs, 3*(3), 172–177. doi:10.1111/1471-3802.00012

Long, S., Aust, D., Abowd, G. D., & Atkeson, C. (1996). Cyberguide: Prototyping context-aware mobile applications. In *CHI '96 Conference Companion*, (pp. 293-294).

Loomis, J. M., Golledge, R. G., & Klatzky, R. L. (2001). GPS-based navigation system for the visually impaired. In Barfield, W., & Caudell, T. (Eds.), *Fundamentals of wearable computers and augmented reality* (pp. 429–446). Mahwah, NJ: Lawrence Erbaum Associates.

Lynch, K. (1960). *The image of the city*. Cambridge, MA: MIT Press.

Miyake, Y., Yohei, O., & Ernst, P. (2004). Two types of anticipation in synchronization tapping. *Acta Neurologica, 64*, 415–426.

Montello, D. R. (1993). Scale and multiple phychologies of space. In Frank, A., & Campari, I. (Eds.), *Spatial information theory: A theoretical basis for GIS* (pp. 312–321). Berlin/ Heidelberg, Germany & New York, NY: Springer.

Noma, H., & Miyasato, T. (1998). Design for locomotion interface in a large scale virtual environment, ATLAS. *ATR Locomotion Interface for Active Self Motion, ASME-DSC, 64*, 111–118.

Pausch, R., Crea, T., & Conway, M. (1992). A literature survey for virtual environments: Military flight simulator visual systems and simulator sickness. *Presence (Cambridge, Mass.), 1*(3), 344–363.

Petrie, H. (1995). User requirements for a GPS-based travel aid for blind people. In Gill, J. M., & Petrie, H. (Eds.), *Orientation and navigation systems for blind persons* (pp. 1–2). UK: February. RNIB.

Copyright © 2011, IGI Global. Copying or distributing in print or electronic forms without written permission of IGI Global is prohibited.

Raubal, M., & Worboys, M. (1999). A formal model for the process of wayfinding in built environments. In C. Freksa & D. M. Mark (Eds.), *Spatial information theory (Proceedings of COSIT 99).* (pp. 381–399). Berlin/Heidelberg, Germany & New York, NY: Springer.

Rieser, J. J. (1989). Access to knowledge of spatial structure at novel points of observation. *Journal of Experimental Psychology. Learning, Memory, and Cognition,* *15*(6), 1157–1165. doi:10.1037/0278-7393.15.6.1157

Sabelman, E. E., Burgar, C. G., Curtis, G. E., Goodrich, G., Jaffe, D. L., Mckinley, J. L., et al. Apple, L. G. (1994). *Personal navigation and wayfinding for individuals with a range of disabilities.* Project report: Device development and evaluation. Retrieved from http://guide.stanford.edu/Publications/dev3.html

Schultheis, M., & Rizzo, A. (2001). The application of virtual reality technology for rehabilitation. *Rehabilitation Psychology,* *46*(3), 296–311. doi:10.1037/0090-5550.46.3.296

Semwal, S. K., & Evans-Kamp, D. L. (2000). *Virtual environments for visually impaired.* Paper presented at the 2nd International Conference on Virtual worlds, Paris, France.

Sibert, L., Templeman, J., Page, R., Barron, J., McCune, J., & Denbrook, P. (2004). *Initial assessment of human performance using the gaiter interaction technique to control locomotion in fully immersive virtual environments. (Technical Report).* Washington, DC: Naval Research Laboratory.

Siegel, A. W., & White, S. H. (1975). The development of spatial representations of large-scale environments. In Rees, H. W. (Ed.), *Advances in child development and behavior* (*Vol. 10*, pp. 9–55). New York, NY: Academic Press.

Slater, M., Usoh, M., & Steed, A. (1995). Taking steps: The influence of a walking metaphor on presence in virtual reality. *ACM Transactions on Computer-Human Interaction,* *2*(3), 201–219. doi:10.1145/210079.210084

Sorrows, M. E., & Hirtle, S. C. (1999). The nature of landmarks in real and electronic spaces. In C. Freksa & D. M. Mark (Eds.), *Spatial information theory (Proceedings of COSIT 99),* (pp. 37–50). Berlin/Heidelberg, Germany & New York, NY: Springer.

Standen, P. J., Brown, D. J., & Cromby, J. J. (2001). The effective use of virtual environments in the education and rehabilitation of students with intellectual disabilities. *British Journal of Educational Technology,* *32*(3), 289–299. doi:10.1111/1467-8535.00199

Copyright © 2011, IGI Global. Copying or distributing in print or electronic forms without written permission of IGI Global is prohibited.

Sternberg, S. (1969). The discovery of processing stages: Extensions of Bonders' method. *Acta Psychologica, 30*, 216–315. doi:10.1016/0001-6918(69)90055-9

Strothotte, T., Fritz, S., Michel, R., Raab, A., Petrie, H., Johnson, V., et al. Schalt, A. (1996). Development of dialogue systems for the mobility aid for blind people: Initial design and usability testing. *ASSETS '96*, Vancouver, British Columbia, Canada, (pp. 139-144).

Tobler, W. (1976). The geometry of mental maps. In Golledge, R. G., & Rushton, G. (Eds.), *Spatial choice and spatial behavior* (pp. 69–82). Columbus, OH: Ohio State University Press.

Tolman, E. (1948). Cognitive maps in rats and men. *Psychological Review, 55*, 189–208. doi:10.1037/h0061626

Tversky, B. (1993). Cognitive maps, cognitive collages, and spatial mental models. In *Spatial Information Theory: A Theroretical Basis for GIS, COSIT '93*, (pp. 14–24).

Ungar, S., Blades, M., & Spencer, S. (1996). The construction of cognitive maps by children with visual impairments. In Portugali, J. (Ed.), *The construction of cognitive maps* (pp. 247–273). Dordrecht, The Netherlands: Kluwer Academic Publishers. doi:10.1007/978-0-585-33485-1_11

Warren, D., & Strelow, E. (1985). *Electronic spatial sensing for the blind*. Boston, MA: Martinus Nijhoff.

Werner, S., Krieg-Bruckner, B., Mallot, H. A., Schweizer, K., & Freksa, C. (1997). Spatial cognition: The role of landmark, route, and survey knowledge in human and robot navigation. In Jarke, M. (Ed.), *Informatik '97 GI Jahrestagung* (pp. 41–50). Berlin/Heidelberg, Germany & New York, NY: Springer.

ADDITIONAL READING

Espinosa, M., & Ochaita, E. (1998). Using tactile maps to improve the practical spatial knowledge of adults who are blind. *Journal of Visual Impairment & Blindness, 92*(5), 338–345.

Lahav, O. (2003). *Blind Persons' Cognitive Mapping of Unknown Spaces and acquisition of Orientation Skills, by Using Audio and Force-Feedback Virtual Environment*. Doctoral dissertation, Tel-Aviv University, Israel (Hebrew).

Copyright © 2011, IGI Global. Copying or distributing in print or electronic forms without written permission of IGI Global is prohibited.

KEY TERMS AND DEFINITIONS

Bi-Dimensional Correlation Coefficients: Bi-dimensional regression is applied to calculate the bi-dimensional correlation coefficients.

Blindness: Legal blindness (which is actually a severe visual impairment) refers to a best-corrected central vision of 20/200 or worse in the better eye or a visual acuity of better than 20/200 but with a visual field no greater than 20° (e.g., side vision that is so reduced that it appears as if the person is looking through a tunnel).

Cognitive Load: A person has a limited amount of cognitive resources which they must allocate amount all mental tasks being concurrently performed. Cognitive load refers to the total amount of mental activity on working memory at an instance in time.

Constructivist Learning: Within the constructivist paradigm, the accent is on the learner rather than the teacher. It is the learner who interacts with his or her environment and thus gains an understanding of its features and characteristics. The learner constructs his own conceptualisations and finds his own solutions to problems, mastering autonomy and independence. According to constructivism, learning is the result of individual mental construction, whereby the learner learns by dint of matching new against given information and establishing meaningful connections, rather than by internalising mere factoids to be regurgitated later on.

Landmark-Route-Survey Theory: The longest standing model of large-scale space representation is the Landmark, Survey, Route (or LRS) model (Siegel and White 1975). LRS theory states that we first identify landmarks in an environment, add route knowledge between landmarks as we traverse the environment and finally add survey (or configurational) knowledge as we become familiar with the environment. Once survey knowledge has been added, we have the capability to propose novel, previously un-traversed paths between landmarks.

Locomotion Interface: Locomotion interface should cancel the user's self motion in a place to allow the user to go to anywhere in a large virtual space on foot.

Presence: Presence is a multi-dimensional concept that involves psychological processes.

Simulator Sickness: In informal usage, "simulator sickness" tends to refer to the generic experience of feeling sick as a result of exposure to computer-generated stimuli.

Virtual Environment: VE provides for creation of simulated objects and events with which people can interact. The definitions of VE, although wide and varied, include a common statement that VE creates the illusion of participation in a synthetic environment rather than going through external observation of such an environment.

Copyright © 2011, IGI Global. Copying or distributing in print or electronic forms without written permission of IGI Global is prohibited.

Chapter 8
Statistical Analysis of Facial Expression on 3D Face Shapes

Jacey-Lynn Minoi
Universiti Malaysia Sarawak, Malaysia

Duncan Gillies
Imperial College London, UK

ABSTRACT

The aim of this chapter is to identify those face areas containing high facial expression information, which may be useful for facial expression analysis, face and facial expression recognition and synthesis. In the study of facial expression analysis, landmarks are usually placed on well-defined craniofacial features. In this experiment, the authors have selected a set of landmarks based on craniofacial anthropometry and associate each of the landmarks with facial muscles and the Facial Action Coding System (FACS) framework, which means to locate landmarks on less palpable areas that contain high facial expression mobility. The selected landmarks are statistically analysed in terms of facial muscles motion based on FACS. Given that human faces provide information to channel verbal and non-verbal communication: speech, facial expression of emotions, gestures, and other human communicative actions; hence, these cues may be significant in the identification of expressions such as pain, agony, anger, happiness, et cetera. Here, the authors describe the potential of computer-based models of three-dimensional (3D) facial expression analysis and the non-verbal communication recognition to assist in biometric recognition and clinical diagnosis.

DOI: 10.4018/978-1-60960-541-4.ch008

Copyright ©2011, IGI Global. Copying or distributing in print or electronic forms without written permission of IGI Global is prohibited.

INTRODUCTION

Facial expressions provide important information to channel non-verbal communications. The human face contains not only information about the identity, gender and age of a person but also their cognitive activity, emotional states, personality and intensions. The ability to discriminate accurately between expressed emotions is an important part of interaction and communication with others. It is also useful in helping listeners to elicit the intended meaning of spoken words. Research conducted by Mehrabian (1968) revealed that although humans have verbal language, messages shown on the face provide extra information supplementing verbal communication. The author stated that 55% of effective face-to-face human communication depends on facial expressions, while only 45% relies on languages and non-verbal body gestures (such as goodbye, pointing, drooping the head and etc.).

Interestingly, humans can recognize the different facial expressions of an unfamiliar person and recognize a familiar person regardless of the person's facial expression. In the interaction between human and machines, a duality exists making it possible to automatically recognize faces and facial expressions in natural human-machine interfaces. These interfaces may be useful in behavioural science, robotic and medical science applications. For example, robotics for clinical practice could benefit from the ability to recognize facial expressions. Even though humans have acquired powerful capabilities of language, the role of facial expressions in communication remains substantial.

Here, we discuss the quantitative analysis of facial expression data using a collection of 3D face surface datasets. Each surface is recorded in an array of surface points in 3-dimensional space. Fiducial landmark points were selected based on craniofacial anthropometry (Kolar & Slater, 1997) and Facial Action Coding System (FACS) frameworks (Ekman & Friesen, 1978). Three-dimensional face data is preferred as it contains additional geometric data used to eliminate some of the intrinsic problems associated with 2D faces systems. Furthermore, 3D geometry of a face is invariant to changes in lighting and head pose conditions.

In this paper, we discuss quantitative analysis of facial expressions from a collection of 3D face surface dataset. Each 3D surface was annotated with the same set of chosen landmarks. The movement of landmark points on palpable features as well as non-palpable facial features are analysed according to the point motions. The spread and the variance of those landmarks with different subjects and facial expressions were studied and analysed. From the gathered information, we conduct facial expression analysis and recognition, and face recognition on the selected landmarks and dense surfaces.

Copyright © 2011, IGI Global. Copying or distributing in print or electronic forms without written permission of IGI Global is prohibited.

Motivation

Current face analysis and identification are primarily based on classifying faces in a set scenario often involving neutral expression and frontal face pose. Such scenarios make the process of identifying an individual a lot simpler. However, in a real environment, subjects do not limit or restrict their facial expressions, and current recognition systems will be confused by data variance in subspaces that make detecting and identifying an individual and their expressions very difficult.

In medical and clinical face applications, some of the research try to identify subtle changes in face associated with growth and ageing. Andresen et al. (2000) work compares the changes of mandible of children over time. Hutton (2004) used a statistical model to analyse a natural way of expressing growth changes with age. This technique is useful in identifying abnormal growth in faces. Simulating age changes can also be useful in the search for missing children. Hammond (2007) works on face shape modelling in dysmorphology.

Analysing facial actions, recognition emotions and synthesizing face shapes are common topics in face expression research nowadays. To develop robust and efficient applications, a face application should be able to deal with a large variety of face variations. As facial expression variation is known as the most difficult problem in face analysis and recognition, a novel framework is needed to address this problem.

Landmark-based facial analysis has been of interest to many face recognition researchers as the number of face datasets and the resolution of face images and 3D models increases. Fiducial landmarks aim at reducing high dimensionality problems. By using them, recognition computation may become faster and more efficient (Riopka & Boult, 2003; Phillips, Moon, Rizvi & Rauss, 2000). Landmarking also allow a more effective search within a face space. Precise landmarks are essential for effective recognition performance (Beumer, Bazen, & Veldhuis, 2005) and face analysis. This suggests that the placement of landmarks and their geometry should be meaningful to enable reliable face shape comparison. Hence, we proposed landmark selections on high expressions mobility. The following list the research questions to the issues in landmarking:

- Which landmark placements have maximum face and facial muscle motion information?
- Is it adequate to only use craniofacial landmarks?
- How are the facial, muscle-based, landmarks selected?
- Is the error between corresponding landmarks minimal when repeating similar landmarking processes on similar faces?

Copyright © 2011, IGI Global. Copying or distributing in print or electronic forms without written permission of IGI Global is prohibited.

LITERATURE IN BRIEF

Facial Expression Models

In the 20th century, many studies relating to facial expressions and inter-human communication have been carried out especially among psychologist and cognitive scientists can influence the meaning and generation of facial expressions. Evident results have shown that spontaneous facial actions are organised without being taught which be seen in the uniformity for expression patterns created by blind infants and children (Charlesworth & Kreutzer, 1973). Overall, the notion that certain fundamental expressions are innate has received robust support from cross-cultural research. Following the studies of a large number of literature and pre-literature societies, Ekman and Friesen (1971) reported that people of all races, including isolated tribes, are able to recognize facial expressions based on emotions, in particular anger, disgust, fear happiness, sadness and surprise. In later studies, this report may contradict in such that the recognition emotion-based facial expression does not automatically extend across races, for example a sincere smile and a sarcastic smile may be perceived differently by the Asians and the British. However, after further studies, the six basic emotions, which Ekman, Levenson, and Friensen (1983) claims to be universal across cultures and human ethnicities (Ekman, 1982; Levenson, Ekman, Heider & Friensen, 1992), became widely accepted as the emotion-based facial expressions. These facial expressions do not include other non emotion-based facial expressions such as winking, smiling sarcastically, anxiety expression and etc.

Cohn (2006) divided facial expression measurement approaches into judgement-based and sign-based methods. Judgement-based methods involve the interpretation of facial expressions in terms of predefined emotions and mental categories. Sign-based methods concern just facial motion and deformation, and are independent of any interpretation. Results are simply coded into visual classes. The judgement-based methods infer what underlies a displayed facial expression change.

The most commonly used expression descriptors in judgement-based approaches (Cohn, 2006) are emotion-based facial expressions. The different types of models for emotion-based facial expressions can be found in (Ekman, Sorenson, & Friesen, 1969; Plutchik, 1980; Russell, 1980). Ekman's emotion-based facial expressions are still limited and they do not include expressions of agreement, boredom, pain and sleepiness, which mean that it does not always display the expression that reflect a person's emotion (Ekman et al., 1983). Thus, these basic emotions may not be sufficient for an automated facial expression analysis system.

Plutchik (1980) extended the universal expressions by introducing an emotion wheel. He suggested eight primary emotions: acceptance, anger, participation,

Copyright © 2011, IGI Global. Copying or distributing in print or electronic forms without written permission of IGI Global is prohibited.

disgust, fear, joy, sadness, and surprise, and by mixing these primary emotions suggested twenty-four secondary emotions. For example, the combination of joy and acceptance produces love. Unfortunately, this theory is based only on the inner state of the person and similar to Ekman's basic emotions, may not also be sufficient to fully describe facial expressions (Valstar, 2008).

Russell (1980) proposed a systematic method of classifying all emotions within a two-dimensional space. Emotions ranging from sadness to happiness, and boredom to frantic excitement lie around two bipolar factors called valence and arousal. The emotions are incorporated with intensity and they can be correlated. Similar to prior emotion models, this theory also does not guaranteed to describe all facial expressions.

The aforementioned judgement-based approaches are based on feelings. In contrast, the Facial Action Coding System (FACS) model is independent of any feeling and interpretation. This framework associates facial expression changes with the actions of the facial muscles. Since FACS is based on facial muscles, it is suitable to describe all facial expressions regardless of whatever emotions the person has.

The generation of facial expressions is complex as it involves facial muscles and interaction between the muscles and the skull bone structures. All these components contribute to the different expressions and other changes of facial appearance caused by mastication, speech, yawning and so on. In a face, there are twenty-six main muscles. Muscles are made up of fibrous tissue, which produces movement by contraction or relaxation, either singly or in combination. Only limited range of movements make facial expressions (Faigan, 1990).

FACS Framework

The FACS was first proposed by (Ekman & Friesen, 1978) with an aim to explain and to measure the behaviour of facial muscles in creating facial expressions. The contraction of one or more muscles on the face is known as an Action Unit (AU). Action units describe specific small facial movements. There are twenty-eight AUs to describe facial expressions. Each facial expression is described by one AU or a combination of two or more AUs. An AU also contains a file-point scale intensity score of a facial expression (Ekman, Friensen & Hager, 2002). These score information does not convey any mental activity information or facial behaviour.

According to Lander (2000), AUs are easier to understand by those who do not have any knowledge of facial muscle movements. In the study of facial expressions, FACS framework is the most popular method used for analysing facial activities. There are more than 7000 different AUs combinations that have been derived (Scherer & Ekman, 1984) and some of them may produce similar face appearances. Table 1 shows the AU rules that represent emotions based facial expressions.

Copyright © 2011, IGI Global. Copying or distributing in print or electronic forms without written permission of IGI Global is prohibited.

Table 1. The description of AUs on Ekman's emotion-based expressions

Emotions	Action Units (AUs)
Happiness	6, 12, 25, 26
Sadness	1, 4, 6, 7, 11, 15, 17, 25, 26
Surprise	1, 2, 5, 26, 27
Anger	2, 4, 5, 7, 10, 17, 22, 23, 24, 25, 26, 27
Disgust	9, 10, 16, 17, 25, 26
Fear	1, 2, 4, 5, 20, 25, 26, 27

Facial Expression Analysis and Recognition Systems

The extensive literature on face recognition and facial expression recognition is discussed in Zhao, Chellappa, and Rosenfeld (2003) and Fasel and Luettin (2002). Most face recognition deals with recognition a person under minimal expression change and only works well with well-framed images with neutral expression. There are many successful methods that have been developed but none of these would work simultaneously for both face and facial expression recognition.

Chang, Bowyer and Flynn (2003) applied existing face recognition techniques to recognise a person in databases containing a set of different faces and facial expressions, which were taken over a time lapse. The results showed that the recognition rate without any expression was around 90%. However, when facial expressions were included, the recognition rate dropped in between 25% to 50%. Recent studies done by Givens, Beveridge, Draper and Bolme (2003) and Chang et al. (2003) reported that facial expression change is one of the most important factors affecting recognition.

There are a number of literature reviews that can be found on automatic recognition of facial expression (Samal & Iyergar, 1992; Fasel & Luettin, 2002; Suwa, Sugie & Fujimura, 1978; Pantic & Rothkrantz, 2000). Principle Component Analysis (PCA) can be used to model variation (Turk & Pentland, 1991) in facial recognition. It is the commonly used linear algebra technique that can address the total variation of data set efficiently. Tian, Kanade and Cohn (2005) listed two approaches that can be used to extract facial features for facial expression analysis: geometric feature-based methods and appearance-based methods. The geometric features are based on the shape (e.g. the curvature, saddle, valley, peak, colour, texture) and locations in terms of the 2D *(x-, y-)* or 3D *(x-, y-, z-)* coordinates of facial features of the corners of the eyes, the tip of the nose, the corners of the mouth and the chin. The appearance-based methods extract information by applying filters (such as Gabor wavelets) to images of either the whole face or sections of it. The extracted infor-

Copyright © 2011, IGI Global. Copying or distributing in print or electronic forms without written permission of IGI Global is prohibited.

mation from these approaches is represented in feature vectors. The feature vectors contain facial action information that can be used to analyse emotion-based facial expression and facial muscle actions (Pantic & Rothkrantz, 2000; Tian et al., 2005).

In recognising facial expressions, classifiers such as neutral networks (Tian, Kanade & Cohn, 2001; Tian, Kanade & Cohn, 2002), support vector machines (SVM) (Bartlett et al., 2001; Ford, 2002), statistical pattern recognition (Cohn, Zlochower, Lien & Kanade, 1999) or Bayesian network (Cohn et al., 2003) are commonly applied. A number of expression recognition systems use rule-based classification from facial action (Pantic & Rothkrantz, 2000; Cohn et al., 2001). This classification is based on the FACS framework, where AUs are recognised.

In our experiment, we used both approaches by firstly analysing facial expressions using landmark points (that is the geometric feature-based method) and then employed principle component analysis (PCA) to extract the overall appearance of the 3D face for recognition purposes.

Landmarking Reviews

Landmarks are defined as characteristic points that can be used to establish correspondence between different objects within populations of the same class (Dryden & Mardia, 1998). There are various synonyms for landmarks, such as points, nodes, vertices, anchor points, fiducial markers, model points, key points, etc. There are three basic groups of landmarks:

1. **Anatomical (traditional) landmarks:** Anatomical landmarks are points that have a unique identifiable place on the object for example, the corners of the eyes and the tip of the nose. Those points can be located easily regardless of the orientation of the object. The landmarks may be independent of any coordinate system or dependent on a particular orientation or a coordinate system. For example, he points at the corners of the eyes are independent of the position and the orientation of the face. Points on the mandible, such as the chin may rotate relative to the rest of the face as the jaw moves.

2. **Fuzzy landmarks (Mathematical landmarks):** Fuzzy landmarks are points corresponding to an average estimation of the location within the identifiable area on the object (Valstar, 2008; Wang, Pan & Wu, 2007). They can be points that are mathematically calculated and located on the object. As fuzzy landmarks are often located on featureless structure, there is a possibility of high placement error (Valstar, 2008). Fuzzy landmarks are usually used on smooth surfaces where there are insufficient anatomical landmarks (Lele & Richtsmeier, 2001). High curvature points or extremum points are the examples of fuzzy landmarks. Areas around the nose and eyebrows on a face have high

Copyright © 2011, IGI Global. Copying or distributing in print or electronic forms without written permission of IGI Global is prohibited.

curvature points and hence can be used as landmarks. The placement of fuzzy landmarks can be improved by taking the average of multiple landmarkings.

3. **Constructed landmarks (Pseudo landmarks):** Constructed landmarks are points on the object at positions defined using a combination of anatomical landmarks and geometric information. Constructed landmarks can be placed manually or computed automatically. For example, landmarks around the cheek areas are constructed using the location of two or more traditional landmarks. Midpoints between the two traditional landmarks are identified and their locations are recorded as a constructed landmark. The error in locating constructed landmarks depends on the error in the location of each of the traditional landmarks used in the construction (Lele & Richtsmeier, 2001).

The studies that use landmark data ensure that the selected landmarks are homologous. Homologous landmarks are those that share a common cause or descent. This means that each landmark placed on an object will have a corresponding landmark on another object. The choice of landmark points depends greatly on the study of interest and on the basis of scientific understanding of the object.

Landmarking are used in face registration, face recognition and facial expression analysis. In face registration, landmark points should be placed on prominent anatomical facial features and at extreme points so they can be used to coarsely align all faces together. The cited landmarks are often craniofacial landmarks, which are on the both corners of the eyes and mouth, the tip of the nose and the chin (Tao & Veldhuis, 2006; Hutton, 2004; Papatheodorou & Rueckert, 2005).

Besides using all the surface points or pixel data, a selection of landmarks can also be used in face recognition application (Goldstein, Harmon, & Lesk, 1971; Brunelli & Poggio, 1993; Craw, Costen, Kato & Akamatsu, 1999). Landmark-based recognition is performed in the same way as geometric recognition. For example, three-dimensional landmark positions can produce a simple polyhedral representation of a face, as illustrated in Figure 1 (b) from a dense surface point map of a face as shown in Figure 1 (a).

Landmark-based face recognition has been of interest to many face recognition researchers as the number of face data sets and the resolution of face images and 3D models increases. Fiducial landmarks aim to reduce high dimensionality problem. By using them, recognition computation may become faster and more efficient (Shi, Samal, & Marx, 2006; Phillips et al., 2000). Precise landmark selections are essential for effective face recognition performance (Riopka & Boult, 2003; Beumer et al., 2005). The selected landmarks are also similar to the craniofacial landmarks (Kaya & Kobayashi, 1971; Goldstein et al., 1971; Shi et al., 2006; Ferrario, Sforza, Pizzini, Vogel & Miani, 1993).

Copyright © 2011, IGI Global. Copying or distributing in print or electronic forms without written permission of IGI Global is prohibited.

Figure 1. (a) Three-dimensional polyhedral face shape (b) Polyhedral face shape based on a set of landmarks

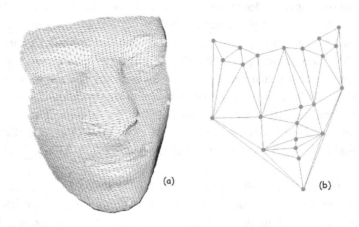

(a)   (b)

In facial expression analysis, the anatomy and physics of facial muscles is important (Ensotelos & Dong, 2008; Wang et al., 2007; Pighin, Hecker, Lischinski & Szeliski, 1998). Facial muscles movements correspond to the generation of different facial expression. Facial expression analysis and landmark-based expression recognition therefore needs landmarks that carry information about the expression movements. Landmark points are chosen to characterise actions of the different facial muscles. Similar to prior, the selected lamdmarks are craniofacial landmarks or at least around the craniofacial landmarks (Cohn et al., 1999; Essa & Pentland, 1997; Black & Yacoob, 1995; Pighin, Szeliski & Salesin, 1999; Terzopoulos & Waters, 1993). Blanz, Basso, Poggio and Vetter (2003) worked with landmarks placed at the bottom half of the face around the cheeks and mouth. However, these landmarks are manually drawn on the face of the subject.

In the study of facial expressions, more landmarks are required and they can be constructed on the basis of craniofacial landmarks as they are obvious and distinct to be identified by the human eyes, and also placed on mobile areas that contain high expression information. Unfortunately, most expression analysis applications have not thoroughly studied the process of placing landmarks or verifying that placements effectively or located on facial muscles.

Copyright © 2011, IGI Global. Copying or distributing in print or electronic forms without written permission of IGI Global is prohibited.

OUR APPROACH

Three-Dimensional Face Datasets

We acquired 3D face shapes from Imperial College London (Papatheodorou and Rueckert, 2005). The Imperial College's faces were captured using a VisionRT 3D camera system. Each of the raw face was pre-processed using rigid and non-rigid registration methods. The pre-processing step aims to regularise the surfaces and to correct flaws in the raw geometric data caused by hair, clothing boundaries and reconstruction errors. The steps included cropping face regions, removing holes and spikes and standardising the triangulated meshes to a set of corresponding vertices.

The subjects in the Imperial College London database were mostly students within an age range of 18-35 years. Each subject was acquired in several different head positions and three facial expression poses. The facial expressions were smiling, frowning and neutral. Each raw reconstructed face model has between 8,000 and 12,000 polygon points. In total, the face dataset has 57 subjects.

Landmark-Based Analysis Approaches

In the first part of the experiment, using the selected a number of landmarks, which are placed on both distinct features based on the craniofacial anthropometry landmark and on areas around those craniofacial features, we analysed the placement of the landmarks in terms of facial muscle motion based on FACS framework. In practice, the landmark points must be easy to identify and also mobile in the different facial expressions. Locating prominent facial features such as at the corners of the eyes and mouth, and the tip of the nose, would be easier, in comparison to identifying areas where no palpable features are visible and available. The areas around the forehead, cheek and mouth make an important contribution to facial expression analysis.

A set of craniofacial landmarks is used as the basis to construct landmarks on facial muscles. The most commonly used craniofacial landmarks are the corners of the eyes, the bridge of the nose, the tip of the nose, the corners of the mouth and the chin. Since we are dealing with 3D face surfaces, we have included features that are not distinct in 2D images but are seen on 3D face surfaces. They are the glabella, subnasal, the top and bottom of the eyes and the mouth. In total, we chose thirteen craniofacial landmarks.

From the selected craniofacial landmarks, we construct pseudo landmarks. The pseudo landmark positions were selected by analysing the rules of FACS. Mathematical formulae using a distance measure were used to locate the constructed landmarks. The pseudo landmarks are not clear anatomically because they are placed on AU

Copyright © 2011, IGI Global. Copying or distributing in print or electronic forms without written permission of IGI Global is prohibited.

areas around the eyebrows and eyes, the cheeks and the mouth. These areas have no palpable features, but linearly-based pseudo landmarks can be computed on the basis of the selected craniofacial landmarks. For example, one pseudo landmark on the cheek is located by drawing a vertical line through the middle of the eyes to meet the horizontal line at the subnasal level (see landmark 30 and 31). These landmark points are constructed in the neutral expression face surfaces. They will move relative to the craniofacial basis with expression changes. We selected twenty pseudo landmarks that incorporate the AU rules. In total, we have selected thirty-three landmark points (as shown in Figure 2). Each of the landmarks is manually placed on each of the 3D face surfaces.

The variation of the gathered points were statistically analysed and the facial appearance were concluded based on the geometric variation and facial expression variation. The geometric variation includes positional variation of facial features. The inclusion of different genders and races may also increases geometric variation. The facial expression variation shows the dispersion of the landmarks across the expression data.

The experiment was designed to determine the best placement of landmarks for distinguishing the different facial expressions. Identifying landmarks that are mobile in facial muscle movements is a good strategy for characterising expressions. Mobility of the different landmark points is also an important factor in their ability to discriminate expression information. The discrimination power of landmarks is also tested in the context of face recognition experiment.

METHODS AND RESULTS

Experiment 1

We randomly asked ten volunteers to manually place the landmarks on the same face surfaces. This is to analyse the simplicity to locate the chosen landmarks. The landmarking consistency result in the landmarking showed about 0.97mm (which is based on the precision measure in standard deviation from the mean) given the resolution of each surface of 5090 mesh points. All the volunteers did the landmarking without having to repeat the landmarking process due to error in placing the landmark points. When asked about the difficulty of identifying the pseudo landmarks, all the test volunteers said that the landmarks were easy to locate.

Copyright © 2011, IGI Global. Copying or distributing in print or electronic forms without written permission of IGI Global is prohibited.

Figure 2. The proposed selected landmarks

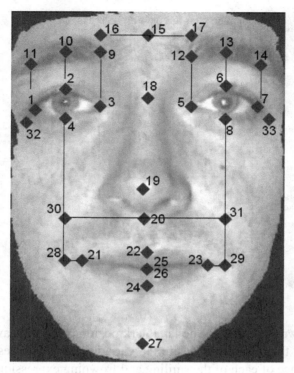

Experiment 2

Based on the chosen thirty-three landmarks, the next experiment is to test the variations of those landmark points across the different facial expressions. The aim is to study the amount of expression information conveyed by each landmark point.

Figure 3 illustrates the movement of the *(x-, y-, z)* landmarks across the different facial expressions. The numbers represent the landmark's numbering in sequence and the different coloured symbols signify the different types of expressions. All of the thirty-three landmarks are weighted against the overall mean. The spread of landmarks across expressions can also be viewed in a 2-dimensional space as shown in Figure 4.

The smiling, neutral and frowning expressions were analysed against the overall mean expressions. The placements of the craniofacial and pseudo landmarks are analysed using positional variance. The variation of landmarks is compared to the neural face. We used the variance measure to identify those points or areas that do not contribute to expressions. The dispersion of the thirty-three landmarks was measured statistically across all expressions of the fifty subjects. The variance for

Copyright © 2011, IGI Global. Copying or distributing in print or electronic forms without written permission of IGI Global is prohibited.

Figure 3. The spread of landmarks in 3-dimensional space

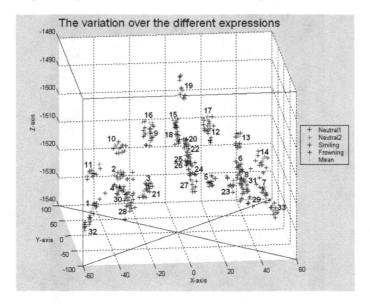

each landmark was computed. The landmark positions are then averaged and the mean is used as the origin to measure the variation across expressions. Figure 5 shows the variance of each of the smiling and frowning expression. It can be seen that the high variances are on landmark 21 and landmark 23 which are placed on both corners of the mouth.

Figure 6 illustrates the landmark variance across all expressions against neutral expression. The bar represents the variance of each landmark point on neutral faces, and the upper and lower limits are the variances for smiling and frowning expressions. High variance of facial feature changes can be seen on areas around the mouth and cheeks (landmark 21 to landmark 29). Landmarks around the eyes and eyebrows also show significant change of expressions (see landmark 1 to landmark 14). The variance can also be sorted in an increasing order as shown in Figure 7.

From the analysis of expressions, we have identified two main types of variations: geometric variation and facial expression variation. The geometric variation includes positional variation of facial features. The inclusion of different genders and races increases geometric variation. One of the results of the geometric variation show that Chinese faces have a smaller nose and shorter nose bridge in comparison to Caucasian faces.

Copyright © 2011, IGI Global. Copying or distributing in print or electronic forms without written permission of IGI Global is prohibited.

Figure 4. The spread of landmarks viewed in 2-dimensional

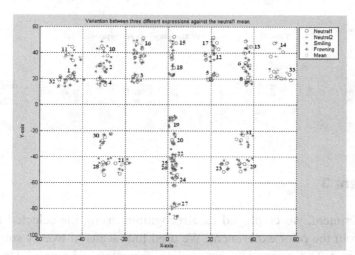

Facial expression variation is illustrated in Figure 8. It illustrates the dispersion of the landmarks across the expression data particularly around the mouth. Here, there is an obvious variation between smiling and frowning.

Not all the craniofacial and pseudo landmarks contain high expression information. The inside corner of the left and right eyes (landmark 3 and landmark 5) and the tip of the nose (landmark 19) have the least positional change of expression variance and the variances are as shown in Figure 7.

Figure 5. Facial expression variances

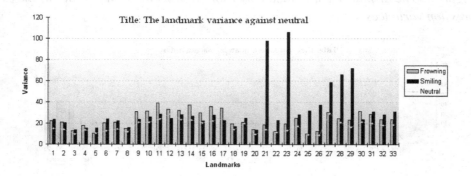

Copyright © 2011, IGI Global. Copying or distributing in print or electronic forms without written permission of IGI Global is prohibited.

Figure 6. The variance of facial expressions against neutral faces

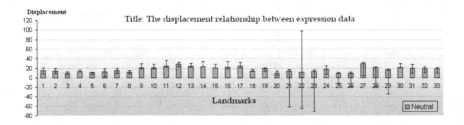

Experiment 3

In this experiment, we employed face recognition using the selected landmarks extracted from the prior experiment. We used four scans of twenty subjects from the face dataset. The expressions are smiling, frowning and neutral. Here, we discard one expression for testing and the remaining faces are used for training. The experiment was divided into two groups – Group 1 used the whole 5090 points on the surface and Group 2 used the thirty-three landmark points (see Figure 9). We employed PCA and the Euclidean distance measurement for recognition purposes.

Table 2 and Table 3 show the recognition results for Group 1 and Group 2. Each recognition probe was tested with 2 and 19 eigenvectors. In sub-experiment 1, the unseen neutral face data is used as the query set while the in the second sub-experiment, a frowning face is used as the query data and finally the third sub-experiment used smiling faces. It is shown that the placement of landmarks can influence the recognition rate.

Figure 7. The displacement of landmarks sorted in an increasing order of the expression variances

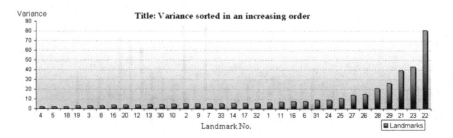

Copyright © 2011, IGI Global. Copying or distributing in print or electronic forms without written permission of IGI Global is prohibited.

Figure 8. The spread of mean landmarks against smiling and frowning landmarks in x-y plane

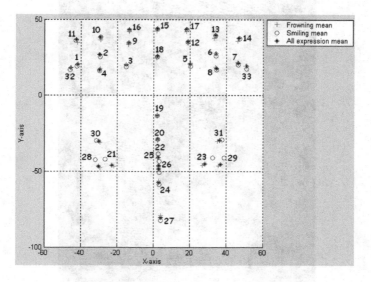

DISCUSSIONS AND CONCLUSION

These experiments were designed to determine the best placement of landmarks for distinguishing different facial expressions. They showed that there is a noticeable difference in the displacement of landmarks under different expressions. The results from the statistical analysis are as follows:

1. There are significant variations in some landmark positions due to facial expressions. The corners of the mouths and some of the pseudo landmarks are highly mobile and could have significant discriminant power in recognising expressions.
2. The tip of the nose, the inside corners of the eyes and the bottom eyes do not contribute much to the facial expressions. This could be due to the minimal facial muscle activity around the area. As for the tip of the nose, there is no facial muscle available. The variation is caused by the neighbouring facial muscles and the pulling of the skin.
3. Facial expressions are similar for all individuals. This is shown by the fact that the calculated expression mean is quite close to the overall neutral mean.
4. Smiling and frowning can be easily distinguished by landmark movements. Around the mouth areas, especially at both corners, the landmarks would move up when smiling and move down when frowning.

Copyright © 2011, IGI Global. Copying or distributing in print or electronic forms without written permission of IGI Global is prohibited.

Figure 9. Landmark points on pre-processed 3D face surface

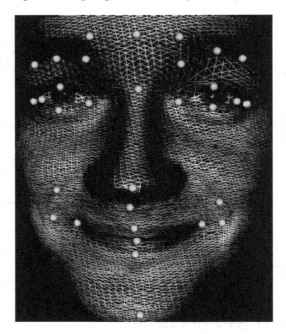

Identifying landmarks that are mobile in facial muscle movements is a good strategy for characterising facial expressions. Mobility of the different landmark points can be an important factor in their ability to discriminate different expressions. This may be useful to analyse the expressions created by people with cerebral palsy, autism, brainstem stroke, traumatic brain injury, schizophrenia and other disorders. And this could assist clinical diagnosis.

Table 2. Recognition rate results for Group 1 (5090 landmark points)

Eigenvectors	Sub-experiment 1	Sub-experiment 2	Sub-experiment 3
2	90.00%	10.00%	10.00%
19	100.00%	10.00%	25.00%

Table 3. Recognition rate results for Group 2 (33 landmark points)

Eigenvectors	Sub-experiment 1	Sub-experiment 2	Sub-experiment 3
2	65.00%	5.00%	50.00%
19	95.00%	10.00%	65.00%

Copyright © 2011, IGI Global. Copying or distributing in print or electronic forms without written permission of IGI Global is prohibited.

To conclude, we investigated both dense surface point models and the use of a small set of anatomical landmarks that best describe facial expression using the FACS and craniofacial anthropometry frameworks. We found that with good placement of landmarks, it is possible to distinguish different facial expressions. We demonstrated that landmarks should optimally be placed in particular regions such as the cheeks and eyebrows. We had also investigated face recognition using landmarks. We found that landmark-based recognition gave high recognition performance only on faces with very high expression changes, for example smiling faces.

REFERENCES

Andresen, P. R., Bookstein, F. L., Conradsen, K., Ersbll, B. K., Marsh, J. L., & Kreiborg, S. (2000). Surface-bounded growth modeling applied to human mandibles. *IEEE Transactions on Medical Imaging, 19*(11), 1053–1063. doi:10.1109/42.896780

Bartlett, M., Braathen, B., Littlewort, G. F., Hershey, J., Fasel, I., & Marks, T. … Movellan, J. R. (2001). *Automatic analysis of spontaneous facial behaviour: A final project report*. (Technical Report INC-MPLab-TR-2001.08), Machine Perception Lab, University of California.

Beumer, G., Bazen, A., & Veldhuis, R. (2005). *On the accuracy of ears in face recognition and the importance of reliable registration*. IEEE Benelux Signal Processing Symposium, (pp. 85–88).

Black, M. J., & Yacoob, Y. (1995). Recognizing facial expressions in image sequences using local parameterized models of image motion. *International Journal of Computer Vision, 25*(1), 23–48. doi:10.1023/A:1007977618277

Blanz, V., Basso, C., Poggio, T., & Vetter, T. (2003). Reanimating faces in images and video. *Annual Conference of the European Association for Computer Graphics, 22*(3), 641–650.

Brunelli, R., & Poggio, T. (1993). Face recognition: Features versus templates. *IEEE Transactions on Pattern Analysis and Machine Intelligence, 15*(10), 1042–1052. doi:10.1109/34.254061

Chang, K., Bowyer, K., & Flynn, P. (2003). *Face recognition using 2d and 3d facial data*. Workshop on Multimodal User Authentication, (pp. 25–32).

Charlesworth, W. R., & Kreutzer, M. A. (1973). *Facial expression of infants and children. Darwin and facial expression: A century of research in review*. New York, NY: Academic.

Copyright © 2011, IGI Global. Copying or distributing in print or electronic forms without written permission of IGI Global is prohibited.

Cohn, J. (2006). *Foundations of human computing: Facial expression and emotion.* ACM International Conference on Multimodal Interfaces, 1, 610–616.

Cohn, J., Kanade, T., Moriyama, T., Ambadar, Z., Xiao, J., Gao, J., & Imamura, H. (2001). *A comparative study of alternative facs coding algorithms.* (Technical Report CMU-RI-TR-02-06), Robotics Institute Carnegie Mellon University.

Cohn, J., Zlochower, A. J., Lien, J. J., & Kanade, T. (1999). Automated face analysis by feature point tracking has high concurrent validity with manual facs coding. *Psychophysiology, 36,* 35–43. doi:10.1017/S0048577299971184

Craw, I., Costen, N., Kato, T., & Akamatsu, S. (1999). How should we represent faces for automatic recognition? *IEEE Transactions on Pattern Analysis and Machine Intelligence, 21*(8), 725–736. doi:10.1109/34.784286

Dryden, I. L., & Mardia, K. V. (1998). *Statistical shape analysis.* John Wiley and Sons.

Ekman, P. (1982). *Emotion in the human face.* Cambridge University Press.

Ekman, P., Friensen, W. V., & Hager, J. C. (2002). *Facial action coding system: A human face.* Salt Lake City.

Ekman, P., & Friesen, W. V. (1971). Constants across cultures in the face and emotion. *Journal of Personality and Social Psychology, 17,* 124–129. doi:10.1037/h0030377

Ekman, P., & Friesen, W. V. (1978). *Facial action coding system: A technique for the measurement of facial movement.* Palo Alto, CA: Consulting Psychologists Press.

Ekman, P., Levenson, R. W., & Friensen, W. V. (1983). Autonomic nervous system activity distinguishes among emotions. *Science, 221,* 1208–1210. doi:10.1126/science.6612338

Ekman, P., Sorenson, E. R., & Friesen, W. V. (1969). Pan-cultural elements in facial emotion. *Science, 164,* 86–88. doi:10.1126/science.164.3875.86

Ensotelos, N., & Dong, F. (2008). Building highly realistic facial modeling and animation: A survey. *The Visual Computer, 24*(1), 13–30. doi:10.1007/s00371-007-0175-y

Essa, I. A., & Pentland, A. P. (1997). Coding analysis interpretation and recognition of facial expressions. *IEEE Transactions on Pattern Analysis and Machine Intelligence, 19*(7), 757–763. doi:10.1109/34.598232

Faigan, G. (1990). *The artist's guide to facial expressions.* Watson-Guphill Publications.

Copyright © 2011, IGI Global. Copying or distributing in print or electronic forms without written permission of IGI Global is prohibited.

Fasel, B., & Luettin, J. (2002). *Automatic facial expression analysis: A survey.* (IDIAP Research Report, 99-19).

Ferrario, V. F., Sforza, C., Pizzini, G., Vogel, G., & Miani, A. (1993). Sexual dimorphism in the human face assessed by Euclidean distance matrix analysis. *Journal of Anatomy, 183,* 593–600.

Ford, G. (2002). *Fully automatic coding of basic expressions from video.* (Technical Report INC-MPLab-TR-2002.03), Machine Perception Lab, University of California.

Givens, G., Beveridge, R., Draper, B., & Bolme, D. (2003). *A statistical assessment of subject factors in the PCA recognition of human faces.* Workshop on Statistical Analysis in Computer Vision.

Goldstein, A. J., Harmon, L. D., & Lesk, A. B. (1971). Identification of human faces. *Proceedings of the IEEE, 59*(5), 748–760. doi:10.1109/PROC.1971.8254

Hammond, P. (2007). The use of 3D face shape modelling in dysmorphology. *Journal of Archives of Disease in Childhood, 93,* 1120–1126.

Hutton, T. (2004). *Dense surface models of the human faces.* Unpublished doctoral dissertation, University College London.

Kaya, Y., & Kobayashi, K. (1971). *A basis study on human face recognition.* Orlando, FL: Academic Press.

Kolar, J. C., & Salter, E. M. (1997). *Craniofacial anthropometry: Practical measurement of the head and face for clinical, surgical and research use.* Charles C Thomas Publisher.

Lander, J. (2000). Flex your facial muscles. *gamasurtra.com.* Retrieved from http://www.gamasutra.com/features/20000414/lander_pfv.htm

Lele, S. R., & Richtsmeier, J. T. (2001). *An invariant approach to statistical analysis of shape, interdisciplinary statistics.* Chapmand and Hall/CRC Press.

Levenson, R. W., Ekman, P., Heider, K., & Friensen, W. V. (1992). Emotion and autonomic nervous system activity in the Minangkabau of West Sumatra. *Journal of Personality and Social Psychology, 62,* 972–988. doi:10.1037/0022-3514.62.6.972

Mehrabian, A. (1968). Communication without words. *Psychology Today, 2*(4), 53–56.

Pantic, M., & Rothkrantz, J. M. L. (2000). Expert system for automatic analysis of facial expression. *Image and Vision Computing Journal, 18*(11), 881–905. doi:10.1016/S0262-8856(00)00034-2

Copyright © 2011, IGI Global. Copying or distributing in print or electronic forms without written permission of IGI Global is prohibited.

Papatheodorou, T., & Rueckert, D. (2005). *Evaluation of 3D face recognition using registration and PCA.* International Conference on Audio and Video-based Biometric Person Authentication, (pp. 35-46).

Phillips, P. J., Moon, H., Rizvi, S. A., & Rauss, P. J. (2000). The feret evaluation methodology for face recognition algorithms. *IEEE Transactions on Pattern Analysis and Machine Intelligence, 22*(10), 1090–1104. doi:10.1109/34.879790

Pighin, F., Hecker, J., Lischinski, D., & Szeliski, R. (1998). *Synthesizing realistic facial expressions from photographs. SIGGRAPH Computer graphics* (pp. 75–84). Orlando, FL: ACM Press.

Pighin, F., Szeliski, R., & Salesin, D. (1999). Resynthesizing facial animation through 3D model-based tracking. *IEEE International Conference on Computer Vision, 1*, 143–150.

Plutchik, R. (1980). *Emotion: A psychoevolutionary synthesis.* New York, NY: Harper and Row.

Riopka, T., & Boult, T. (2003). *The eyes have it.* ACM SINGMM Multimedia Biometrics Methods and Applications Workshop, (pp. 9–16).

Russell, J. (1980). A circumplex model of effect. *Journal of Personality and Social Psychology, 39*, 1161–1178. doi:10.1037/h0077714

Samal, A., & Iyergar, P. A. (1992). Automatic recognition and analysis of human faces and facial expressions: A survey. *Pattern Recognition, 25*(1), 102–141. doi:10.1016/0031-3203(92)90007-6

Scherer, R., & Ekman, P. (1984). *Approaches to emotion.* Hillsdale, NJ: Lawrence Erlbaum Associates.

Shi, J., Samal, A., & Marx, D. (2006). How effective are landmarks and their geometry for face recognition? *Computer Vision and Image Understanding, 102*, 117–133. doi:10.1016/j.cviu.2005.10.002

Suwa, M., Sugie, N., & Fujimura, K. (1978). *A preliminary note on pattern recognition of human emotional expression.* International Joint Conference on Pattern Recognition, (pp. 408–410).

Tao, Q., & Veldhuis, R. N. J. (2006). *Verifying a user in a personal face space.* Conference on Control, Automation, Robotics and Vision.

Copyright © 2011, IGI Global. Copying or distributing in print or electronic forms without written permission of IGI Global is prohibited.

Terzopoulos, D., & Waters, K. (1993). Analysis and synthesis of facial image sequences using physical and anatomical models. *IEEE Transactions on Pattern Analysis and Machine Intelligence*, *15*(6), 569–579. doi:10.1109/34.216726

Tian, Y. L., Kanade, T., & Cohn, J. (2001). Recognising action units for facial expression analysis. *IEEE Transactions on Pattern Analysis and Machine Intelligence*, *23*(2), 1–19. doi:10.1109/34.908962

Tian, Y. L., Kanade, T., & Cohn, J. (2002). *Evaluation of Gabor-wavelet-based facial action unit recognition in image sequences of increasing complexity*. IEEE International Conference on Automatic Face and Gesture Recognition.

Tian, Y. L., Kanade, T., & Cohn, J. (2005). Facial expression analysis. In *Springer handbook of face recognition*.

Turk, M., & Pentland, A. (1991). Eigenfaces for recognition. *Journal of Cognitive Neuroscience*, *1*(3), 71–86. doi:10.1162/jocn.1991.3.1.71

Valstar, M. F. (2008). *Timing is everything, a spatio-temporal approach to the analysis of facial action*. Unpublished doctoral dissertation, Imperial College London.

Wang, Y., Pan, G., & Wu, Z. (2007). *3D face recognition in the presence of expression: A guidance-based constraint deformation approach*. IEEE Conference on Computer Vision and Pattern Recognition.

Zhao, W., Chellappa, R., & Rosenfeld, A. (2003). Face recognition: A literature survey. *IEEE Transactions on Pattern Analysis and Machine Intelligence*, *24*(1).

ADDITIONAL READING

Belhumeur, P. N., Hespanha, J. P., & Kriegman, D. J. (1997). Eigenfaces vs fisherfaces: recognition using class specific linear projection. *IEEE Transactions on Pattern Analysis and Machine Intelligence*, *19*(7), 711–720. doi:10.1109/34.598228

Besl, P. J., & McKay, N. D. (1992). A method for registration of 3d shapes. *IEEE Transactions on Pattern Analysis and Machine Intelligence*, *14*(2), 239–256. doi:10.1109/34.121791

Blanz, V., Romdhani, S., & Vetter, T. (2002). Face identification across different poses and illuminations with a 3d morphable model. In Conference on *Automatic Face and Gesture Recognition*, 202–207.

Copyright © 2011, IGI Global. Copying or distributing in print or electronic forms without written permission of IGI Global is prohibited.

Blanz, V., & Vetter, T. (1999). A morphable model for the synthesis of 3d faces. In *ACM SIGGRAPH*, 187–194.

Bookstein, F. L. (1989). Principle warps: thin-plate splines and the decomposition of deformation. *IEEE Transactions on Pattern Analysis and Machine Intelligence*, *11*(6), 567–585. doi:10.1109/34.24792

Bronstein, A., Bronstein, M., & Kimmel, R. (2005). Three-dimensional face recognition. *International Journal of Computer Vision*, *64*, 5–30. doi:10.1007/s11263-005-1085-y

Cohen, Sebe, N., Cozman, F., Cirelo, M., & Huang, T. (2003). Coding, analysis, interpretation and recognition of facial expressions. *Journal of Computer Vision and Image Understanding Special Issue on Face Recognition.*

Cootes, T., & Lanitis, A. (2004). *Statistical models of appearance for computer vision. Technical Report*. Draft.

Cootes, T., Taylor, C., Cooper, D., & Graham, J. (1998). Active appearance models. *European Conference on Computer Vision*, 484–498.

Cootes, T., Taylor, C. J., Cooper, D. H., & Graham, J. (1995). Active shape models - their training and application. *Computer Vision and Image Understanding*, *61*(1), 38–59. doi:10.1006/cviu.1995.1004

Farkas, L. G. (1994). Anthropometry of the head and face. Raven Press, New York, 2 edition.

Farkas, L. G., Hajnis, K., & Posnick, J. C. (1993). Anthropometric and anthroposcopic findings of the nasal and facial regions in cleft patients before and after primary lip and palate repair. *The Cleft Palate-Craniofacial Journal*, *30*, 1–12. doi:10.1597/1545-1569(1993)030<0001:AAAFOT>2.3.CO;2

Gauthier, I., & Logothetis, N. (2000). Is face recognition so unique after all? *Journal of Cognitive Neuropsychology*, *17*, 125–142. doi:10.1080/026432900380535

Kitani, E. C., Thomaz, C. E., & Gillies, D. F. (2006). A statistical discriminant model for face interpretation and reconstruction. *Brazilian Symposium on Computer Graphics and Image Processing*, 247–254.

Kolar, J.C. & Salter, E.M.(1997). Craniofacial anthropometry: practical measurement of the head and face for clinical, surgical and research use: Charles C Thomas Publisher.

Copyright © 2011, IGI Global. Copying or distributing in print or electronic forms without written permission of IGI Global is prohibited.

Kolda, T.G. & Bader, B.W.(2008). Tensor decompositions and applications. to be appeared in SIAM Review.

Minoi, J. L. (2009). *Geometric expression invariant 3D face recognition using statistical discriminant models*, PhD Thesis Imperial College, UK

Minoi, J. L., Amin, S. H., Thomaz, C. E., & Gillies, D. F. (2008). Synthesizing Realistic Expressions in 3D Face Data Sets, *2nd IEEE International Conference on Biometrics - Theory, Applications and Systems (BTAS 2008), IEEE*, 253-258.

Minoi, J. L., & Gillies, D. F. (2007). 3d facial expression analysis and deformation. *Symposium on Applied Perception in Graphics and visualization*, 138–138, Tubigen, Germany: ACM.

Minoi, J. L., & Gillies, D. F. (2008). Sub-tensor decomposition for expression variant 3d face recognition. *IEEE International Conference on Geometric Modeling and Imaging*, 108–113.

O'Toole, A., Price, T., Vetter, T., Bartlett, J., & Blanz, V. (1999). Three-dimensional shape and two-dimensional surface textures of human faces: The role of averages in attractiveness and age. *Image and Vision Computing Journal*, *18*(1), 9–19.

Papatheodorou, T. (n.d.) *3d face recognition using rigid and non-rigid registration*. PhD Thesis, Imperial College.

Thomaz, C. E., Kitani, E. C., & Gillies, D. F. (2006). A maximum uncertainty lda-based approach for limited size problems - with applications to face recognition. [September.]. *Journal of the Brazilian Computer Society*, *12*(2), 7–18. doi:10.1007/BF03192391

Yin, L., Wei, X., Longo, P., & Bhuvanesh, A. (2006). Analyzing facial expressions using intensity-variant 3d data for human computer interaction. *International Conference on Pattern Recognition*, 1248–1251.

Copyright © 2011, IGI Global. Copying or distributing in print or electronic forms without written permission of IGI Global is prohibited.

Chapter 9
The Role of Augmented E-Learning Systems for Enhancing Pro-Social Behaviour in Socially Impaired Individuals

Jonathan Bishop
Glamorgan Blended Learning Ltd, UK

ABSTRACT

E-learning systems generally rely on good visual and cognitive abilities, making them suitable for individuals with good levels of intelligence in these areas. A group of such individuals are those with non-systemising impairments (NSIs), such as people with autism spectrum conditions (ASCs). These individuals could benefit greatly from technology that allows them to use their abilities to overcome their impairments in social and emotional functioning in order to develop pro-social behaviours. Existing systems such as PARLE and MindReading are discussed, and a new one, the Visual Ontological Imitation System (VOIS), is proposed and discussed. This chapter details an investigation into the acceptability of these systems by those working in social work and advocacy. The study found that VOIS would be well received, although dependency on assistive technology and its impact on how others view NSIs still need to be addressed by society and its institutions.

DOI: 10.4018/978-1-60960-541-4.ch009

Copyright ©2011, IGI Global. Copying or distributing in print or electronic forms without written permission of IGI Global is prohibited.

INTRODUCTION

E-learning systems have formed part of visions of a deschooled, 'wired' society where the full potential of learners is realised (Buckingham, 2002). In fact, e-learning now accounts for 85 percent of the training provided in some organisations (Ettinger, Holton, & Blass, 2006). Much of this technology relies on good visual and cognitive abilities making it suitable to individuals with strengths in these areas. There has been an advance of augmented e-learning systems, which attempt to enhance the learners' capabilities, since the beginning of the 21st century. One of these, PARLE, described by Bishop (2003) will be discussed later in this chapter, but there are others that have come about since then, such as that proposed by Kaliouby, Picard, and Baron-Cohen (2006). Such technologies are often not only augmented in that they enhance human capabilities, but also can be considered to be unified communication (UC) systems as they are often multimodal, using voice, text and video for example, to reduce human difficulties with communication (Dewing, 2009). According to Dewing (2009) these UC systems are attractive to organisations wanting to improve communications, but as much as 55 per cent of decision-makers with responsibility for UC said that "there is confusion about the value of UC." There appears to be value in such systems for individuals with strengths in visual communications, who may be deficit in other aspects of their abilities, such as in relating to others socially and empathetically. Such individuals can be considered to have non-systemising impairments (NSIs), which consist of a range of documented conditions that medical and educational professionals have described in detail. The Diagnostic and Statistical Manual of Mental Disorders has classified one group of NSIs, namely Autism Spectrum Conditions (ASCs), as Autism Disorder and Asperger Syndrome (AS). Both these NSIs are diagnosable according to DSM-IV if the individual has qualitative impairments in social interaction and restricted repetitive & stereotyped patterns of behaviour, interests and activities. The later, AS, differs in that it is also a requirement for the individual to show no clinically significant general delay in language and no clinically significant delay in the development of age-appropriate self-help skills, non-social adaptive behaviour and curiosity about the environment in childhood. An ASC can be seen to be a condition where on receiving a social or emotional stimulus the individual with this particular NSI has difficulty in utilising the information and whose mind may not be able to deal with large amounts of these types of stimuli due to deficits in response flexibility. Response flexibility in this context refers to the ability of an individual to shift response strategies or patterns with a change in environmental contingencies (Ragozzino, 2007). Another group of NSIs are Emotional-Behavioural Conditions (EBCs), which are characterised by the individual generating excessive emotional and physical stimuli above the normal amount a typical person is able

Copyright © 2011, IGI Global. Copying or distributing in print or electronic forms without written permission of IGI Global is prohibited.

to deal with causing response inflexibility. The ASCs will be explored primarily in this chapter and the role of augmented e-learning systems using unified communications in assisting individuals with such NSIs will be explored in detail. There is a potential role for affordable UC systems such as these in the education marketplace as the adoption of the technologies grows and prices come down. Dewing (2009) estimates that UC market across North America, Europe, and Asia Pacific will have a compound annual growth rate (CAGR) of 35.9% through 2015, growing from $1.2 billion in 2008 to $14.5 billion.

Contextualising Non-Systemising Impairments

Prevalence of autism and related ASCs is substantially greater than previously recognised, with 1 per cent of the child population having an NSI in the form of autism and it is recommended that services in health, education, and social care will need to recognise the needs of children with such conditions (Baird et al., 2006). It is well known that NSIs such as Asperger Syndrome score average to above average on intelligence quotient (IQ) tests (Williams, 1995). This suggests that intelligence is an area that should be investigated in relation to NSIs and can shape the way augmented e-learning systems can be designed to assist people with such impairments.

Wheelwright et al. (2006) discussed how measuring the empathising and systemising abilities of individuals is predictive of their ASC. The study found that empathising is largely but not completely independent of systemising and that the weak but significant negative correlation may indicate a trade-off between them. It also concluded that ASCs involve impaired empathising alongside intact or superior systemising. The study further suggested that the basis of these dimensions should be investigated, something that will be addressed by this chapter. This research appears to be saying that individuals with ASCs while appearing intelligent on measures to do with modelling systems and concepts also appear less intelligent with regards to dealing with social and emotional contact with others. This view of NSI individuals being 'differently-abled' contrasts with the medical model, where authors such Bushwick (2001) argue that individuals with ASCs are abnormal.

Gardner (1983) explored the possibility of there being multiple intelligences. While social and emotional intelligence were not among his identified intelligences, which are the areas in which people with autism appear to be deficit, his theory did include logical-mathematical and spatial intelligence, essential for systemising, where people with ASCs appear to be strong. Nardi (2001) argues that spatial intelligence is linked to visual ability indicating that visual-spatial intelligence includes seeing visual images of all kinds and carrying out tasks such as map navigation. Pease and Pease (1998) have suggested that men are stronger in this area than women, which appears to be supported by Baron-Cohen's (2002) view of autism as an ex-

Copyright © 2011, IGI Global. Copying or distributing in print or electronic forms without written permission of IGI Global is prohibited.

treme male brain (EMB) phenomenon if the Systemising Quotient is a measure of cognitive and spatial intelligence. First-hand accounts from people with ASCs have shown that they have high visual and olfactory ability (Grandin, 1995). A study by Westervelt, Ruffolo, and Tremont (2005) found a strong correlation between the ability to perform mental tasks and olfactory ability, suggesting that an individual that has good olfactory ability may also have strong cognitive intelligence, creating a strong link between these in addition to the strong link between visual ability and spatial intelligence identified by Nardi (2001).

If the Systemising Quotient is a measure of cognitive and spatial intelligence then it might be expected that the Empathising Quotient is a measure of social and emotional intelligence. This would support the work of Pease & Pease (1998) arguing that the typical woman has greater social abilities than men, which concurs with the EMB theory of Baron-Cohen (2002) that NSI individuals with autism have less social ability than the average person.

A study by Jabbi, Swart, and Keysers (2007) showed a strong link between the perception of positive and negative emotions and gustatory perception, suggesting that an individual with effective emotional intelligence also has good gustatory ability. Individuals with ASCs are known to have extreme emotional reactions to different tastes (Frith, 1991), suggesting they are weaker in gustatory ability and emotional intelligence.

A further relevant intelligence explored by Gardner (1983) was bodily-kinaesthetic intelligence. It is well known that individuals with ASCs have a high tolerance of pain and other reduced sensitivity (Siegel, 2003) and often have difficulties with the motor skills involved in writing in addition to having an unusual way of walking along with compulsive finger, hand, arm and leg movements (Aquilla, Yack, & Sutton, 2005), suggesting a difference in physical-kinaesthetic intelligence to typical individuals.

Taking this into account with Bishop's (2007) idea of there being five cognitions that impact on ones behavior, it suggests that these five intelligences shapes our ability to create cognitions and store and access them in our memory. The cognitions of 'belief' and 'value' are probably stores in 'declarative memory' and 'goals' and 'plans' in 'procedural memory'. Where NSIs may have difficulty is with interests, which the author believes might be stored in a separate memory bank which he calls 'dunbar memory'. This is named after Robin Dunbar, a British anthropologist who hypothesised that people can only hold in memory 150 people at a time. It may be that NSIs with an ASC have difficulty access this type of memory or that it is smaller in size than for NTs.

Copyright © 2011, IGI Global. Copying or distributing in print or electronic forms without written permission of IGI Global is prohibited.

Emotion and Idiom Recognition Difficulties in NSI Individuals

People with an Autism Spectrum Conditions tend to have literal interpretations of what others say to them (Attwood, 1998). For example, they may interpret the statement 'I could die for a cup of tea' as an extreme thing for someone to do to quench their thirst. This can cause great difficulties in social situations where such idioms are frequently used, making the individual feel stupid and socially inadequate.

A related difficulty for individuals with ASC is an inability to adequately respond to closed-ended questions or statements. They may interpret a comment such as 'it's nice weather today' as a statement of fact and not as an invitation to engage in casual conversation. In such situations, the individual usually responds with single-word answers and may even disagree with the statement without understanding that this could be offensive.

In human-to-human communication, emotions are communicated mainly through facial expressions, bodily gestures and the tone in which something is said. Socially impaired individuals can feel excluded from social situations through the inability to recognise, interpret or respond to these various affects.

A study by Klin, Jones, Schultz, Volkmar, and Cohen (2002) found that individuals with ASCs focus twice as much attention on the mouths and bodies of people as on eyes in social situations. The study also found that when those with ASCs concentrated on the eyes of others they were not able to interpret the affect being communicated and those who concentrate on the mouth did so as a way of coping when others express idioms or irony in which the verbal and non-verbal messages are contradicting.

Diagnosis and Treatment

Often, the only way an individual with an NSI can obtain help and support is through seeking a medical diagnosis from their physician. This convention of using the medical model of disability to classify people and then treat the symptoms of the impairment as opposed to making changes in social structure is in most cases accepted as the norm. Diagnosis is often the first step in a long struggle for individuals with non-systemising impairments as illustrated in a study conducted by the National Autistic Society (Barnard, Prior, & Potter, 2000), which found that children diagnosed with ASC are on average 20 times more likely to be excluded from school than their peers.

Non-systemising impairments are most often diagnosed using the Diagnostic and Statistical Manual of Mental Disorders, Fourth Edition (DSM-IV). Ameringen, Mancini, and Farvolden (2003) emphasised the importance of diagnosing and treating non-systemising impairments in children and adolescents to ensure that as many

Copyright © 2011, IGI Global. Copying or distributing in print or electronic forms without written permission of IGI Global is prohibited.

youth as possible have the opportunity to enjoy education at all levels and become full participants and contributors to society.

Medical Treatment

Medical treatment is usually only conducted when the impaired individual is unable to overcome their disability through social skills training. A study by Blades (2000) into the effect of change of diet on children diagnosed with ASC found that inclusion of a probiotic in a child's diet decreased the symptoms of ASC, including the need for strict routines. A number of studies have investigated the role of anticonvulsant medication in treating NSI individuals. However, Martino and Tuchman (2001) stressed that there is only anecdotal evidence to suggest that there is a beneficial role for anticonvulsants in children with ASC. The role of affective anticonvulsants in children with ASC with or without seizures is not established. In addition, Keller (2001) indicates that little research has been conducted into the role of antidepressants in alleviating non-systemising impairments and that it is not known whether such drugs act directly to affect mechanisms that mediate social functioning, or via clinical improvement of depression.

Towards an Inclusive Solution

The medical model of disability has come under a significant attack from academics in the last 40 years, who have suggested that it is society that disables impaired individuals and that disability is something imposed on top of such impairments by the way disabled people are isolated and excluded from full participation in society (Oliver, 1993). The diagnosis and treatment approach of the medical model of disability is very limited in helping socially impaired individuals understand themselves and colleagues so that they can fully participate in society. Oliver advocates a 'social model' approach to understanding disability, which suggests that society is excluding NSIs and not the impairments themselves. However, having their impairment classed as a medical condition is often the only way NSIs can attempt to acquire the support they need from employers, educators and governmental organisations. The medical model puts the responsibility on the impaired individual to seek treatment and adapt to their environment through developing coping strategies, meaning the NSI individual is treated in the same way as their peer group with no concessions made to take into account the difficulties they face.

Frith (1991) questions this approach in individuals with an ASC, indicating that in the workplace, nondisclosure of their impairment to employers can lead to employees with ASCs losing their jobs. For example, a change in working hours may seem like an acceptable proposal to the employer, but a lack of understanding

Copyright © 2011, IGI Global. Copying or distributing in print or electronic forms without written permission of IGI Global is prohibited.

or knowledge of the impairment may make such a request for change in routine seem completely unacceptable to an employee with ASC.

In the past two decades, there have been a significant number of policy initiatives aimed at disabled individuals, from employment rights to access to goods and services (Burchardt, 2000). The Disability Discrimination Act 1995 (DDA) introduced by the UK Government gave these policies statutory recognition making it an offence to unfairly discriminate against individuals with an impairment. The Special Educational Needs and Disability Act 2001 (SENDA) extended the DDA to education establishments making it a requirement for them to make the appropriate adjustments to allow individuals with impairments to access all educational services made available to individuals without impairments. The 2005 amendment to the DDA introduced by the UK Government gave greater rights to NSIs as there is no longer a requirement that their impairment be recognised. New rights applied to all public authorities except, it might be argued, the ones where NSIs are overly underrepresented, such as the UK House of Commons and House of Lords. The subsequent Equality Act 2010 harmonised the law relating to equality and created the concept of 'protected characteristics' of which disability, sex, and sexual orientation are some.

The Role of Augmented E-Learning Systems

Lupton and Seymour (2000) argue that technology offers the potential to assist individuals with physical disabilities by augmenting or substituting particular bodily functions, thus making it possible for them to participate in previously inaccessible activities and domains. Parsons and Mitchell (2002) recommend that e-learning systems should only be used in a blended learning environment, where the individual with an NSI works in collaboration with other people and not to circumvent real–world social interaction altogether.

According to the UK Parliament new media technology, such as information and communications technologies (ICTs) have an increasingly central role in supporting the learning of individuals both through e-learning and the Internet as a major source of information (Education and Skills Committee, 2006). These new media technologies have been reshaped by developers to act as augmented e-learning systems, which enhance the capabilities of people with NSIs. Some of these have been explored in detail by Hartley (2006), though the ones most relevant to people NSIs, are explored below, namely, mobile technologies, agent-guided education systems and Web 2.0-based environments.

Copyright © 2011, IGI Global. Copying or distributing in print or electronic forms without written permission of IGI Global is prohibited.

Mobile Technologies

Mobile technologies for learning primarily consist of Personal Digital Assistants (PDAs), mobile phones and smartphones, but there are also other devices that share their characteristics in size, form or function (Trinder, 2005). Recent research has found that of those users with third generation (3G) mobile phones 77 per cent of them use it for video and text-based services (Carlsson, Walden, & Veijalainen, 2003). A mobile phone system that can increase social ability in NSIs that uses such features is the Portable Affect Recognition Learning Environment (PARLE). The PARLE System (Bishop, 2003) uses a mobile augmented reality application, much like the Wikitude AR Travel Guide developed six years later, to capture the emotions of someone a person with an NSI is talking to and to decode its meaning into something they can understand. PARLE uses semantic querying of a computer database via an Internet-based mobile phone in real-time during social situations to translate idioms, aphorisms and common phrases into more meaningful expressions along with explanations and suggested responses. For example, if during a conversation the individual with an NSI was asked, 'cat got your tongue?' this would be translated into an open-ended question such as, 'you appear quiet, how come?' This translation would make more sense to a person with an ASC who may have interpreted the original statement literally. Using 3G hardware with video, sound and text transmission, a mobile educational agent allows real-time interpretations of conversations to be delivered to the socially impaired individual as depicted in Figure 1.

The system has been tested on individuals with ASCs and General Social Phobia (GSP) and while those with GSP found it focussed on areas they have little diffi-

Figure 1. Processes of the PARLE system

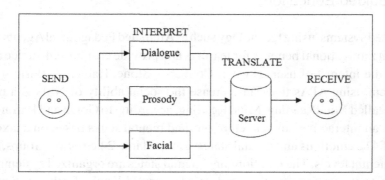

Copyright © 2011, IGI Global. Copying or distributing in print or electronic forms without written permission of IGI Global is prohibited.

culty with, the individuals with ASCs gave a positive response to it, indicating that they would use it in social situations.

The Mobile Phone Application Market

The mobile phone has been among the most impressive techno-cultural phenomena of the current millennium (Susani, 2009). The mobile market is now highly developed with mass availability of portable video receiving and transmission systems, from Apple's iPhone to Windows-based Ultra Mobile PCs (UMPCs) with integrated cameras. The market for mobile applications is developing fast. The magazine, *.net*, which is the world's best-selling journal for web designers, says that while the current trend towards *'app stores'* is a step backwards for open standards, the move towards HTML5 should mean the eventual dilution of device-specific applications (Anonymous, 2010). Indeed while app stores solve the age-old problem of consumers not knowing where to find mobile phone applications and then to know whether they work with their particular phone (Paulos, Joki, Vora, & Burke, 2007), the mobile Web based around open standards could give the e-learning industry the way into making learning technologies available through all mobile phones. The competitiveness of the mobile phone market is driving down prices and users are adopting phones that support applications as a preferred option. A variety of mobile phone applications are on the rise, many of which utilise physical location to express the context of information (Ofstad, Nicholas, Szcodronski, & Choudhury, 2008), suggesting context aware systems are becoming socially acceptable. The role of mobile phone applications for promoting healthy lifestyles is becoming more considered, with the communication of health messages aimed at the modification of lifestyle behaviours and also in the monitoring of patient health data through mobile applications being adopted (Blake, 2008).

Agent-Guided Education

Agent based systems, using technology such as Animated Pedagogical Agents (APAs) offer great motivational benefits for learners and provide customised advice and can maintain the interest of users (Lester, Converse, Stone, Kahler, & Barlow, 1997). One system using APAs that can increase the social ability of NSIs is a piece of software called MindReading. Mind Reading, according to Golan and Baron-Cohen (2006), is an interactive guide to emotions and mental states based on a taxonomic system of 412 emotions and mental states, grouped into 24 emotion groups, and six developmental levels. The emotions and mental states are organized systematically, according to the emotion groups and developmental levels. Each emotion group is introduced and demonstrated by a short video clip giving some clues for later

Copyright © 2011, IGI Global. Copying or distributing in print or electronic forms without written permission of IGI Global is prohibited.

analysis of the emotions in this group. Each emotion is defined and demonstrated in six silent films of faces, six voice recordings, and six written examples of situations that evoke this emotion. The system uses an APA to guide individuals though the learning programmes in the package, as depicted in Figure 2.

Web 2.0

Web 2.0 refers to tools such as blogs, wikis, photo and video sharing, and social networking technologies that are changing how learners understand and make sense of the world (Solomon & Schrum, 2007). The adoption of such technologies is increasing at a vast rate, although research has shown some gender disparities, where in some countries for example 76 percent of weblog authors are men and 24 percent are women (Golkar, 2005). Contemporary studies have looked on some of these technologies as fitting into classes, where the technical aspects of them place them in specific genres of online community (Bishop, 2009).

According to Richardson (2006) photograph sharing tools such as the website Flickr are good for introducing learners not only to digital images and publishing,

Figure 2. MindReading and its animated pedagogical agent

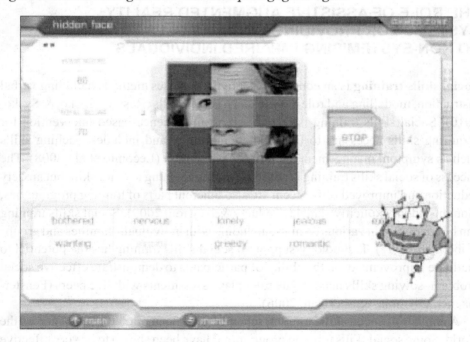

Copyright © 2011, IGI Global. Copying or distributing in print or electronic forms without written permission of IGI Global is prohibited.

but also to the social conversations and collaborative opportunities the Web offers. Through using such technologies educators can allow their learners to be creative and produce photographs that document a classroom or field project or activity and allow more people to share in their learning. Teehan (2006) further argues that such websites can be used for scrapbooking and the telling of digital stories. Another Internet technology that allows learners to be creative and share their creations is podcasting. According to King and Gura (2007) podcasting, which is a method of digitally producing and distributing audio, can allow educators to facilitate the development of speaking and listening skills in learners and be used in activities such as report writing where students would normally only use the written word, allowing them to make presentations and engage in debates. The creation and sharing of video is another digitally based method for blending Internet technologies with classroom or field activities.

According to Bishop (2004) an effective means of allowing learners to express their learning after formal lessons and practical activities are through allowing them to complete Weblogs. The use of Weblogs in educational contexts is further supported by Mcintosh (2006) who agrees that they can be used as learning logs and reflective journals.

THE ROLE OF ASSISTIVE AUGMENTED REALITY SYSTEMS FOR PROVIDING SOCIAL SKILLS TRAINING TO NON-SYSTEMISING IMPAIRED INDIVIDUALS

Social skills training is an educational activity that uses methods including verbal instruction, modelling and role-play to teach social skills (Results, Sysko, & Sysko, 2010). Social skills training is recognised as an evidence-based intervention for acquiring skills necessary to live in the community and includes teaching skills such as symptom management and relapse prevention (Lecomte et al., 2008). The success of social skills training is not solely due to learning a motor skill, but anxiety reduction and improved self-esteem are also inherent parts of training programmes, though seldom explicitly stated (Kindness & Newton, 2009). Social skills training can be conducted in various formats, including with individuals, families and groups (Liberman, 2007). Technology-supported social skills training has the potential to facilitate improvements in the ability of participants to demonstrate effective social problem–solving skills in analogue role–play assessments with live peers (Fenstermacher, Olympia, & Sheridan, 2006).

A number of social skills training schemes have been piloted and run across the world. Some social skills training programmes have been shown to be very effective for assisting individuals with the most severe of emotional recognition impairments,

Copyright © 2011, IGI Global. Copying or distributing in print or electronic forms without written permission of IGI Global is prohibited.

such as SZ (Thorup et al., 2006) and others such as the Quantum Opportunity Pro-gramme (QOP) has offered financial incentives and mentoring for participation in programmes aimed at improving both social skills and market readiness of other affected groups (Verry, 2001).

Individuals with ASCs have a sense of being, or ontological outlook, that does not take account of the social or affective states of others in the way a typical person is able to. The role of technology in helping people with Autistic Spectrum Conditions (ASCs) to appreciate affective states has been explored by Kaliouby et al. (2006), reviewing technologies such as PARLE in providing an assistive e-learning solu-tion to socially-impaired individuals (NSIs). The study found that the technology is available to support prosthetic devices that allow people with autism to receive information on the mental states of those people they are communicating with.

Technology has come a long way since Bishop (2003) first proposed the Por-table Affect Recognition Learning Environment. Mobile Internet technologies such as '3G' are now widely available at reasonable prices. Consumer electronics now include affordable visual solutions such as video glasses, which can be combined with sensor-based systems such as Nintendo's Wii.

The Visual Ontological Imitation System (VOIS)

The inclusion agenda suggests that society should be disabling barriers for people with social and emotional impairments and encouraging them to take part in social situations (Oliver, 1993). The diversity agenda says that society should stop try-ing to cure people with disabilities and accept their differences (Griffin & Pollak, 2008). A new system for achieving this, which builds on PARLE, could be the Visual Ontological Imitation System, VOIS, which is pronounced 'Voice'. VOIS, like PARLE, is a server-side driven mobile phone application that gives people with non-systemising impairments the augmented ability to take part in social situations they would normally find difficult or confusing. VOIS would allow NSIs to over-come their anxiety in social situations by providing socially contextual information on how they should react and alleviate concerns about other's true meanings. VOIS allows NSIs to receive information in real-time through video-based devices such as headsets or mobile phones, which means they are able to make decisions using their systemising capabilities in situations where individuals with a high Empathis-ing Quotient would have little difficulty but where they do.

As can be seen from Figure 3 the primary user of the system interacts with a user interface, such as a mobile phone, personal digital assistant, a VR-headset with audio/video inputs/outputs, or in the future an interface linked directly to the human neural system. The interface captures audio and video ('Data Capture') and decodes its content and meaning using previously published algorithms ('Data Decoding')

Copyright © 2011, IGI Global. Copying or distributing in print or electronic forms without written permission of IGI Global is prohibited.

Figure 3. Application cycles of VOIS

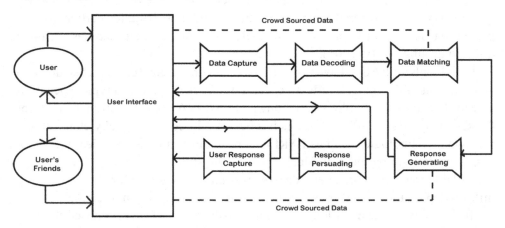

in a similar way to Bishop (2003) and Kaliouby, Teeters, and Picard (2006). Using publicly available algorithms based on the three affect inputs of PARLE (e.g. Ioannou et al., 2007 for facial, Eyben et al., 2009 for prosody, and Yoo, et al., 2011 for dialogue), then there would be a potential 6,292 affective states. The data from the algorithms is then matched against database records, which are pre-programmed and in addition added to by users of the system ('Data Matching') using the sematic querying approach of Bishop (2003). This produces a natural language query that is displayed to the user under the guise of an avatar called 'Parley', which is fed into an advice agent ('Response Generating') who recommends appropriate responses under the guise of an avatar called 'Paige', which interacts with them to convince them of the appropriate choice to make ('Response Persuading') using the approach in Bishop (2009). Their actual response is then captured ('User Response Capture') including through the microphone and a camera facing them and their friends as part of an online social network are able to recommend alternative responses which are fed back into the system for the 'Paige' agent to use.

The VOIS system could in its current form, using the continuum proposed by Milgram and Kishino (1994), be considered to be a mixed reality system somewhere between augmented reality and augmented virtuality in its various modes of delivery as implied in Figure 4.

Exploring Opinions of New Media Interventions

Using a focus group, a qualitative method that supports spontaneous reactions and group dynamics (Nielsen, 1993), a study was carried out to investigate the opinions of educators and disability advocates on the role of new media technology for in-

Copyright © 2011, IGI Global. Copying or distributing in print or electronic forms without written permission of IGI Global is prohibited.

Figure 4. VOIS on the IPhone

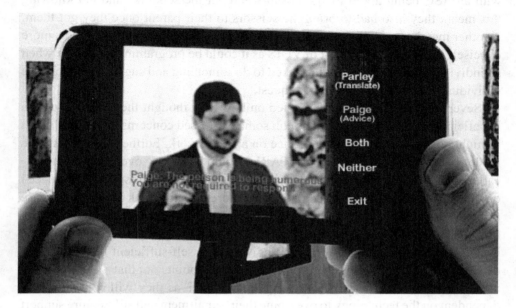

tervening to assist NSIs, in order to evaluate whether a system like VOIS would be recommended by social workers and educationalists for use by individuals with an NSI. According to Kuniavsky (2003) focus groups allow the participants to share their view of issues and assumptions that lie at the core of their experiences and relate them to specific situations.

The focus groups consisted of 8 members of the charity, RCT People's First, an organisation based in Wales that provides training to individuals with disabilities so they can themselves provide advocacy training on disability issues to organisations wanting to improve their equality practices.

The participants in the study were shown three scenarios (see Appendix A) of technology used for people with ASCs and asked to comment on the appropriateness of the systems and how they could be utilised and be adapted for more effective usage in education. Scenario 1 is drawn from the study by Bishop (2003) scenario 2 from the study by Bishop (2007) and scenario 3 has been constructed from content available at http://www.autismwiki.com.

RESULTS

A member of the focus group suggested that PARLE could be adapted to provide prompts when certain questions are asked. They gave the example of an individual

Copyright © 2011, IGI Global. Copying or distributing in print or electronic forms without written permission of IGI Global is prohibited.

with an ASC being asked to "go upstairs and get the scissors" and not knowing this meant they also had to bring the scissors to their parent once they got them. Another member said that non-NSIs need to learn how to present statements more concisely. This could form part of VOIS as it could be programmed to notice when an individual with an NSI is being asked to do something and suggest questions the individual could ask to clarify the request.

Several group members commented on how they thought the system could be beneficial to people with ASCs, though some expressed concerns about how much it might cost to subscribe to the service on a 3G network. Further comments were made about how technology such as PARLE could be used to overcome communication difficulties, though the group felt there should be some responsibility placed on the non-NSI individuals to communicate more effectively as it may be the case that they are not listening to NSII in addition to the problems that PARLE solves. Indeed, French (1993) suggests that assistive technology can become a burden because others will see the impaired individual as self-sufficient believing their disability to be removed by the technology. French points out that visual aids will not make someone who is visually impaired sighted, as they will continue to be dependent on the technology to overcome their impairment and still require support for some activities.

The group felt that organisations, including themselves need to "adapt the way we work with people" to take account of differences in the way people communicate, which suggests that VOIS may not be an appropriate solution as it attempts to change the impaired person rather than the society they are in.

With regard to scenario 2, the group were a bit concerned that MindReading did not have the additional support for an NSII to develop coping strategies to deal with the new social abilities they have. The group also felt that while technologies such as PARLE and MindReading can help individuals with ASCs overcome their difficulties, others in society, such as teachers and lecturers should receive additional training to deal with the differences that NSIs have. This again suggests that VOIS, while providing similar benefits to PARLE and MindReading, is not the full solution as society needs to adapt to take account of people with NSIs. However, it also provides an opportunity for VOIS to be further developed to enhance the emotional capabilities of NSIs.

With regard to scenario 3, the group all felt that the AutismWiki website was particularly relevant to advocacy organisations such as theirs. Several commented how if individuals with disabilities are able to communicate their experiences through new media technology others without those impairments might be better able to understand them. This suggests that VOIS could be enhanced to make use of Web 2.0 technologies so that users can share their experiences through a more social

Copyright © 2011, IGI Global. Copying or distributing in print or electronic forms without written permission of IGI Global is prohibited.

form of learning and help fine-tune the system to take account of new phrases and more obscure emotions and facial expressions.

DISCUSSION

New media technologies have formed part of visions of a deschooled, 'wired' society where the full potential of learners is realised and of this technology relies on good visual and cognitive abilities making it suitable to individuals with strengths in these areas. Some individuals with such strengths may be deficit in other aspects of their abilities, such as in relating to others socially and emphatically. These non-systemising impairments (NSIs) consist of a range of documented conditions, which medical and educational professionals have described in detail. Some NSIs, such as Autism Spectrum Conditions (ASCs), can be seen as conditions where on receiving a social or emotional stimulus the individual with the condition has difficulty in utilising the information and whose mind may not be able to deal with large amounts of these types of stimuli due to deficits in response flexibility.

A new e-learning system was developed that took into account these premises called the Visual Ontological Imitation System. VOIS allows people with NSIs to receive information in real-time that allows the individual to make decisions using their systemising capabilities on situations where individuals with a high Empathising Quotient would have little difficulty but where they do.

A study using a focus group was carried out to evaluate the opinions of those that support disabled people and their attitude towards new media technologies, specifically those that assist NSIs, as a way of evaluating the social acceptability of VOIS. A member of the focus group suggested that VOIS could provide prompts when certain questions are asked based on modifications of the PARLE system's features. Several group members commented on how they thought the system could be beneficial to people with ASCs, though some expressed concerns about how much it might cost to subscribe to the service on a 3G network. Alternatives, such as placing it on a Micro-SD card, could make the system more efficient and then only require a download of the interfacing application for the specific platform it is on that supports it (e.g. Windows Phone, Android). Further comments were made about how technology such as VOIS could be used to overcome communication difficulties, though the group felt there should be some responsibility placed on the non-NSI individuals to communicate more effectively as it may be the case that they are not listening to the person with an NSI in addition to the problems that PARLE solves. The group also felt that while technologies such as PARLE and MindReading can help individuals with ASCs overcome their difficulties, others in society, such as teachers and lecturers should receive additional training to deal

Copyright © 2011, IGI Global. Copying or distributing in print or electronic forms without written permission of IGI Global is prohibited.

with the differences that NSIs have. Several commented how if individuals with disabilities are able to communicate their experiences through new media technology others without those impairments might be better able to understand them. A future version of VOIS could make use of the Circle of Friends technology (Bishop, 2008) by allowing the NSIs to tag the video clips they capture with what they think they mean and then have their neurotypical friends validate it to say whether they got it right or not. This crowd-sourced data could then be fed into the system and geo-coded to increase the cultural sensitivity of the system and the semantic functionality of it. The server could use an API-based system to connect to the mobile phone application and allow authorised providers to develop applications for other devices, with the interface possibly being renamed the 'Versatile Ontological Imitation System' to take account of this. The use of Web 2.0 technologies would allow for the database to be expanded by including new idioms and facial expressions not previously considered.

Limitations and Directions for Future Research

This chapter has proposed a system for educating NSIs through an augmented environment. Future research could explore this system in more detail and discover whether in a supportive environment it can help NSIs, particularly autism spectrum conditions overcome their difficulties and play a greater role in society, or whether the focus should turn to the neurotypical individuals and the development of e-learning systems that promote tolerant attitudes and acceptance of different social and emotional practices and abilities. The outcome of this debate could lead to a decision as to whether it would be ethical to pursue the development of a nanotechnology based version of VOIS, which could be implanted into the NSI individual to increase their competencies and ability to function in social situations. The VOIS system, based on current research into emotion recognition may have biases, such as on gender, sexuality or culture, which need to be taken into account in future implementations. For example, by taking into account other contemporary research, such as 'Queer Theory' it may be possible to conclude that there is a link between the 'male' and 'female' characteristics identified by Baron-Cohen (2002) and sexual orientation, which VOIS may not be able to differentiate between. The author's anecdotal evidence of having female friends orientated to the same sex having more systemising biases than other women they know, and male same-sex orientated friends being more emotionally-driven than other men, may suggest that there is an overlap between gender and sexuality and systemising/empathising abilities, which could have an impact on the effectiveness of VOIS in integrating NSIs into society by providing too generic information. It has been known since the dawn of post-cognitivist psychology that the location in which someone is based affects

Copyright © 2011, IGI Global. Copying or distributing in print or electronic forms without written permission of IGI Global is prohibited.

their responses to questions, so the geo-coding part of the crowd-sourcing aspect of VOIS could be used to calculate the most effect response for the NSI individual to make. Further research needs to be done to establish the links between gender, sexual orientation, disability and systemising/emphasising abilities, to discover whether VOIS has any application in managing tensions between these groups, so that there is a greater appreciation and tolerance of and between diverse groups in society. Should additional types of affect such as those above be added to VOIS in addition to the three ones in PARLE, then there could be nearly quarter of a million affective states from which accurate and precise recommendations could be made. This could grow into the millions as the crowd sourcing algorithm is expanded to collect information on newer antecedents that are found to affect emotional perception and response.

REFERENCES

Ameringen, M. V., Mancini, C., & Farvolden, P. (2003). The impact of anxiety disorders on educational achievement. *Journal of Anxiety Disorders*, *17*(5), 561–571. doi:10.1016/S0887-6185(02)00228-1

Anonymous,. (2010, April 1). Breaking the Web? There's an app for that. *Net Magazine*, *200*, 14.

Aquilla, P., Yack, E., & Sutton, S. (2005). Sensory and motor differences for individuals with Asperger syndrome: Occupational therapy assessment and intervention. In Stoddart, K. P. (Ed.), *Children, youth and adults with Asperger syndrome: Integrating multiple perspectives*. London, UK: Jessica Kingsley Publishers.

Attwood, T. (1998). *Asperger's syndrome: A guide for parents and professionals*. Jessica Kingsley Pub.

Baird, G., Simonoff, E., Pickles, A., Chandler, S., Loucas, T., Meldrum, D., & Charman, T. (2006). Prevalence of disorders of the autism spectrum in a population cohort of children in South Thames: The special needs and autism project (SNAP). *Lancet*, *368*(9531), 210–215. doi:10.1016/S0140-6736(06)69041-7

Barnard, J., Prior, A., & Potter, D. (2000). *Inclusion and autism: Is it working?* London, UK: National Autistic Society.

Baron-Cohen, S. (2002). The extreme male brain theory of autism. *Trends in Cognitive Sciences*, *6*(6), 248–254. doi:10.1016/S1364-6613(02)01904-6

Copyright © 2011, IGI Global. Copying or distributing in print or electronic forms without written permission of IGI Global is prohibited.

Bishop, J. (2003). The Internet for educating individuals with non-systemising impairments. *Journal of Computer Assisted Learning, 19*(4), 546–556. doi:10.1046/j.0266-4909.2003.00057.x

Bishop, J. (2004). *The potential of persuasive technology for educating heterogeneous user groups.* Unpublished MSc thesis, University of Glamorgan, Pontypridd.

Bishop, J. (2007). *An investigation into how the European Union affects the development and provision of e-learning services.* Unpublished manuscript.

Bishop, J. (2007). Increasing participation in online communities: A framework for human–computer interaction. *Computers in Human Behavior, 23*(4), 1881–1893. doi:10.1016/j.chb.2005.11.004

Bishop, J. (2008). Understanding and facilitating the development of social networks in online dating communities: A case study and model. In Romm-Livermore, C., & Setzekorn, K. (Eds.), *Social networking communities and e-dating services: Concepts and implications.* Hershey, PA: IGI Global.

Bishop, J. (2009). Enhancing the understanding of genres of web-based communities: The role of the ecological cognition framework. *International Journal of Web Based Communities, 5*(1), 4–17. doi:10.1504/IJWBC.2009.021558

Blades, M. (2000). Autism: An interesting dietary case history. *Nutrition & Food Science, 30*(3), 137–140. doi:10.1108/00346650010319741

Blake, H. (2008). Innovation in practice: Mobile phone technology in patient care. *British Journal of Community Nursing, 13*(4), 160–165.

Buckingham, D. (2002). *The electronic generation? Children and new media. Handbook of new media: Social shaping and consequences of ICTs.* Sage Publications.

Burchardt, T. (2000). The dynamics of being disabled. *Journal of Social Policy, 29*(4), 645–668. doi:10.1017/S0047279400006097

Bushwick, N. L. (2001). Social learning and the etiology of autism. *New Ideas in Psychology, 19*(1), 49–75. doi:10.1016/S0732-118X(00)00016-7

Carlsson, C., Walden, P., & Veijalainen, J. (2003). Mobile commerce. *Proceedings of the 36th Annual Hawaii International Conference on System Sciences, 2003,* (p. 87).

Dewing, H. (2009). *Market overview: Sizing unified communications.* London, UK: Forrester Reports.

Copyright © 2011, IGI Global. Copying or distributing in print or electronic forms without written permission of IGI Global is prohibited.

Ettinger, A., Holton, V., & Blass, E. (2006). E-learner experiences: What is the future for e-learning? *Industrial and Commercial Training, 38*(4), 208. doi:10.1108/00197850610671991

Eyben, F., Wöllmer, M., & Schuller, B. (2009). openEAR: Introducing the munich open-source emotion and affect recognition toolkit.

Fenstermacher, K., Olympia, D., & Sheridan, S. M. (2006). Effectiveness of a computer-facilitated, interactive social skills training program for boys with attention deficit hyperactivity disorder. *School Psychology Quarterly, 21*(2), 197. doi:10.1521/scpq.2006.21.2.197

French, S. (1993). *What's so great about independence?* (pp. 44–48).

Frith, U. (1991). *Autism and Asperger syndrome.* Cambridge University Press. doi:10.1017/CBO9780511526770

Gapen, M. A. (2009). *Facial non-systemising impairments in individuals with PTSD symptoms.* Unpublished doctoral dissertation, Emory University.

Gardner, H. (1983). *Frames of mind: The theory of multiple intelligences.* Basic Books.

Golan, O., & Baron-Cohen, S. (2006). Systemizing empathy: Teaching adults with Asperger syndrome or high-functioning autism to recognize complex emotions using interactive multimedia. *Development and Psychopathology, 18*(2), 591–617. .doi:10.1017/S0954579406060305

Golkar, S. (2005). Politics in weblogs: A safe space for protest. *Iran Analysis Quarterly*, 49-59.

Grandin, T. (1995). *Thinking in pictures: And other reports from my life with autism.* Doubleday.

Griffin, E., & Pollak, D. (2008). Student experiences of neurodiversity in higher education: INSIghts from the BRAINHE project. *Dyslexia (Chichester, England), 14*(4).

Hartley, J. (2006). Teaching, learning and new technology: A review for teachers. *British Journal of Educational Technology, 38*(1), 42–62. doi:10.1111/j.1467-8535.2006.00634.x

Ioannou, S., caridakis, G., Karpouzis, K., & Kollias, S. (2007). Robust feature detection for facial expression recognition. Journal on image and video processing, 2007(2), 5

Copyright © 2011, IGI Global. Copying or distributing in print or electronic forms without written permission of IGI Global is prohibited.

Jabbi, M., Swart, M., & Keysers, C. (2007). Empathy for positive and negative emotions in the gustatory cortex. *NeuroImage*, *34*(4), 1744–1753. .doi:10.1016/j. neuroimage.2006.10.032

Kaliouby, R., Picard, R., & Baron-Cohen, S. (2006). Affective computing and autism. *Annals of the New York Academy of Sciences*, *1093*, 228–248. .doi:10.1196/ annals.1382.016

Kaliouby, R., Teeters, A., & Picard, R. W. (2006). *An exploratory social-emotional prosthetic for autism spectrum disorders*. International Workshop on Wearable and Implantable Body Sensor Networks, BSN 2006. 2.

Keller, M. (2001). Role of serotonin and noradrenaline in social dysfunction: A review of data on reboxetine and the social adaptation self-evaluation scale (SASS). *General Hospital Psychiatry*, *23*(1), 15–19. doi:10.1016/S0163-8343(00)00115-8

Kindness, K., & Newton, A. (2009). Patients and social skills groups: Is social skills training enough? *Behavioural and Cognitive Psychotherapy*, *12*(3), 212–222.

King, K. P., & Gura, M. (2007). *Podcasting for teachers: Using a new technology to revolutionize teaching and learning*. Information Age Publishing.

Klin, A., Jones, W., Schultz, R., Volkmar, F., & Cohen, D. (2002). Visual fixation patterns during viewing of naturalistic social situations as predictors of social competence in individuals with autism. *Archives of General Psychiatry*, *59*(9), 809. doi:10.1001/archpsyc.59.9.809

Kuniavsky, M. (2003). *Observing the user experience: A practitioner's guide to user research*. London, UK: Morgan Kaufmann Publishers.

Lecomte, T., Leclerc, C., Corbière, M., Wykes, T., Wallace, C. J., & Spidel, A. (2008). Group cognitive behavior therapy or social skills training for individuals with a recent onset of psychosis? Results of a randomized controlled trial. *The Journal of Nervous and Mental Disease*, *196*(12), 866. doi:10.1097/NMD.0b013e31818ee231

Lester, J. C., Converse, S. A., Stone, B. A., Kahler, S. E., & Barlow, S. T. (1997). *Animated pedagogical agents and problem-solving effectiveness: A large-scale empirical evaluation*.

Liberman, R. P. (2007). Dissemination and adoption of social skills training: Social validation of an evidence-based treatment for the mentally disabled. *Journal of Mental Health (Abingdon, England)*, *16*(5), 595–623. doi:10.1080/09638230701494902

Lupton, D., & Seymour, W. (2000). Technology, selfhood and physical disability. *Social Science & Medicine*, *50*(12), 1851–1862. doi:10.1016/S0277-9536(99)00422-0

Copyright © 2011, IGI Global. Copying or distributing in print or electronic forms without written permission of IGI Global is prohibited.

Martino, A. D., & Tuchman, R. F. (2001). Antiepileptic drugs: Affective use in autism spectrum disorders. *Pediatric Neurology, 25*(3), 199–207. doi:10.1016/S0887-8994(01)00276-4

Mcintosh, E. (2006). Podcasting and wikis. In Freedman, T. (Ed.), *Coming of age: An introduction to the new World Wide Web*. Ilford, UK: Terry Freedman Ltd.

Milgram, P., & Kishino, F. (1994). A taxonomy of mixed reality visual displays. *IEICE Transactions on Information and Systems, 77*(12), 1321–1329.

Nardi, D. (2001). *Multiple intelligences & personality type: Tools and strategies for developing human potential*. Telos Publications.

Nielsen, J. (1993). *Usability engineering*. San Francisco, CA: Morgan Kaufman.

Ofstad, A., Nicholas, E., Szcodronski, R., & Choudhury, R. R. (2008). Aampl: Accelerometer augmented mobile phone localization. *Proceedings of the First ACM International Workshop on Mobile Entity Localization and Tracking in GPS-Less Environments*, (pp. 13-18).

Oliver, M. (1993). *Social work: Disabled people and disabling environments*. Jessica Kingsley Pub.

Parsons, S., & Mitchell, P. (2002). The potential of virtual reality in social skills training for people with autistic spectrum disorders. *Journal of Intellectual Disability Research, 46*(5), 430–443. doi:10.1046/j.1365-2788.2002.00425.x

Paulos, E., Joki, A., Vora, P., & Burke, A. (2007). AnyPhone: Mobile applications for everyone. *Proceedings of the 2007 Conference on Designing for User eXperiences,* 1.

Pease, B., & Pease, A. (1998). *Why men won't listen and women can't read maps*. Mona Vale, NSW: Pease Training International.

Ragozzino, M. E. (2007). The contribution of the medial prefrontal cortex, orbitofrontal cortex, and dorsomedial striatum to behavioral flexibility. *Annals of the New York Academy of Sciences, 1121*, 355–375. .doi:10.1196/annals.1401.013

Results, V., Sysko, H. B., & Sysko, H. B. (2010). Antecedent assessment and intervention: Supporting children and adults with developmental disabilities in community settings. *Education & Treatment of Children, 33*(1).

Richardson, W. (2006). *Blogs, wikis, podcasts, and other powerful web tools for classrooms*. Corwin Press.

Siegel, B. (2003). *Helping children with autism learn: Treatment approaches for parents and professionals*. USA: Oxford University Press.

Copyright © 2011, IGI Global. Copying or distributing in print or electronic forms without written permission of IGI Global is prohibited.

Solomon, G., & Schrum, L. (2007). *Web 2.0: New tools, new schools*. Intl Society for Technology.

Susani, M. (2009). Mobile interaction design in the age of experience ecosystems. *Human-Computer Interaction: Design Issues, Solutions, and Applications,* 131.

Teehan, K. (2006). *Digital storytelling: In and out of the classroom*. London, UK: LuLu Inc.

Thorup, A., Petersen, L., Jeppesen, P., Øhlenschlæger, J., Christensen, T., & Krarup, G. (2006). Social network among young adults with first-episode schizophrenia spectrum disorders. *Social Psychiatry and Psychiatric Epidemiology, 41*(10), 761–770. doi:10.1007/s00127-006-0098-3

Trinder, J. (2005). Mobile technologies and systems. In *Mobile learning: A handbook for educators and trainers*. London, UK: Routledge.

Verry, D. (2001). *Economics and finance of lifelong learning*. London, UK: Organization for Economic Co-operation and Development.

Westervelt, H. J., Ruffolo, J. S., & Tremont, G. (2005). Assessing olfaction in the neuropsychological exam: The relationship between odor identification and cognition in older adults. *Archives of Clinical Neuropsychology: The Official Journal of the National Academy of Neuropsychologists, 20*(6), 761–769. doi:.doi:10.1016/j.acn.2005.04.010

Wheelwright, S., Baron-Cohen, S., Goldenfeld, N., Delaney, J., Fine, D., & Smith, R. (2006). Predicting autism spectrum quotient (AQ) from the systemizing quotient-revised (SQ-R) and empathy quotient (EQ). *Brain Research, 1079*(1), 47–56. .doi:10.1016/j.brainres.2006.01.012

Williams, C., & Wood, R. L. (2009). Impairment in the recognition of emotion across different media following traumatic brain injury. *Journal of Clinical and Experimental Neuropsychology,* 1-11. doi:10.1080/13803390902806543

Williams, K. (1995). Understanding the student with Asperger syndrome: Guidelines for teachers. *Focus on Autism and Other Developmental Disabilities, 10*(2), 9. doi:10.1177/108835769501000202

Yoo, H., & Min-Yong, K., & Kwon, Ohbyung. (2011). Emotional index measurement method for context-aware service. *Expert Systems with Applications, 38*, 785–793. doi:10.1016/j.eswa.2010.07.034

Copyright © 2011, IGI Global. Copying or distributing in print or electronic forms without written permission of IGI Global is prohibited.

KEY TERMS AND DEFINITIONS

Visual Ontological Imitation System (VOIS): Versatile Ontological Imitation System; Associated in the manuscript with: augmented e-learning system, PARLE.

Portable Affect Recognition Learning Environment (PARLE): VOIS, MindReading.

Autism Spectrum Condition (ASC): Emotional-Behaviour Condition, General Social Phobia.

Non-Systemising Impairments (NSIs): Associated in the manuscript with: autism spectrum condition, emotional-behaviour condition, general social phobia.

Web 2.0: Social networking; Associated in the manuscript with: Weblog, podcasting.

Weblog: Online community ; Associated in the manuscript with: Web 2.0.

Podcasting: Also known as: *audio blogging ;* Weblog; Associated in the manuscript with: Web 2.0.

Empathising Quotient (EQ): Emotional intelligence, social intelligence; Associated in the manuscript with: systemising quotient.

Systemising Quotient (SQ): Spatial intelligence, cognitive intelligence; Associated in the manuscript with: empathising quotient.

Nanotechnology: augmented reality; Associated in the manuscript with: augmented e-learning system.

Augmented E-Learning System: augmented reality; Associated in the manuscript with: PARLE, VOIS

Copyright © 2011, IGI Global. Copying or distributing in print or electronic forms without written permission of IGI Global is prohibited.

APPENDIX A

Scenario 1: A student at Bryn Celeynnog Comprehensive School took part in a trial of a newly designed e-learning system called PARLE. The student, having Asperger Syndrome, was part of the 'ASC' category and was asked to complete a survey on the system. The student used PARLE to convert phrases they found offensive or confusing into more concise and understandable definitions. Analysing their attitudes in the survey found that the technology enables socially impaired individuals to learn the meaning of emotions and understand more about how they communicate with their peers. The study concluded that governmental organisations, education providers and society as a whole need to adopt a cohesive approach to communication to ensure socially impaired individuals are fully included in society.

Scenario 2: A student at the University of Glamorgan, who was diagnosed with Asperger Syndrome took part in a year-long trial a year later that was organised by the University of Cambridge of a newly released e-learning system called MindReading that is intended to teach people with autistic spectrum disorders how to recognise emotions. The student was part of the unsupported condition of the trial, where he was asked to use the system at his home without the support of a tutor. After using the system for a sustained period the student began experiencing symptoms of paranoia when applying what the e-learning system taught, and was later diagnosed as suffering from a psychotic disorder. The student was paid expenses to undertake the trial, and the e-learning system is now available.

Scenario 3: Guillermo Gomez, an individual with Asperger Syndrome, lives a life of solitude in an upstairs apartment, supported by Social Security and paying $157 per month in rent. He also works part-time at a video-editing suite, a job he considers very easy-going job where his skills are valued. Guillermo shares his experience with others through Autism Wiki, a website for people with autism spectrum conditions to collaborate on knowledge-based activities.

Chapter 10
The Outdoor Wireless Healthcare Monitoring System for Hospital Patients Based on ZigBee

Xiaoxin Xu
Zhejiang University, China

Mingguang Wu
Zhejiang University, China

Bin Sun
China JiLiang University, China

Jianwei Zhang
China JiLiang University, China

Cheng Ding
HangZhou Meacon Automatic Technology Co., Ltd, China

ABSTRACT

Advances in embedded computing systems have resulted in the emergence of Wireless Sensor Networks (WSNs), which provide unique opportunities for sensing physical environments. ZigBee-compliant WSN platforms have been proposed for healthcare monitoring, smart home, industrial monitoring and sensor, and other applications. In this chapter, the authors, using TI CC2430 and CC2431 chipsets with Z-Stack, designed an outdoor patients' healthcare monitoring system for tracking patients and helping doctors and nurses to keep tabs on patients' health remotely. Furthermore, several important techniques are elaborated, including reliable communication,

DOI: 10.4018/978-1-60960-541-4.ch010

Copyright ©2011, IGI Global. Copying or distributing in print or electronic forms without written permission of IGI Global is prohibited.

localization algorithm, and backup power, which can enhance the system performance. Finally, some suggestions for future development are presented.

INTRODUCTION

Wireless Sensor Networks (WSNs) platforms (Yang, 2006) for remote healthcare monitoring are hot research topics in recent years. A number of systems have been reported for wireless healthcare monitoring. The CodeBlue (Lorincz et al. 2004) project creates a WSN system for per-hospital and in-hospital emergency care, disaster response, and stroke patient rehabilitation. Scalable Medical Alert and Response Technology (SMART) (Waterman 2005) is an easy deployment system for monitoring and tracing patients.

In this paper, we design an outdoor wireless healthcare monitoring system with ZigBee WSN technology. ZigBee is the first industrial standard WSN technology based on IEEE 802.15.4 (ZigBee, 2006) that provides short range, low power and low data rate communication, and supports mesh networking and multi-hopping. Compared with Bluetooth, ZigBee has less transmission rate, but it has longer communication range and less power consumption. Hence, ZigBee is more convenient for outdoor healthcare monitoring system.

In the outdoor monitoring area, numerous ZigBee-based WSN nodes are deployed, collecting and transmitting information from multiple subjects. Yet, they are inevitably interference by other types of radio devices, such as Bluetooth, WiFi, etc. The ambient radio interference will affect the communication between ZigBee nodes. In this case, some data inevitability lost during the communication between two nodes. But in our outdoor patients' healthcare monitoring system, these data, especially the physiological data mustn't be lost. So, in this paper we will propose a reliable data transmission method to prevent data from losing in our healthcare monitoring system.

Patient tracking is very important in our outdoor healthcare monitoring system. When emergency occurs, it is necessary to identify the patient's position. Although, a location engine is embedded onto the TI CC2431 chipset, it is not suitable for our application. Hence, we mix the location engine and localization algorithm based on Manhattan distance to locate our patients.

Power supply is the third key point in our system. Typically, when a ZigBee device wore by a patient exhausts its power, doctors and nurses may loose tab on the patient. However in our system when this case happens, the backup battery will be activated that can provide power to keep the basic monitoring on the patient.

Copyright © 2011, IGI Global. Copying or distributing in print or electronic forms without written permission of IGI Global is prohibited.

BACKGROUND

Zigbee

The name of ZigBee comes from the zigzagging path a bee (a data packet) takes to get from flower to flower (or node to node) (Niagara, 2005). ZigBee is primarily intended low power and low duty-cycle sensors. ZigBee nodes can active for less than 1% of the time. For instance, an off-line node can connect to a network in about 30 ms. Waking up a sleeping node takes about 15 ms, as does accessing a channel and transmitting data. Our healthcare system will get benefit from this technology. In large outdoor monitoring area, not all of nodes should work all the times. These nodes could go to sleep, and wake up until a new task coming.

As an IEEE 802.15.4 based standard, ZigBee is described by referring to the 7-layer OSI model for layered communication systems. But not all of the 7 layers are defined, ZigBee Alliance only specifies four layers (Physical, Data Link, Network, and Application), as well the Application Layer (APL) that allows end-developers design custom applications that use the services provided by the lower layers. It should be noted that the ZigBee Alliance choose to use an already existing data link and physical layers specification. These are published IEEE 802.15.4 (IEEE Standard 2003) standards for low-rate personal area networks. The network and application layer are defined by the alliance itself.

Localization Algorithm Based on Manhattan Distance

The localization algorithm based on Manhattan distance is one of the Received Signal Strength Indication localization algorithms. On the basis of the detection signal strength, we choose the signal difference of a Reference Node and the Mobile Device as a distance metric. And the difference function is Manhattan distance. We denote the signal victor of Mobile Device i as RSSI_mob_i, and the signal victor of Reference Node j as RSSI_ref_j (its dimension is m), the equation of Manhattan difference value is:

$$Diff\_Manht_i = \sum_{j=1}^{m} \left| RSSI\_mob\_i - RSSI\_ref\_j \right| \qquad (1)$$

In certain extent, the signal difference of a Reference Node and the Mobile Device reflect their distance. The smaller of the difference value, the shorter of their distance. And their correlation is stronger. We use the weighted centroid function to calculate the position of the patient who wears Mobile Device (Shen, Wang & Sun, 2005). The equation is:

Copyright © 2011, IGI Global. Copying or distributing in print or electronic forms without written permission of IGI Global is prohibited.

$$(X_{est}, Y_{est}) = \left(\frac{M_1^{-\alpha} X_1 + M_2^{-\alpha} X_2 + \dots\dots M_N^{-\alpha} X_N}{M_1^{-\alpha} + M_2^{-\alpha} + \dots\dots M_N^{-\alpha}}, \frac{M_1^{-\alpha} Y_1 + M_2^{-\alpha} Y_2 + \dots\dots M_N^{-\alpha} Y_N}{M_1^{-\alpha} + M_2^{-\alpha} + \dots\dots M_N^{-\alpha}} \right)$$

(2)

In above function X_{est} and Y_{est} is the estimate position of our patient with Localization algorithm based on Manhattan distance. $(X_1 \dots X_n, Y_1 \dots Y_n)$ are the Coordinates of Reference Node which are involved in localization calculation. M_i is the Manhattan difference value of Mobile Device i. is the weighting coefficient of one Mobile Device's difference Value.

MAIN FOCUS OF THE CHAPTER

Native Effects in ZigBee Network Communication

In open space ZigBee network communication quality are mainly affect by radio interference, especially channel overlap, frame length, communication distance. All of these native effects could raise the packets error rate (PER) during communication. These factors on a descending order are radio channel overlap > frame length > communication distance (Li et al. 2008). The PER of channel overlap will reduce with the range extended from ZigBee devices to other type of radio devices. But increase of frame length and distance of two ZigBee Devices cause the PERs of communication rapidly rise. Packets error will lead to data invalid and may cause the monitoring system false alarm which will affect nurses' routine work. We should try our best to find out a high reliable data transmission scheme and avoid this happening. But very few Monitoring system articles talk about the strategies to overcome the negative effects in wireless communication.

Defects of Location Engine Localization Algorithm

CC2431 embeds location engine, and its localization algorithm is based on RSSI. It is suggested to deploy three to eight Reference Nodes to calculate the position of a Mobile Device. Therefore, in some extreme case if one Mobile Device unfortunately could not find the nearest three Reference Nodes in the open air, it could not locate itself by location engine.

The parameters input to location engine are shown in Table 1. From this table we could find that an exact measurement of parameters A and n_index are very difficult. But these parameters significantly affect localization accuracy. So we need improve the location engine algorithm to fit our outdoor healthcare monitoring system

Copyright © 2011, IGI Global. Copying or distributing in print or electronic forms without written permission of IGI Global is prohibited.

Table 1. Hardware inputs parameters (CC2431 2010)

Name	Description
A	The absolute RSSI value in dBm one meter apart for a transmitter.
n_index	This value represent the signal propagation exponent, this value depends on the environment.
RSSI	Received Signal Strength Indicator this value is measured in dBm. The location engine using the absolute value as input.
X, Y	These values represent the X and Y coordinates relative to a fixed point. The values are in meters and the accuracy is 0.25 meters.

Battery Causes Potential Risks

Researchers usually pay more attention on developing more portable remote monitoring devices and little focus on power supply. But it hides potential risks. Battery run out sometimes is a very dangerous satuation in outdoor area for patients. Not like indoors they can exchange a new battery immediately. If there's no backup battery available, doctors and nurses may lose tab on them for a while. If patients feel discomfort, heart attack or sudden cerebral hemorrhage and lose communication with their doctors in this case. They will miss the best time to make emergency rescue and even lost their lives.

SOLUTIONS AND RECOMMENDATIONS

Outdoor Wireless Health Care Monitoring System Architecture

The architecture of outdoor wireless healthcare monitoring system is shown in Figure 1. The whole system can be divided into two parts: ZigBee-compliant WSN platform and Host Servers. The WSN platform consists of a Gateway, Reference Nodes, and Mobile Devices. The Gateway and Reference Nodes are deployed in outdoor space. The Gateway communicates with Host Servers via Ethernet, GPRS or WiFi. It delivers messages between Host Servers and Reference Nodes or Mobile Devices. Reference Nodes provide reference coordinates and the value of Manhattan difference (denote as M-value) for Mobile Devices. And route messages to the Gateway. Our patients can wear Mobile Devices walking under open sky. The Mobile Device transmits ECG, heart rate, SpO2, blood pressure, temperature and position messages to the Gateway. Host Servers will store, analyze, display patients' physiological and localization information, as well as configure the ZigBee wireless network.

Copyright © 2011, IGI Global. Copying or distributing in print or electronic forms without written permission of IGI Global is prohibited.

Figure 1. Outdoor wireless healthcare monitoring system architecture @ outdoor wireless healthcare monitoring system for hospital patients based on ZigBee

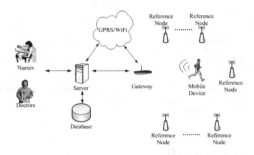

Gateway

The Gateway organizes the ZigBee network and delivers messages between Host Servers and Reference Nodes or Mobile Devices. When the Gateway is power up, it creates a ZigBee network, and permit Reference Nodes or Mobile Devices to join the network. After that the Gateway loops scan each thread. If there is any message via GPRS or WiFi over the air, or comes from Ethernet, the Gateway will read these data and verify them. If the Gateway confirm the message is correct, it will retransmit it in the ZigBee network, or it requests Host Servers to resent it. If the message comes from ZigBee network, the Gateway will also check the message to ensure all bits in the message are correct. And then it will classify the message according their cluster identification (cluster ID). Pack these data and up load to the Host Servers.

Reference Node

A Reference Node provides reference coordinates the M-value and route path for Mobile Devices. When the program is startup, the Reference Node will join ZigBee network immediately. Then it will loop scan all threads. If any message is received, it will be verified at once. If the message without any error bit, it will be classified by its cluster ID. If the cluster ID is a coordinate request message, the Reference Node will send its own coordinates which is stored in flash as a response. If the data in flash is null, the Reference Node will return a default coordinate $(X,Y) = (16383.75, 16383.75)$. If the cluster ID is a coordinate configure message, Reference Node will write a new coordinate in flash. If the cluster ID is a localization request message, the Reference Node will broadcast its position and M-value in one-hop, and receive position and M-value messages from other Reference Nodes nearby. Then it obtains RSSI values, fresh its RSSI base from these messages and calculate

Copyright © 2011, IGI Global. Copying or distributing in print or electronic forms without written permission of IGI Global is prohibited.

a new M-value for next position request. The details of localization algorithm will talk about in section V.

Mobile Device

We adopt TI CC2431 chipsets for Mobile Devices which embedded location engine instead of TI CC2430 chipsets in Reference Node or Gateway.

When its program works, the Mobile Device will join the ZigBee network, and the loop scan all threads. When the Mobile Device receives patient's ECG, heart rate, SpO2, blood pressure and temperature information from other sensors in Mobile Device, it will classify the information and sent them into their own process. After that the Mobile Device will build these information into several messages and transmit them to the Gateway. When it receives localization information, it will calculate its position with received coordinates, RSSI values and Reference Nodes' M-values nearby. There is an alarm button on the Mobile Device. In case of emergency, patient press this button, program will stop other processes and sent the alarm message first to call nurses or doctors for help.

RELIABLE DATA TRANSMISSION

To keep high quality communications, we set ZigBee devices transmission in a different channel with WiFi devices. And deploy ZigBee devices in proper range. Finally, we made a reliable data transmission scheme by using timed response mechanism based on the original code and their complement code check as seen in Figure 2. We suppose ZigBee device A transmits a message to ZigBee device B. Before ZigBee device A transmits the message, it writes these data into buffer first. If ZigBee device A doesn't receive a response within apscAckWaitDuration seconds from ZigBee device B, it repeats the process of transmitting these data up to a maximum of apscMaxFrameRetries times. If a response is not received after apscMaxFrameRetries retransmissions, the APS sub-layer shall assume the transmission has failed and notify the next higher layer of the failure (ZigBee, 2010). In this case, the next higher layer retransmits these data. If ZigBee device A receives a retransmission request, it transmits the message again. If ZigBee device A receives the acknowledgement, it deletes the message from the buffer. When ZigBee device B receives the message, it divides the message into first half and second half. The first half is the original data and the second half is the complement of the first half. If the first half XOR the second half is zero, it means the message is correct. ZigBee device B responses an acknowledgement to ZigBee device A and writes the message into buffer. If the result not equals zero, there must be some error bits in the

Copyright © 2011, IGI Global. Copying or distributing in print or electronic forms without written permission of IGI Global is prohibited.

Figure 2. Reliable data transmission scheme @ outdoor wireless healthcare monitoring system for hospital patients based on ZigBee

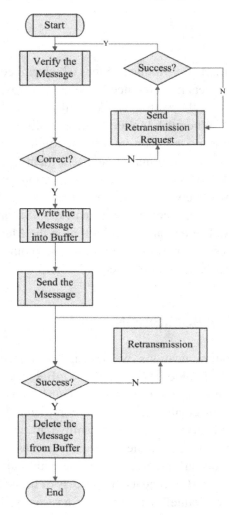

message. ZigBee device B requests ZigBee device A to retransmit the message. If ZigBee device B don't receive the message with apscAckWaitDuration seconds from ZigBee device A, it repeats the process of transmitting this request until receive the message again. After verify the message, ZigBee device B transmits the message to the next hop from the routing list.

Copyright © 2011, IGI Global. Copying or distributing in print or electronic forms without written permission of IGI Global is prohibited.

Figure 3. Localization request @ outdoor wireless healthcare monitoring system for hospital patients based on ZigBee

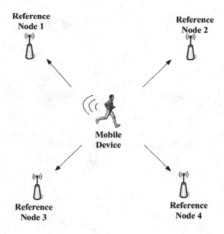

LOCALIZATION ALGORITHM

Hybrid Localization Algorithm

The hybrid localization algorithm mixes location engine algorithm with localization algorithm based on Manhattan distance. Basic steps of the algorithm are as follow:

Step 1:

A Mobile Device broadcasts a localization request to one-hop Reference Nodes nearby (Figure 3).

Step 2:

Reference Nodes obtain the value of RSSI from request, and this value is denoted as RSSI_mob_i, where i is the short address of the Mobile Device. And then these Reference Nodes broadcast their own M-value and coordinate for all ZigBee devices in one-hop. If M-value doesn't exist, then M=NULL. Every Reference Nodes will obtain RSSI values of other Reference Nodes nearby, refresh its own RSSI database and calculate a new M-value according to the equation:

$$M_i = \sum \left| RSSI\_mob\_i - RSSI\_ref\_j \right| \tag{3}$$

Copyright © 2011, IGI Global. Copying or distributing in print or electronic forms without written permission of IGI Global is prohibited.

Figure 4. RSSI database build & calculate m-value @ outdoor wireless healthcare monitoring system for hospital patients based on ZigBee

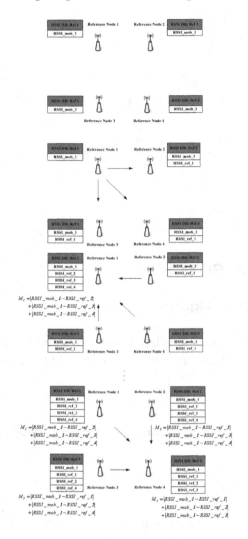

In this equation i is the short address of the Mobile Device and j is the short address of a Reference Node (Figure 4).

Step 3:

After received M-values and coordinates, the Mobile Device calculates the position based on Manhattan distance with the equation:

Copyright © 2011, IGI Global. Copying or distributing in print or electronic forms without written permission of IGI Global is prohibited.

Figure 5. Experimental result @ outdoor wireless healthcare monitoring system for hospital patients based on ZigBee

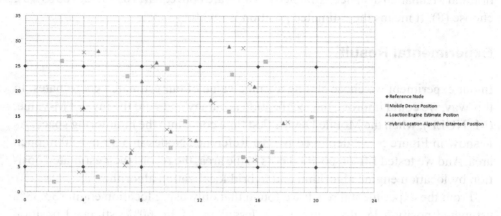

$$\left(X_{manht}, Y_{manht}\right) = \left(\frac{M_1^{-\alpha} X_1 + M_2^{-\alpha} X_2 + \ldots\ldots M_N^{-\alpha} X_N}{M_1^{-\alpha} + M_2^{-\alpha} + \ldots\ldots M_N^{-\alpha}}, \frac{M_1^{-\alpha} Y_1 + M_2^{-\alpha} Y_2 + \ldots\ldots M_N^{-\alpha} Y_N}{M_1^{-\alpha} + M_2^{-\alpha} + \ldots\ldots M_N^{-\alpha}}\right)$$
(4)

In this function β is a weighting coefficient. If in this function Mi (i∈(1, 2, ..., N))=NULL, then

$$(X_{manht}, Y_{manht}) = (16383.75, 16383.75).$$
(5)

After that, we use a limiting amplitude wave filter to process these obtain RSSI values. If the number of valid RSSI values is larger than 3, then sent these RSSI values with their related coordinates and environment factors A and n_index into the location engine and calculate the estimated position denote as (X_{loc}, Y_{loc}). If the number of valid RSSI values, then

$$(X_{loc}, Y_{loc}) = (16383.75, 16383.75).$$
(6)

We mix these two estimated position with the equations:

$$(X_{Est}, Y_{Est}) = \begin{cases} \left(\beta X_{Loc} + (1-\beta) X_{Manht}, Y_{Loc} + (1-\beta) Y_{Mahth}\right) & (8) \\ (16383.75, 16383.75), \end{cases}$$
(7)

In these equations β is a weight factor. If the location engine estimated position $(X_{loc}, Y_{loc}) = (16383.75, 16383.75)$, β=0. If Manhattan distance estimated position

Copyright © 2011, IGI Global. Copying or distributing in print or electronic forms without written permission of IGI Global is prohibited.

$(X_{manht}, Y_{manht}) = (16383.75, 16383.75)$, $\beta=1$. If both location engine estimated position and Manhattan distance estimated position are both equal (16383.75, 16383.75), choose (8). It means the estimated position is invalid.

Experimental Result

In our experiment we chose sliding average value of our estimated coordinates. In this way, we could improve the localization accuracy and void the invalid M-value. (M=NULL), when the Mobile Device first time come into the monitoring space. As is show in Figure 5, we deployed twelve Reference Nodes in a 30 m ×20 m open area. And we tested fifteen position dots in the area, the record their estimated position by location engine algorithm and hybrid localization algorithm.

From the experimental result we found that only using location engine 33.33% estimated position localization error is less than 2.5 m. 60% estimated position localization error is less than 3 m. 86.67% estimated position localization error is less than 3.5 m. 100% estimated position localization error is less than 4 m. The localization error in edge area is larger than in the central. When we use the hybrid localization algorithm, the accuracy of localization has improved. 26.67% estimated position localization error is less than 2 m. 73.33% estimated position localization error is less than 2.5 m. 93.33% estimated position localization error is less than 3 m. 100% estimated position localization error is less than 3.5 m. The accuracy of estimated position localization in edge area generally increase 0.4-0.6m. The accuracy of estimated position localization in central area generally increase 0.2-0.3m.

POWER SUPPLY

To keep high reliable power supply to Mobile Devices, we adopt backup power strategy. In this way, when the main battery could not supply enough power for the device, the backup batter works for helping doctors and nurse to keep basic monitoring for patients.

There are two different types of battery in our Mobile Device. One is lithium battery which supplies the Mobile Device working in normal situation. The other is button cell battery. Usually it doesn't work. When the lithium battery exhausts its power, the button cell battery turns to supply power and transmit a battery exhausted message to Host servers. But the button cell battery only supply CC2431 chipsets and alarm button module to help doctors or nurses keep basic monitoring on patients. When the patient goes back to hospital, nurses will change the lithium battery.

Copyright © 2011, IGI Global. Copying or distributing in print or electronic forms without written permission of IGI Global is prohibited.

FUTURE RESEARCH DIRECTIONS

With the technology development, wireless monitoring system will be composed of Body Sensor Network (BSN), 3G wireless network and cloud computing platform in future. Body Sensors will be simple, smart and wearable device. They are based on WSN technology and acquisition physiological data. BSN is connected to mobile phone and transmit these data to cloud computing platform via 3G network. Cloud computing platform translate these data into health information and send back to the mobile phone after data analysis and mining. These information will remind people aware physical problems in daily life.

In the future, we will keep pace with information and electric technology trends and develop ZigBee mobile device based on mobile phone. We will provide audio, video and more sophisticated monitoring services relying on 3G networks.

CONCLUSION

In this chapter, we proposed an outdoor patients' healthcare monitoring system contained Reference Nodes, Mobile Devices, a Gateway and Host servers for tracking patients, helping doctors and nurses to keep tabs on their patients' healthy remotely. A reliable data transmission strategy which was based on timed response mechanism, original code and complement code check was pointed out in our work. We improved through a hybrid model of the location engine and Manhattan distance localization algorithm to overcome defects of location engine localization algorithm and improve localization accuracy. At last, we introduced a backup power strategy to help doctors and nurses keep basic monitoring on patients in detail.

REFERENCES

CC2431 Location Engine. (2010). Retrieved from http://focus.ti.com/analog/docs/litabsmultiplefilelist.tsp?literatureNumber=swra095&docCategoryId=1&familyId=367

IEEE Standard for Part 802.15.4. (2003). *Wireless Medium Access Control (MAC) and Physical Layer (PHY) specifications for Low Rate Wireless Personal Area Networks (LR-WPANs)*. Washington DC.

Copyright © 2011, IGI Global. Copying or distributing in print or electronic forms without written permission of IGI Global is prohibited.

Li, Y.-Z., Wang, L., Wu, X.-M., & Zhang, Y.-T. (2008). Experimental analysis on radio transmission and localization of a Zigbee-based wireless healthcare monitoring platform. In the *Proceedings of 5th International Conference on Information Technology and Application in Biomedicine, in conjunction with The 2nd International Symposium & Summer School on Biomedical and Health Engineering* (pp. 488-490). Shenzhen. *China, ISBN-7,* 9781424422555.

Lorincz, K., Malan, D. J., Fulford-Jones, T. R. F., Nawoj, A., Clavel, A., & Shnayder, V. ... Moulton, S. (2004). *Sensor networks for emergency response: Challenges and opportunities*. Pervasive Computing Conference (pp. 16-23). ISBN: 15361268

Niagara, F. (2005). ZigBee networks open the door to more wireless medical devices. *Medical Design, 92*(4), 57–64.

Shen, X., Wang, Z., & Sun, Y. (2005). *Connectivity and RSSI based localization scheme for wireless sensor networks*. Paper presented at the meeting of Computer Science ICIC 2005, Hefei, China.

Waterman, J., Curtis, D., Goraczko, M., Shih, E., Sarin, P., & Pino, E. ...Stair, T. (2005). Demonstration of SMART (Scalable Medical Alert Response Technology). In the *Proceedings of AMI2005 Annual Symposium*, (pp. 1182–1183).Washington, DC. ISBN: 1942-597X

Yang, G. Z. (2006). *Body sensor network*. Berlin, Germany: Springer. doi:10.1007/1-84628-484-8

ZigBee Alliance. (2006). *ZigBee specification 2006. (ZigBee Alliance Document 053474r13)*. CA: San Ramon.

ZigBee Alliance. (2007). *ZigBee-2007 layer PICS and stack profiles*. Retrieved from http://www.zigbee.org/zigbee/en/spec_download/spec_download.asp?AccessCode=1249307135

ADDITIONAL READING

Aghera, P., Krishnaswamy, D., Fang, D., Coskun, A., & Rosing, T. (2010). *DynAHeal: Dynamic energy efficient task assignment for wireless healthcare systems*. Paper presented at the meeting of Design, Automation and Test in Europe Conference and Exhibition, Dresden, Germany.

Alasaarela, E., Nemana, R., & DeMello, S. (2009). *Drivers and challenges of wireless solutions in future healthcare*. Paper presented at the meeting of International Conference on eHealth, Telemedicine, and Social Medicine, Cancun, Mexico.

Copyright © 2011, IGI Global. Copying or distributing in print or electronic forms without written permission of IGI Global is prohibited.

Alshehab, A., Kobayashi, N., Ruiz, J., Kikuchi, R., Shimamoto, S., & Ishibashi, H. (2008). A study on intrabody communication for personal healthcare monitoring system. *Telemedicine and e-Health, 14*(8), 851-857.

Archer, N., Bajaj, H., & Zhang, H. Y. (2008). Supply management for home health-care services. *INFOR, 46*(2), 137–145.

Bava, M., Cacciari, D., Sossa, E., Zangrando, R., & Zotti, D. (2009). *Information security risk assessment in healthcare: The experience of an Italian paediatric hospital.* Paper presented at the meeting of 2009 1st International Conference on Computational Intelligence, Communication Systems and Networks, Indore, India.

Chen, S. L., Lee, H. Y., Chen, C. A., Huang, H. Y., & Luo, C. H. (2009). Wireless body sensor network with adaptive low-power design for biometrics and healthcare applications. *IEEE Systems Journal, 3*(4), 398–409. doi:10.1109/JSYST.2009.2032440

Dagtas, S., Natchetoi, Y., Wu, H., & Shapiro, A. (2007). *An integrated wireless sensing and mobile processing architecture for assisted living and healthcare applications.* Paper presented at the meeting of 5th International Conference on Mobile Systems, Applications and Services, San Juan, Puerto Rico.

Dinesen, B., & Toft, E. (2009). Telehomecare challenge collaboration among healthcare professionals. *Wireless Personal Communications, 51*(4), 711–724. doi:10.1007/s11277-009-9767-3

Fariborzi, H., Moghavvemi, M., & Mehrkanoon, S. (2007). *The design of an intelligent wireless sensor network for ubiquitous healthcare.* Paper presented at the meeting of 2007 International Conference on Intelligent and Advanced Systems, Kuala Lumpur, Malaysia

Gama, Ó., Carvalho, P., Afonso, J. A., & Mendes, P. M. (2008). *Quality of service support in wireless sensor networks for emergency healthcare services.* Paper presented at the meeting of 30th Annual International Conference of the IEEE Engineering in Medicine and Biology Society, Vancouver, BC, Canada.

Ho, C., Evans, J., Mark, M., Rabaey, J., Koplow, M., & Miller, L. …Wright, P. (2009). *Technologies for an autonomous wireless home healthcare system.* Paper presented at the meeting of 2009 6th International Workshop on Wearable and Implantable Body Sensor Networks, Berkeley, CA.

Jafari, R., Bajcsy, R., Glaser, S., Gnade, B., Sgroi, M., & Sastry, S. (2007). *Platform design for health-care monitoring applications.* Paper presented at the meeting of 2007 Joint Workshop on High Confidence Medical Devices, Software, and Systems and Medical Device Plug-and-Play Interoperability, Cambridge, MA.

Copyright © 2011, IGI Global. Copying or distributing in print or electronic forms without written permission of IGI Global is prohibited.

Kew, H. P., & Jeong, D. U. (2009). *Wearable patch-type ECG using ubiquitous wireless sensor network for healthcare monitoring application.* Paper presented at the meeting of 2nd International Conference on Interaction Sciences: Information Technology, Culture and Human, Seoul, Republic of Korea.

Lee, H., Park, K. S., Lee, B. Y., Choi, J. S., & Elmasri, R. (2008). *Issues in data fusion for healthcare monitoring.* Paper presented at the meeting of 1st International Conference on Pervasive Technologies Related to Assistive Environments, Athens, Greece.

Li, H. B., Takahashi, T., Toyoda, M., Mori, Y., & Kohno, R. (2009, Dec). Wireless body area network combined with satellite communication for remote medical and healthcare applications. *Wireless Personal Communications, 51*(4), 697–709. doi:10.1007/s11277-009-9765-5

Li, Z., & Zhang, G.-L. (2007). *A physical activities healthcare system based on wireless sensing technology.* Paper presented at the meeting of 13th IEEE International Conference on Embedded and Real-Time Computing Systems and Applications, Daegu, Republic of Korea.

Martin, T., Jones, M., Edmison, J., & ShenoyTowards, R.. (2003). *Towards a design framework for wearable electronic textiles.* Paper presented at the meeting of Seventh IEEE International Symposium on Wearable Computers White Plains, NY.

Park, S., Mackenzie, K., & Jayaraman, S. (2002). *The wearable motherboard: a framework for personalized mobile information processing (PMIP).* Paper presented at the meeting of the 39th Design Automation Conference, New Orleans, LA.

Ren, Y. L., Werner, R., Pazzi, N., & Boukerche, A. (2010). Monitoring patients via a secure and mobile healthcare system. *IEEE Wireless Communications, 17*(1), 59–65. doi:10.1109/MWC.2010.5416351

Sammon, M. J., Karmin, L. S. B., Peebles, E., & Seligmann, D. D. (2007). *MACCS: An industrial study of hands-free wireless communications for mobile healthcare workers.* Paper presented at the meeting of 5th International Conference on Mobile Systems, Applications and Services, San Juan, Puerto Rico.

Song, W. J., Cho, M. K., Ha, I. S., & Choi, M. K. (2006). *Healthcare system architecture, economic value, and policy models in large-scale wireless sensor networks.* Paper presented at the meeting of 25th International Conference on Computer Safety, Reliability, and Security, Gdansk, Poland.

Toninelli, A., Montanari, R., & Corradi, A. (2009). Enabling secure service discovery in mobile healthcare enterprise networks. *IEEE Wireless Communications, 16*(3), 24–32. doi:10.1109/MWC.2009.5109461

Copyright © 2011, IGI Global. Copying or distributing in print or electronic forms without written permission of IGI Global is prohibited.

Varshney, U., Boric-Lubecke, O., & Lubecke, V. M. (2002). Using wireless technologies in healthcare. *International Journal of Mobile Communications, 4*(3), 354–368.

Wagner, S. (2008). *Zero-configuration of pervasive healthcare sensor networks.* Paper presented at the meeting of 2008 3rd International Conference on Pervasive Computing and Applications, Alexandria, Egypt.

Xiao, S., Dhamdhere, A., Sivaraman, V., & Burdett, A. (2009). Transmission power control in body area sensor networks for healthcare monitoring. *IEEE Journal on Selected Areas in Communications, 27*(1), 37–48. doi:10.1109/JSAC.2009.090105

Xuemei, L., Liangzhong, J., & Jincheng, L. (2008). *Home healthcare platform based on wireless sensor networks.* Paper presented at the meeting of 5th International Conference on Information Technology and Applications in Biomedicine, ITAB 2008 in conjunction with 2nd International Symposium and Summer School on Biomedical and Health Engineering, IS3BHE 2008, Shenzhen, China.

Yu, W. D., Gummadikayala, R., & Mudumbi, S. (2008). *A web-based wireless mobile system design of security and privacy framework for u-healthcare.* Paper presented at the meeting of 2008 10th IEEE Intl. Conf. on e-Health Networking, Applications and Service, Singapore, Singapore.

Zao, J. K., Fan, S.-C., Yang, B.-S., Hsu, S.-H., Cheng, H.-C., & Liu, M.-L. … Teng, F-Y. (2008). *Custos: Remote on-demand healthcare aided with wireless sensors and mobile phones.* Paper presented at the meeting of 2008 IEEE International Conference on Systems, Man and Cybernetics, Singapore, Singapore.

KEY TERMS AND DEFINITIONS

ZigBee: A low-power, low-cost, mesh networking wireless communication protocol.

Wireless Monitoring System: Monitoring system based on WSN technology and help doctors and nurses to remote healthcare.

Mobile Device: A wearable remote healthcare device acquisition patient's physiological data and send them to host servers.

Reliable Data Transmission Scheme: Timed response mechanism based on the original code and their complement code check.

Location Engine: A kind of hardware which embedded in CC2431 can calculate its position based on RSSI & Reference coordinates.

Hybrid Localization Algorithm: A localization algorithm mix location engine algorithm with localization algorithm based on Manhattan distance.

Backup Battery: Only supply additional power to CC2431 chipsets for basic healthcare monitoring after lithium battery run out.

Copyright © 2011, IGI Global. Copying or distributing in print or electronic forms without written permission of IGI Global is prohibited.

Compilation of References

Abowd, G. D., Atkeson, C. G., Hong, J., Long, S., Kooper, R., & Pinkerton, M. (1997). Cyberguide: A mobile context aware tour guide. *Wireless Networks*, *3*(5), 421–433. doi:10.1023/A:1019194325861

Aires, K. R., Santana, A. M., & Medeiros, A. A. D. (2008). Optical flow using color information: Preliminary results. *Proceedings of the 2008 ACM Symposium on Applied Computing*. Fortaleza, Ceara, Brazil: ACM.

Alarifi, S. A. (2008). *An exploratory study of higher education virtual campuses in Second Life*. Nottingham, UK: University of Nottingham.

American Psychiatric Association. (2000). *Diagnostic and statistical manual for mental disorders* (4th ed.-text revision), (pp. 70-71). Washington, DC: American Psychiatric Association.

Ameringen, M. V., Mancini, C., & Farvolden, P. (2003). The impact of anxiety disorders on educational achievement. *Journal of Anxiety Disorders*, *17*(5), 561–571. doi:10.1016/S0887-6185(02)00228-1

Andresen, P. R., Bookstein, F. L., Conradsen, K., Ersbll, B. K., Marsh, J. L., & Kreiborg, S. (2000). Surface-bounded growth modeling applied to human mandibles. *IEEE Transactions on Medical Imaging*, *19*(11), 1053–1063. doi:10.1109/42.896780

Aquilla, P., Yack, E., & Sutton, S. (2005). Sensory and motor differences for individuals with Asperger syndrome: Occupational therapy assessment and intervention. In Stoddart, K. P. (Ed.), *Children, youth and adults with Asperger syndrome: Integrating multiple perspectives*. London, UK: Jessica Kingsley Publishers.

Ashraf, A. B., Lucey, S., Cohn, J. F., Chen, T., Ambadar, Z., Prkachin, K. M., & Solomon, P. E. (2009). The painful face–pain expression recognition using active appearance models. *Image and Vision Computing*, *27*(12), 1788–1796. doi:10.1016/j.imavis.2009.05.007

Attwood, T. (2006). *The complete guide to Asperger's syndrome*. London, UK: Jessica Kingsley Publisher.

Attwood, T. (1998). *Asperger's syndrome: A guide for parents and professionals*. Jessica Kingsley Pub.

Copyright ©   , IGI Global. Copying

Ausburn, L. J., & Ausburn, F. B. (2004). Desktop virtual reality: A powerful new technology for teaching and research in industrial teacher education. *Journal of Industrial Teacher Education, 41*(4). Retrieved October 05, 2009, from http://scholar.lib.vt.edu/ejournals/JITE/v41n4/ausburn.html

Autism Society. (2008). *What causes autism.* Retrieved October 5, 2009, from http://www.autism- society.org/ site/ PageServer?pagename= about_whatcauses

Baig, M. A. (n.d.). Traditional v/s virtual learning environment. Retrieved October 26, 2009, from http://sites.google.com/site/virtualearningorg/Home/virtual-learning-environment/next

Baird, G., Simonoff, E., Pickles, A., Chandler, S., Loucas, T., Meldrum, D., & Charman, T. (2006). Prevalence of disorders of the autism spectrum in a population cohort of children in South Thames: The special needs and autism project (SNAP). *Lancet, 368*(9531), 210–215. doi:10.1016/S0140-6736(06)69041-7

Balogh, J., Michael, C., & Giangola, J. (2004). *Voice user interface design: Minimizing cognitive load.* Addison Wesley Professional.

Bao, L., & Intille, S. S. (2004). *Activity recognition from user-annotated acceleration data.* Pervasive Conference 2004, (pp. 1–17).

Bardram, J. E., & Nørskov, N. (2008). A context aware patient safety system for the operating room. In *Ubicomp '08: Proceedings of the 10th international conference on ubiquitous computing* (pp. 272–281). New York, NY: ACM.

Barnard, J., Prior, A., & Potter, D. (2000). *Inclusion and autism: Is it working?* London, UK: National Autistic Society.

Baron-Cohen, S. (2002). The extreme male brain theory of autism. *Trends in Cognitive Sciences, 6*(6), 248–254. doi:10.1016/S1364-6613(02)01904-6

Bartlett, M. S., Littlewort, G., Fasel, I., & Movellan, J. R. (2003). Real time face detection and facial expression recognition: Development and applications to human computer interaction. *Computer Vision and Pattern Recognition Workshop, 5,* 53.

Bartlett, M., Braathen, B., Littlewort, G. F., Hershey, J., Fasel, I., & Marks, T. … Movellan, J. R. (2001). *Automatic analysis of spontaneous facial behaviour: A final project report.* (Technical Report INC-MPLab-TR-2001.08), Machine Perception Lab, University of California.

Bauminger, N. (2002). The facilitation of social-emotional understanding and social interaction in high-functioning children with autism: Intervention outcomes. *Journal of Autism and Developmental Disorders, 32*(4), 283–298. doi:10.1023/A:1016378718278

Bax, M., Cockerill, H., & Carroll-Few, L. (2001). Who needs augmentative communication, and when? In Cockerill, H., & Carroll-Few, L. (Eds.), *Communication without speech: Practical augmentative & alternative communication* (pp. 65–71). London, UK: Mac Keith Press.

Berhad, M. I. M. O. S. (2008). *National biometrics technology roadmap.* Ministry of Science, Technology and Innovation, Malaysia. Retrieved December 31, 2009 from http://www.mosti. gov.my/ mosti/ images/ stories/ DICT/ policy/ Biometrics%20Technology%20Roadmap% 20Public% 20Version.pdf

Betz, M., Huq, M., Pipek, V., Rohde, M., Stevens, G., & Englert, R. (2007). An architecture for adaptive and adaptable mobile applications for physically handicapped people. In Stephanidis, C. (Ed.), *Hci (5)* (*Vol. 4554*, pp. 335–344). Springer.

Beumer, G., Bazen, A., & Veldhuis, R. (2005). *On the accuracy of ears in face recognition and the importance of reliable registration.* IEEE Benelux Signal Processing Symposium, (pp. 85–88).

Bezryadin, S., Bourov, P., & Ilinih, D. (2007). *Brightness calculation in digital image processing.* Technologies for Digital Fulfillment, KWI International Inc. Retrieved March 25, 2010, from http://www.kweii.com/site/color_theory/2007_LV/BrightnessCalculation.pdf

Bieber, G., Voskamp, J., & Urban, B. (2009). Activity recognition for everyday life on mobile phones. In Stephanidis, C. (Ed.), *Hci (6)* (*Vol. 5615*, pp. 289–296). Springer.

Biocca, F. (1992). Will simulation sickness slow down the diffusion of virtual environment technology? *Presence (Cambridge, Mass.)*, *1*(3), 334–343.

Bishop, J. (2003). The Internet for educating individuals with non-systemising impairments. *Journal of Computer Assisted Learning*, *19*(4), 546–556. doi:10.1046/j.0266-4909.2003.00057.x

Bishop, J. (2007). Increasing participation in online communities: A framework for human–computer interaction. *Computers in Human Behavior*, *23*(4), 1881–1893. doi:10.1016/j.chb.2005.11.004

Bishop, J. (2009). Enhancing the understanding of genres of web-based communities: The role of the ecological cognition framework. *International Journal of Web Based Communities*, *5*(1), 4–17. doi:10.1504/IJWBC.2009.021558

Bishop, J. (2008). Understanding and facilitating the development of social networks in online dating communities: A case study and model. In Romm-Livermore, C., & Setzekorn, K. (Eds.), *Social networking communities and e-dating services: Concepts and implications.* Hershey, PA: IGI Global.

Bishop, J. (2004). *The potential of persuasive technology for educating heterogeneous user groups.* Unpublished MSc thesis, University of Glamorgan, Pontypridd.

Bishop, J. (2007). *An investigation into how the European Union affects the development and provision of e-learning services.* Unpublished manuscript.

Black, M. J., & Yacoob, Y. (1995). Recognizing facial expressions in image sequences using local parameterized models of image motion. *International Journal of Computer Vision*, *25*(1), 23–48. doi:10.1023/A:1007977618277

Black, K. (2007). *Flying with disability in Second Life.* Retrieved January 15, 2010, from https://lists.secondlife.com/ pipermail/ educators/ 2007-May/ 009309.html

Blades, M. (2000). Autism: An interesting dietary case history. *Nutrition & Food Science*, *30*(3), 137–140. doi:10.1108/00346650010319741

Blake, H. (2008). Innovation in practice: Mobile phone technology in patient care. *British Journal of Community Nursing*, *13*(4), 160–165.

Blanz, V., Basso, C., Poggio, T., & Vetter, T. (2003). Reanimating faces in images and video. *Annual Conference of the European Association for Computer Graphics, 22*(3), 641–650.

Bradski, G., & Kaehler, A. (2008). *Learning OpenCV: Computer vision with the OpenCV library.* O'Reilly Media, Inc. ISBN: 9780596516130

Bradyn, J. A. (1985). A review of mobility aids and means of assessment. In Warren, D. H., & Strelow, E. R. (Eds.), *Electronic spatial sensing for the blind* (pp. 13–27). Martinus Nijhoff.

BrailleNote. (2009). *Braillenotes product information.* Retrieved April 29, 2009, from http://www.humanware.com/en-asia/products/blindness/braillenotes

Bregman, J. D. (2005). Definitions and characteristics of the spectrum. In Zager, D. B. (Ed.), *Autism spectrum disorders: Identification, education and treatment* (3rd ed., pp. 3–46). Routledge.

Brezmes, T., Gorricho, J., & Cotrina, J. (2009). Activity recognition from accelerometer data on a mobile phone. *In Proceedings of the 10th International Work-Conference on Artificial Neural Networks: Part II: Distributed Computing, Artificial Intelligence, Bioinformatics, Soft Computing, and Ambient Assisted Living,* (pp. 796-799). Salamanca, Spain: Springer-Verlag.

Bronstein, I. N., & Semendjajew, K. A. (1979). *Taschenbuch der mathematik.* Verlag Harri Deutsch, Thun and Frankfurt am Main, reprint of the 20th edition.

Brooks, F. P., Jr. (1986). Walk through- a dynamic graphics system for simulating virtual buildings. *Proceedings of 1986 Workshop on Interactive 3D Graphics,* (pp. 9-21).

Brown, D. J., Standen, P. J., & Cobb, S. V. (1998). Virtual environments: Special needs and evaluative methods. In Riva, G., Wiederhold, B. K., & Molinari, E. (Eds.), *Virtual environments in clinical psychology and neuroscience* (pp. 91–102). Amsterdam, The Netherlands: Ios Press.

Brown, P. J. (1996). The stick-e document: A framework for creating context aware applications. In *Proceedings of EP'96, Palo Alto* (pp. 259–272).

Brubaker, S. C., Wu, J., Sun, J., Mullin, M. D., & Rehg, J. M. (2008). Fast asymmetric learning for cascade face detection. *IEEE Transactions on Pattern Analysis and Machine Intelligence, 30,* 369–382. doi:10.1109/TPAMI.2007.1181

Brunelli, R., & Poggio, T. (1993). Face recognition: Features versus templates. *IEEE Transactions on Pattern Analysis and Machine Intelligence, 15*(10), 1042–1052. doi:10.1109/34.254061

Buckingham, D. (2002). *The electronic generation? Children and new media. Handbook of new media: Social shaping and consequences of ICTs.* Sage Publications.

Burchardt, T. (2000). The dynamics of being disabled. *Journal of Social Policy, 29*(4), 645–668. doi:10.1017/S0047279400006097

Burdea, G., & Coiffet, P. (2003). *Virtual reality technology.* New York, NY: John Wiley & Sons.

Burton, A. (2006). *Giving a Powerpoint presentation in Second Life.* Retrieved January 19, 2010, from http://oreilly.com/ pub/h/5239

Bushwick, N. L. (2001). Social learning and the etiology of autism. *New Ideas in Psychology*, *19*(1), 49–75. doi:10.1016/S0732-118X(00)00016-7

Busso, C., Deng, Z., Yildirim, S., & Bulut, M. Lee, C. M., Kazemzadeh, A., ... Narayanan, S. (2004). *Analysis of emotion recognition using facial expression, speech and multimodal information*. International Conference on Multimodal Interfaces.

Butler, D., & White, J. (2008). A slice of second life: Academics, support staff and students navigating a changing landscape, Hello! Where are you in the landscape of educational technology? In *Proceedings of ascilite*, Melbourne.

Calongne, C. M. (2008). Educational frontiers: Learning in a virtual world. *EDUCAUSE Review*, *43*(5).

Capps, L., Kehres, J., & Sigman, M. (1998). Conversational abilities among children with autism and children with developmental delays. *Autism: The International Journal of Research and Practice*, *2*(4), 325–344.

Cardin, S., Thalmann, D., & Vexo, F. (2007). Wearable system for mobility improvement of visually impaired people. *The Visual Computer: International Journal of Computer Graphics*, *23*(2), 109–118. doi:10.1007/s00371-006-0032-4

Carey, T. (2008). *Real life employment through Second Life*. Retrieved March 20, 2010, from http://disabilityvoicespace.org/dnn/ Articles/ Education Employment/ Real Life Employment Through Second Life/ tabid/ 89/ Default.aspx

Carlsson, C., Walden, P., & Veijalainen, J. (2003). Mobile commerce. *Proceedings of the 36th Annual Hawaii International Conference on System Sciences, 2003,* (p. 87).

Cassidy, M. (2007). Flying with disability in second life. *Jesuit Communications Australia, 17*(8).

Catarinucci, L., Colella, R., Esposito, A., Tarricone, L., & Zappatore, M. (2009). A context aware smart infrastructure based on RFID sensor-tags and its application to the healthcare domain. In *ETFA '09: Proceedings of the 14th IEEE International Conference on Emerging Technologies & Factory Automation* (pp. 1356–1363). Piscataway, NJ: IEEE Press.

CC2431 Location Engine. (2010). Retrieved from http://focus.ti.com/analog/docs/litabsmultiplefilelist.tsp?literatureNumber=swra095&docCategoryId=1&familyId=367

Chai, T. Y., Rizon, M., Woo, S. S., & Tan, C. S. (2009). Facial features for template matching based face recognition. *American Journal of Applied Sciences*, *6*(11), 1897–1901. doi:10.3844/ajassp.2009.1897.1901

Chandler, P., & Sweller, J. (1999). *Cognitive load while learning to use a computer program. Applied Cognitive Psychology*. University of New South Wales.

Chang, K., Bowyer, K., & Flynn, P. (2003). *Face recognition using 2d and 3d facial data*. Workshop on Multimodal User Authentication, (pp. 25–32).

Chang, T. S., Ho, C. J., Hsu, D. C., Lee, Y. H., Tsai, M. S., Wang, M. C., & Hsu, J. (2005). *iCane-a partner for the visually impaired*. (pp. 393-402).

Charlesworth, W. R., & Kreutzer, M. A. (1973). *Facial expression of infants and children. Darwin and facial expression: A century of research in review*. New York, NY: Academic.

Chen, X., & Huang, T. (2003). Facial expression recognition: A clustering-based approach. *Pattern Recognition Letters, 24*, 1295–1302. doi:10.1016/S0167-8655(02)00371-9

Chen, C. J., Toh, S. C., & Wan, M. F. (2004). The theoretical framework for designing desktop virtual reality based learning environments. *Journal of Interactive Learning Research, 15*(2), 147–167.

Chen, H., Finin, T., & Joshi, A. (2003, October). An intelligent broker for context aware systems. *Adjunct Proceedings of Ubicomp, 2003*, 183–184.

Cheng, Y. F., Moore, D., McGrath, P., & Fan, Y. L. (2005). Collaborative virtual environment technology for people with autism. *Proceedings of the Fifth IEEE International Conference on Advanced Learning Technologies (ICALT'05)*, (pp. 1-3).

Cheng, Y., Moore, D., McGrath, P., & Fan, Y. (2005). Collaborative virtual environment technology for people with autism. In *Proceedings of the Fifth IEEE International Conference on Advanced Learning Technologies, ICALT'05*, (pp. 247-248). Washington, DC: IEEE Computer Society.

Cheverst, K., Davies, N., Mitchell, K., Friday, A., & Efstratiou, C. (2000). Developing a context aware electronic tourist guide: Some issues and experiences. In *Chi '00: Proceedings of the Sigchi Conference on Human Factors in Computing Systems* (pp. 17–24). New York, NY: ACM.

Chibelushi, C. C., & Bourel, F. (2002). *Facial expression recognition: A brief tutorial overview*. University of Edinburgh, UK. Retrieved February 4, 2010, from http://homepages.inf.ed.ac.uk/rbf/CVonline/LOCAL_COPIES/CHIBELUSHI1/CCC_FB_FacExprRec-CVonline.pdf

Chin, J., Diehl, V., & Norman, K. (1988). Development of an instrument measuring user satisfaction of the human-computer interface. *Proceedings of CHI*, (pp. 213-218).

Cho, J., Mirzaei, S., Oberg, J., & Kastner, R. (2009). *FPGA-based face detection system using Haar classifiers*. International Symposium on Field Programmable Gate Arrays.

Cho, Y., Nam, Y., Choi, Y., & Cho, W. (2008). SmartBuckle: Human activity recognition using a 3-axis accelerometer and a wearable camera. In *Proceedings of the 2nd international Workshop on Systems and Networking Support for Healthcare and Assisted Living Environments* (pp. 1–3). Breckenridge, CO: ACM.

Chuah, K. M., Chen, C. J., & Teh, C. S. (2009). ViSTREET: An educational virtual environment for the teaching of road safety skills to school students. In Zaman, H. B. (Eds.), *Visual informatics: Bridging research and practice* (pp. 392–403). Berlin/ Heidelberg, Germany: Springer-Verlag. doi:10.1007/978-3-642-05036-7_37

Clark-Carter, D., Heyes, A., & Howarth, C. (1986). The effect of non-visual preview upon the walking speed of visually impaired people. *Ergonomics, 29*(12), 1575–1581. doi:10.1080/00140138608967270

Cohen, I., Grag, A., & Huang, T. S. (2000). *Emotion recognition from facial expression using multilevel HMM*. Neural Information Processing Systems.

Cohen, I., Sebe, N., Garg, A., Chen, L. S., & Huang, T. S. (2003). Facial expression recognition from video sequences: Temporal and static modeling. *Computer Vision and Image Understanding, 91*, 160–187. doi:10.1016/S1077-3142(03)00081-X

Cohn, J., Zlochower, A. J., Lien, J. J., & Kanade, T. (1999). Automated face analysis by feature point tracking has high concurrent validity with manual facs coding. *Psychophysiology, 36*, 35–43. doi:10.1017/S0048577299971184

Cohn, J. (2006). *Foundations of human computing: Facial expression and emotion.* ACM International Conference on Multimodal Interfaces, 1, 610–616.

Cohn, J., Kanade, T., Moriyama, T., Ambadar, Z., Xiao, J., Gao, J., & Imamura, H. (2001). *A comparative study of alternative facs coding algorithms.* (Technical Report CMU-RI-TR-02-06), Robotics Institute Carnegie Mellon University.

Colwell, C., Petrie, H., Kornbrot, D., Hardwick, A., & Furner, S. (1998). Haptic virtual reality for blind computer users. In *Proceedings of the 3rd International ACM Conference on Assistive Technologies (ASSETS '98),* (pp. 92–99). Marina del Rey, Calif, USA.

Cooper, G. (2004). *Research into cognitive load theory and instructional design at UNSW.* University of New South Wales. Retrieved from http://www.google.com/scholar?hl=en&lr=&q=cache:BP2uyE_8R1EJ:www.uog.edu/coe/ed451/tHEORY/LoadTheory1.pdf+research+into+cognitive+load+theory+and+instructional+design+at+unsw

Crandall, W., Bentzen, B., Myers, L., & Mitchell, P. (1995). *Transit accessibility improvement through talking signs remote infrared signage, a demonstration and evaluation.* San Francisco, Calif, USA: Tech. Rep., The Smith-Kettlewell Eye Research Institute, Rehabilitation Engineering Research Center.

Craw, I., Costen, N., Kato, T., & Akamatsu, S. (1999). How should we represent faces for automatic recognition? *IEEE Transactions on Pattern Analysis and Machine Intelligence, 21*(8), 725–736. doi:10.1109/34.784286

Crestwood Communication Aids Inc. (2009). *Product: Talk Back 12.* Retrieved October 14, 2009 from http://www.communicationaids.com/talkback12.htm

Crowley, J. L., Coutaz, J., Rey, G., & Reignier, P. (2002). *Perceptual components for context aware computing.* In Ubicomp 2002, International Conference on Ubiquitous Computing, Goteborg (pp. 117–134).

Crozier, S., & Sileo, N. M. (2005). Encouraging positive behavior with social stories. *Teaching Exceptional Children, 37*(6), 26–31.

Crozier, S., & Tincani, M. (2007). Effects of social stories on prosocial of preschool children with autism spectrum disorders. *Journal of Autism and Developmental Disorders, 37*, 1803–1814. doi:10.1007/s10803-006-0315-7

Crozier, S., & Tincani, M. J. (2005). Using a modified social story to decrease disruptive behavior of a child with autism. *Focus on Autism and Other Developmental Disabilities, 20*(3), 150–157. doi:10.1177/10883576050200030301

Darken, R. P., Cockayne, W. R., & Carmein, D. (1997). The omni-directional treadmill: A locomotion device for virtual worlds. *Proceedings of UIST, 97*, 213–221. doi:10.1145/263407.263550

Datcu, D., & Rothkrantz, L. (2007). Facial expression recognition in still picture and video using active appearance models: A comparison approach. *ACM International Conference Proceeding Series, 285.*

D'Atri, E., Medaglia, C. M., Serbanati, A., Ceipidor, U. B., Panizzi, E., & D'Atri, A. (2007). *A system to aid blind people in the mobility: A usability test and its results.* Paper presented at the Second International Conference on Systems, Sainte-Luce, Martinique.

Davis, A. B., Moore, M. M., & Storey, V. C. (2003). Context aware communication for severely disabled users. In *CUU '03: Proceedings of the 2003 Conference on Universal Usability* (pp. 106–111). New York, NY: ACM.

Davis, J. W. (2001). *Hierarchical motion history images for recognizing human motion.* IEEE Workshop on Detection and Recognition of Events in Video, (pp. 39-46).

Dawson, G., Rogers, S., Munson, J., Smith, M., Winter, J., Greenson, J., et al. Varley, J. (2010). Randomized, controlled trial of an intervention for toddlers with autism: The early start Denver model. *Pediatrics, 125*, e17-e23. Retrieved May 6, 2010, from http://pediatrics. aappublications.org/ cgi/ content/ abstract/ peds.2009-0958v1

De Luca, A., Mattone, R., & Giordano, P. R. (2007). *Acceleration-level control of the CyberCarpet.* 2007 IEEE International Conference on Robotics and Automation, Roma, I, (pp. 2330-2335).

Del Valle, P. R., McEachern, A. G., & Chambers, H. D. (2001). Using social stories with autistic children. *Journal of Poetry Therapy, 14*(4), 187–197. doi:10.1023/A:1017564711160

Desbonnet, M., Rahman, A., & Cox, S. L. (1997). A virtual reality based training system for disabled children. In Anogianakis, G. (Eds.), *Advancement of assistive technology* (pp. 139–147). Amsterdam, The Netherlands: IOS Press.

Dewing, H. (2009). *Market overview: Sizing unified communications.* London, UK: Forrester Reports.

Dey, A. K., Abowd, G. D., & Salber, D. (2001). A conceptual framework and a toolkit for supporting the rapid prototyping of context-aware applications. *Human-Computer Interaction, 16*(2-4), 97–166. doi:10.1207/S15327051HCI16234_02

Dickey, M. D. (2005). Brave new (interactive) worlds: A review of the design affordances and constraints of two 3D virtual worlds as interactive learning environments. *Interactive Learning Environments, 13*, 121–137. doi:10.1080/10494820500173714

Dixon, D. R., Garcia, M. J., Granpeesheh, D., & Tarbox, J. (2009). Differential diagnosis in autism spectrum disorders. In Matson, J. L. (Ed.), *Applied behavior analysis for children with autism spectrum disorders* (pp. 83–108). New York, NY: Springer. doi:10.1007/978-1-4419-0088-3_5

Dodson, A. H., Moore, T., & Moon, G. V. (1999). *A navigation system for the blind pedestrian. GNSS 99* (pp. 513–518). Italy: Genoa.

Donato, G., Bartlett, M. S., Hager, J. C., Ekman, P., & Sejnowski, T. J. (1999). Classifying facial action. *Advances in Neural Information Processing Systems*, 8.

Donker, A., & Reitsma, P. (2007). Young children's ability to use a computer mouse. *Computers & Education*, *48*, 602–617. doi:10.1016/j.compedu.2005.05.001

Downs, R. M., & Stea, D. (1977). *Maps in minds: Reflections on cognitive mapping*. New York, NY: Harper and Row.

Downs, R. M., & Stea, D. (1997). Cognitive maps and spatial behaviour: Process and products. In R.M. Downs & D. Stea (Eds,), *Image and environment* (pp. 8-26). Chicago, IL: Aldine.

Dryden, I. L., & Mardia, K. V. (1998). *Statistical shape analysis*. John Wiley and Sons.

Dubuisson, S., Davoine, F., & Masson, M. (2002). A solution for facial expression representation and recognition. *Signal Processing Image Communication*, *17*, 657–673. doi:10.1016/S0923-5965(02)00076-0

Earnshaw, R. A., Gigante, M. A., & Jones, H. (Eds.). (1993). *Virtual reality systems*. Academic Press.

Ekman, P., & Friesen, W. V. (1978). *Facial action coding system: Investigator's guide*. Palo Alto, CA: Consulting Psychologists Press.

Ekman, P. (1982). *Emotion in the human face*. Cambridge University Press.

Ekman, P., & Friesen, W. V. (1971). Constants across cultures in the face and emotion. *Journal of Personality and Social Psychology*, *17*, 124–129. doi:10.1037/h0030377

Ekman, P., & Friesen, W. V. (1978). *Facial action coding system: A technique for the measurement of facial movement*. Palo Alto, CA: Consulting Psychologists Press.

Ekman, P., Levenson, R. W., & Friensen, W. V. (1983). Autonomic nervous system activity distinguishes among emotions. *Science*, *221*, 1208–1210. doi:10.1126/science.6612338

Ekman, P., Sorenson, E. R., & Friesen, W. V. (1969). Pan-cultural elements in facial emotion. *Science*, *164*, 86–88. doi:10.1126/science.164.3875.86

Ekman, P., Friensen, W. V., & Hager, J. C. (2002). *Facial action coding system: A human face*. Salt Lake City.

Elen, R. (2009). *Oxford University's virtual first World War site opens in Second Life*. Retrieved January 20, 2010, from http://brideswell.com/ content/ uncategorized/ oxford- universitys- virtual- first- world- war- site- opens- in- second- life/.

Elzouki, S. Y. A., Fabri, M., & Moore, D. J. (2007). Teaching severely autistic children to recognise emotions: Finding a methodology. In D. Ramduny-Ellis & D. Rachovides (Eds.), *Proceedings of the 21st British Computer Society Human Computer Interaction Group Conference: Vol. 2. Human Computer Interaction 2007*, (pp. 137-140). Lancaster University, UK: British Computer Society.

Ensotelos, N., & Dong, F. (2008). Building highly realistic facial modeling and animation: A survey. *The Visual Computer*, *24*(1), 13–30. doi:10.1007/s00371-007-0175-y

Epstein, F. (2008). Second Life is my wheelchair. *The Metaverse Journal*. Retrieved April 1, 2010, from http://www.metaverse journal.com/ 2008/ 09/ 19/ second- life- is- my- wheel chair/

Ertan, S., Lee, C., Willets, A., Tan, H., & Pentland, A. (1998). *A wearable haptic navigation guidance system*. 2nd International Symposium on Wearable Computer, Pittsburgh, PA, (pp. 164-165).

Essa, I. A., & Pentland, A. P. (1997). Coding analysis interpretation and recognition of facial expressions. *IEEE Transactions on Pattern Analysis and Machine Intelligence, 19*(7), 757–763. doi:10.1109/34.598232

Ettinger, A., Holton, V., & Blass, E. (2006). E-learner experiences: What is the future for e-learning? *Industrial and Commercial Training, 38*(4), 208. doi:10.1108/00197850610671991

Evans, R. (n.d.). Asperger's syndrome – is there real cure for it? *Comeunity: Children's Disabilities and Special Needs,* 1996-2009. Retrieved December 1, 2009, from http://www.comeunity.com/ disability/ autism/ aspergers syndrome.html

Eyben, F., Wöllmer, M., & Schuller, B. (2009). openEAR: Introducing the munich open-source emotion and affect recognition toolkit.

Fabri, M. (2006). *Emotionally expressive avatars for collaborative virtual environments*. Unpublished doctoral thesis, Leeds Metropolitan University, United Kingdom.

Fahy, P., & Clarke, S. (2004). *CASS-a middleware for mobile context aware applications*. In Workshop on Context Awareness, Mobisys.

Faigan, G. (1990). *The artist's guide to facial expressions*. Watson-Guphill Publications.

Falkman, K. W. (2005). *Communicating your way to a theory of mind. The Development of mentalizing skills in children with atypical language development*. Sweden: Göteborg University.

Fasel, B., & Luettin, B. (2003). Automatic facial expression analysis: A survey. *Pattern Recognition, 36*, 259–275. doi:10.1016/S0031-3203(02)00052-3

Fasel, B. (2002). Multiscale facial expression recognition using convolutional neural networks. In *Proceedings of the Third Indian Conference on Computer Vision, Graphics and Image Processing (ICVGIP 2002)*.

Fasel, B., & Luettin, J. (2002). *Automatic facial expression analysis: A survey*. (IDIAP Research Report, 99-19).

Fenstermacher, K., Olympia, D., & Sheridan, S. M. (2006). Effectiveness of a computer-facilitated, interactive social skills training program for boys with attention deficit hyperactivity disorder. *School Psychology Quarterly, 21*(2), 197. doi:10.1521/scpq.2006.21.2.197

Ferrario, V. F., Sforza, C., Pizzini, G., Vogel, G., & Miani, A. (1993). Sexual dimorphism in the human face assessed by Euclidean distance matrix analysis. *Journal of Anatomy, 183*, 593–600.

Fombonne, E. (2003). Modern views of autism. *Canadian Journal of Psychiatry, 48*(8), 503–505.

Ford, G. (2002). *Fully automatic coding of basic expressions from video*. (Technical Report INC-MPLab-TR-2002.03), Machine Perception Lab, University of California.

Franco, L., & Treves, A. (2001). *A neural network facial expression recognition system using unsupervised local processing*. Image and Signal Processing and Analysis.

Freksa, C. (1997). *Spatial and temporal structures in cognitive processes* (pp. 379–387). (LNCS 1337). Berlin/Heidelberg, Germany & New York, NY: Springer.

French, S. (1993). *What's so great about independence?* (pp. 44–48).

Freundschuh, S. M., & Egenhofer, M. J. (1997). Human conceptions of spaces: Implications for geographic information systems. *Transactions in GIS, 2*(4), 361–375.

Frith, U. (1991). *Autism and Asperger syndrome*. Cambridge University Press. doi:10.1017/CBO9780511526770

Fruchterman, J. (1995). Archenstone's orientation tools: Atlas speaks and strider. In J. M. Gill, & H. Petrie (Eds.), *Orientation and navigation systems for blind persons*. Hatfield, UK. 1-2 February 1995. RNIB.

Gabbert, C. (2010). *Using social stories to teach kids with Asperger's disorder*. Bright hub, The Hub for Bright Minds. Retrieved May 7, 2010, from http://www.brighthub.com/ education/ special/ articles/ 29487.aspx

Gapen, M. A. (2009). *Facial non-systemising impairments in individuals with PTSD symptoms.* Unpublished doctoral dissertation, Emory University.

Gapp, K. P. (1995). An empirically validated model for computing spatial relations. In I. Wachsmuth, C. R. Rollinger, & W. Brauer (Eds.), *KI-95: Advances in Artificial Intelligence. 19th Annual German Conference on Artificial Intelligence*, (pp. 245–256). Berlin/Heidelberg, Germany & New York, NY: Springer.

Gardner, H. (1983). *Frames of mind: The theory of multiple intelligences*. Basic Books.

Giess, C., Evers, H., & Meinzer, H. (1998). Haptic volume rendering in different scenarios of surgical planning. In *Proceedings of the 3rd Phantom Users Group Workshop (PUG '98)*, (pp. 19–22). Massachusetts Institute of Technology, Cambridge, MA, USA.

Givens, G., Beveridge, R., Draper, B., & Bolme, D. (2003). *A statistical assessment of subject factors in the PCA recognition of human faces*. Workshop on Statistical Analysis in Computer Vision.

Glaser, B. G. (1992). *Emergence vs forcing: Basics of grounded theory*. Mill Valley, CA: Sociology Press.

Glaser, B. G. (2001). *The grounded theory perspective: Conceptualization contrasted with description*. Mill Valley, CA: Sociology Press.

Glaser, B. G. (2002). *Private conversations in Paris*. Mill Valley, CA: Sociology Press.

Glaser, B. G., & Strauss, A. L. (1967). *The discovery of grounded theory: Strategies for qualitative research*. Aldine.

Golan, O., & Baron-Cohen, S. (2006). Systemizing empathy: Teaching adults with Asperger syndrome or high-functioning autism to recognize complex emotions using interactive multimedia. *Development and Psychopathology, 18*(2), 591–617. .doi:10.1017/S0954579406060305

Golding, A. R., & Lesh, N. (1999). *Indoor navigation using a diverse set of cheap, wearable sensors*. Third International Symposium on Wearable computers, San Francisco, CA, (pp. 29-36).

Goldstein, A. J., Harmon, L. D., & Lesk, A. B. (1971). Identification of human faces. *Proceedings of the IEEE, 59*(5), 748–760. doi:10.1109/PROC.1971.8254

Golkar, S. (2005). Politics in weblogs: A safe space for protest. *Iran Analysis Quarterly*, 49-59.

Golledge, R. G., Klatzky, R. L., Loomis, J. M., Speigle, J., & Tietz, J. (1998). A geographical information system for a GPS based personal guidance system. *International Journal of Geographical Information Science*, *12*(7), 727–749. doi:10.1080/136588198241635

Golledge, R., Klatzky, R., & Loomis, J. (1996). Cognitive mapping and wayfinding by adults without vision. In Portugali, J. (Ed.), *The construction of cognitive maps* (pp. 215–246). The Netherlands: Kluwer. doi:10.1007/978-0-585-33485-1_10

Gorman, P., Lieser, J., Murray, W., Haluck, R., & Krummel, T. (1998). Assessment and validation of force feedback virtual reality based surgical simulator. In *Proceedings of the 3rd Phantom Users Group Workshop (PUG '98)*. MIT, Cambridge, MA, USA.

Gourlay, D., Lun, K. C., Lee, Y. N., & Tay, J. (2000). Virtual reality for relearning daily living skills. *International Journal of Medical Informatics*, *60*, 255–261. doi:10.1016/S1386-5056(00)00100-3

Grandin, T. (1995). *Thinking in pictures: And other reports from my life with autism*. Doubleday.

Graves, A., Fernandez, S., & Schmidhuber, S. (2007). Multi-dimensional recurrent neural networks. *Proceedings of the 17th International Conference on Artificial Neural Networks* (pp. 549-558). Porto, Portugal: Springer-Verlag

Gregory, P., & Simon, M. A. (2008). *Biometrics for dummies*. Wiley Publishing, Inc.

Griffin, E., & Pollak, D. (2008). Student experiences of neurodiversity in higher education: INSIghts from the BRAINHE project. *Dyslexia (Chichester, England)*, *14*(4).

Gu, T., Pung, H. K., & Zhang, D. (2005). A service-oriented middleware for building context aware services. *Journal of Network and Computer Applications*, *28*(1), 1–18. doi:10.1016/j.jnca.2004.06.002

Hagiwara, T., & Myles, B. S. (1999). A multimedia social story intervention: Teaching skills to children with autism. *Focus on Autism and Other Developmental Disabilities*, *14*(2), 82–95. doi:10.1177/108835769901400203

Hall, M., Frank, E., Holmes, G., Pfahringer, B., Reutemann, P., & Witten, I. H. (2009). The weka data mining software: An update. *SIGKDD Explorations*, 11.

Hammond, P. (2007). The use of 3D face shape modelling in dysmorphology. *Journal of Archives of Disease in Childhood*, *93*, 1120–1126.

Hartley, J. (2006). Teaching, learning and new technology: A review for teachers. *British Journal of Educational Technology*, *38*(1), 42–62. doi:10.1111/j.1467-8535.2006.00634.x

Heffner, G. J. (2002). Social stories: An introduction. *BBB Autism*. Retrieved December 17, 2009, from http://www.bbbautism.com/pdf/ article_27_ Social_ Stories.pdf

Heimann, M., Nelson, K. E., Tjus, T., & Gillberg, C. (1995). Increasing reading and communication skills in children with autism through an interactive multi-media computer program. *Journal of Autism and Developmental Disorders*, *25*(5), 459–480. doi:10.1007/BF02178294

Helal, A. S., Moore, S. E., & Ramachandran, B. (2001). *Drishti: An integrated navigation system for visually impaired and disabled*. 5th International Symposium on Wearable Computers, Zurich, Switzerland.

Henricksen, K. (2003). *A framework for context aware pervasive computing applications*. Unpublished doctoral dissertation, School of Information Technology and Electrical Engineering, The University of Queensland.

Herrman, T., & Grabowski, J. (1994). *Sprechen–Psychologie der Sprachproduktion*. Berlin/Heidelberg, Germany: Spektrum Akademischer Verlag.

Heward, W. L. (2006). *Exceptional children: An introduction to special education*. Wisconsin: Pearson Allyn Bacon Prentice Hall.

Hickey-Moody, A., & Wood, D. (2008). *Imagining otherwise: Deleuze, disability & Second Life. ANZCA08 Conference*. Wellington: Power and Place.

Hirose, M., & Yokoyama, K. (1997). Synthesis and transmission of realistic sensation using virtual reality technology. *Transactions of the Society of Instrument and Control Engineers, 33*(7), 716–722.

Hirsch, D. (2009). *Autism spectrum disorders*. WebMD Medical Reference. Retrieved October 06, 2009, from http://www.webmd.com/ brain/ autism/ autism- spectrum- disorders? page=2

Hollerbach, J. M., Xu, Y., Christensen, R., & Jacobsen, S. C. (2000). Design specifications for the second generation Sarcos Treadport locomotion interface. *Haptics Symposium, Proc. ASME Dynamic Systems and Control Division, DSC-Vol. 69-2*, Orlando, Nov. 5-10, 2000, (pp. 1293-1298).

Holmes, B. (2009, December 05). Treat autism early. *New Scientist, 2737*, 7.

Hull, R., Neaves, P., & Bedford-Roberts, J. (1997). Towards situated computing. In *Iswc '97: Proceedings of the 1st IEEE International Symposium on Wearable Computers* (p. 146). Washington, DC: IEEE Computer Society.

iSuppli. (2010, March). *One-third of mobile phones to use accelerometers by 2010, spurred by iPhone and Palm Pre*. Retrieved March 25, 2010, from http://www.isuppli.com/ News/Pages/One-Third-of-Mobile-Phones-to-Use-Accelerometers-by-2010-Spurred-by-iPhone-and-Palm-Pre.aspx

Hutton, T. (2004). *Dense surface models of the human faces*. Unpublished doctoral dissertation, University College London.

IBM. (2008). Virtual worlds user interface for the blind. Retrieved April 10, 2010, from http://services. alphaworks. ibm.com/ virtual worlds/

Icaza, M. D. (2008). *Scripting with mono*. Mono-Project. Retrieved January 20, 2010, from http://www.mono- project.com/ Scripting_ With_ Mono

IEEE Standard for Part 802.15.4. (2003). *Wireless Medium Access Control (MAC) and Physical Layer (PHY) specifications for Low Rate Wireless Personal Area Networks (LR-WPANs)*. Washington DC.

Information Solutions Group. (2008). *Disabled gamers comprise 20% of casual video game audience*. Retrieved September 28, 2009, from http://www.infosolutions group. com/ press_ release_ E.htm

Ioannou, S., caridakis, G., Karpouzis, K., & Kollias, S. (2007). Robust feature detection for facial expression recognition. Journal on image and video processing, 2007(2), 5

Ittelson, W. (1973). Environment and cognition. In *Environment perception and contemporary perceptual theory* (pp. 1–19). New York, NY: Seminar Press.

Iwata, H., & Fujji, T. (1996). Virtual preambulator: A novel interface device for locomotion in virtual environment. *Proceedings of IEEE VRAIS*, *96*, 60–65.

Iwata, H., Yano, H., Fukushima, H., & Noma, H. (2005). CirculaFloor. *IEEE Computer Graphics and Applications*, *25*(1), 64–67. doi:10.1109/MCG.2005.5

Iwata, H., & Yoshida, Y. (1999). Path reproduction tests using a torus treadmill. *Presence (Cambridge, Mass.)*, *8*(6), 587–597. doi:10.1162/105474699566503

Iwata, H., Yano, H., & Tomioka, H. (2006). *Powered shoes*. SIGGRAPH 2006 Conference DVD.

Iwata, H., Yano, H., & Tomiyoshi, M. (2007). *String walker*. Paper presented at SIGGRAPH 2007.

Jabbi, M., Swart, M., & Keysers, C. (2007). Empathy for positive and negative emotions in the gustatory cortex. *NeuroImage*, *34*(4), 1744–1753. .doi:10.1016/j.neuroimage.2006.10.032

Jansson, G., Fanger, J., Konig, H., & Billberger, K. (1998). Visually impaired persons' use of the phantom for information about texture and 3D form of virtual objects. In *Proceedings of the 3rd Phantom Users Group Workshop*, MIT, Cambridge, MA, USA.

Johnson, S. (2008, October 17). There are 5 different types of autism disorders. *ezinearticles.com*. Retrieved August 30, 2009, from http://ezinearticles.com/ ?There-Are-5 -Different- Types-of-Autism- Disorders& id=1592117

Jonsson, E. (2002). *Inner navigation: Why we get lost and how we find our way* (pp. 27–126). New York, NY: Scribner.

Joseph, B. (2007). *Global Kids, Inc's best practices in using virtual worlds for education*. Second Life Education Workshop 2007, Part of the Second Life Community Convention, (pp. 7-14). Chicago, IL: WordPress.

Kalb, C. (2009, January 16). Autism: Kids with autism love this software. *Newsweek*. Retrieved from http://www.newsweek.com/ id/179952

Kaliouby, R., Picard, R., & Baron-Cohen, S. (2006). Affective computing and autism. *Annals of the New York Academy of Sciences*, *1093*, 228–248. .doi:10.1196/annals.1382.016

Kaliouby, R., Teeters, A., & Picard, R. W. (2006). *An exploratory social-emotional prosthetic for autism spectrum disorders*. International Workshop on Wearable and Implantable Body Sensor Networks, BSN 2006. 2.

Kay, L. (1980). Air sonar with acoustical display of spatial information. In Busnel, R. G., & Fish, J. F. (Eds.), *Animal sonar system* (pp. 769–816). New York, NY: Plenum Press.

Kay, J. (2009). *Educational uses of Second Life*. Retrieved March 3, 2009, from http://sl-education. wikispaces.com/ educational uses

Kaya, Y., & Kobayashi, K. (1971). *A basis study on human face recognition*. Orlando, FL: Academic Press.

Keller, M. (2001). Role of serotonin and noradrenaline in social dysfunction: A review of data on reboxetine and the social adaptation self-evaluation scale (SASS). *General Hospital Psychiatry*, *23*(1), 15–19. doi:10.1016/ S0163-8343(00)00115-8

Kemmerling, M., & Schliepkorte, H. (1998). *An orientation and Information System for blind people based on RF-speech-beacons.* Helsinki: TIDE.

Kennedy, R. S., Lane, N. E., Berbaum, K. S., & Lilienthal, M. G. (1993). Simulator sickness questionnaire: An enhanced method for quantifying simulator sickness. *The International Journal of Aviation Psychology, 3*(3), 203–220. doi:10.1207/s15327108ijap0303_3

Kern, N., Schiele, B., & Schmidt, A. (2007). Recognizing context for annotating a live life recording. *Personal and Ubiquitous Computing, 11*(4), 251–263. doi:10.1007/s00779-006-0086-3

Kindness, K., & Newton, A. (2009). Patients and social skills groups: Is social skills training enough? *Behavioural and Cognitive Psychotherapy, 12*(3), 212–222.

King, K. P., & Gura, M. (2007). *Podcasting for teachers: Using a new technology to revolutionize teaching and learning.* Information Age Publishing.

Kitchin, R. M., Blades, M., & Golledge, R. G. (1997). Understanding spatial concepts at the geographic scale without the use of vision. *Progress in Human Geography, 21*(2), 225–242. doi:10.1191/030913297668904166

Kitchin, R. M., & Jacobson, R. D. (1997). GIS and people with visual impairments or blindness: Exploring the potential for education, orientation, and navigation. *Transactions in Geographic Information System, 2*(4), 315–332.

Klin, A., Jones, W., Schultz, R., Volkmar, F., & Cohen, D. (2002). Visual fixation patterns during viewing of naturalistic social situations as predictors of social competence in individuals with autism. *Archives of General Psychiatry, 59*(9), 809. doi:10.1001/archpsyc.59.9.809

Kolar, J. C., & Salter, E. M. (1997). *Craniofacial anthropometry: Practical measurement of the head and face for clinical, surgical and research use.* Charles C Thomas Publisher.

Korpipää, P., Mäntyjärvi, J., Kela, J., Keränen, H., & Malm, E. J. (2003). Managing context information in mobile devices. *IEEE Pervasive Computing / IEEE Computer Society [and] IEEE Communications Society, 2*, 42–51. doi:10.1109/MPRV.2003.1228526

Kotsia, I., & Pitas, I. (2007). Facial expression recognition in image sequences using geometric deformation features and support vector machines. *IEEE Transactions on Image Processing, 16*(1), 172–187. doi:10.1109/TIP.2006.884954

Kovac, J., Peer, P., & Solina, F. (2003). Human skin colour clustering for face detection. In B. Zajc (Ed.), *EUROCON 2003—International Conference on Computer as a Tool*, Ljubljana, Slovenia, Sept. 2003.

Krueger, A., Ludwig, A., & Ludwig, D. (2009). *Universal design: Including everyone in virtual world design. Journal of Virtual Worlds Research- Universal Design, 2(3).* Technology, Economy, and Standards.

Kujawski, J. (2007). *Learning isn't second notch in second life.* Texas A&M University College of Education and Human Development. Retrieved March 16, 2010, from http://tlac.tamu. edu/ articles/ learning_ isn_t_ second_ notch_ in_ second_ life

Compilation of References

Kuniavsky, M. (2003). *Observing the user experience: A practitioner's guide to user research*. London, UK: Morgan Kaufmann Publishers.

Laerhoven, K. V., & Cakmakci, O. (2000). What shall we teach our pants? In *Iswc '00: Proceedings of the 4th IEEE International Symposium on Wearable Computers* (p. 77). Washington, DC: IEEE Computer Society.

Lahav, O., & Mioduser, D. (2003). A blind person's cognitive mapping of new spaces using a haptic virtual environment. *Journal of Research in Special Educational Needs*, *3*(3), 172–177. doi:10.1111/1471-3802.00012

Lander, J. (2000). Flex your facial muscles. *gamasurtra.com*. Retrieved from http://www.gamasutra.com/features/20000414/lander_pfv.htm

Later, L., & Milena, D. (2009). *Proposal for the creation of a disability liasion*. Retrieved March 15, 2010, from http://jira.second life.com/ browse/ MISC-2867

Lau, S. L., Klein, N., Pirali, A., Koenig, I., Droegehorn, O., & David, K. (2008). *Making service creation for (almost) everyone*. Stockholm: In ICT-MobileSummit.

Lau, B. T. (2009). Portable real time needs expression for people with communication disabilities. In D. Versick (Ed.), *Communication in computer and Information Science: Intelligent interactive assistance and mobile multimedia computing* (pp. 85-95). International Conference, Rostock-Warnemunde, Germany, Nov 2009. Berlin/Heidelberg, Germany: Springer-Verlag.

Lau, S. L., & David, K. (2010). Movement recognition using the accelerometer in smartphones. *Proceedings of Future network & Mobilesummit 2010.*

Lawrence, K. (2009). Kansas University department of art enters the virtual world on Second Life. Retrieved January 17, 2010, from http://www.infozine.com/ news/ stories/ op/ stories View/ sid/32117/

Lecomte, T., Leclerc, C., Corbière, M., Wykes, T., Wallace, C. J., & Spidel, A. (2008). Group cognitive behavior therapy or social skills training for individuals with a recent onset of psychosis? Results of a randomized controlled trial. *The Journal of Nervous and Mental Disease*, *196*(12), 866. doi:10.1097/NMD.0b013e31818ee231

Lee, L. W. (2007). Development of multimedia learning resources for children with learning disabilities in an undergraduate special education technology course. *MEDC*, 1. Retrieved October 12, 2009, from http://www.usm.my/education/MEDC/Vol1/4-%20DEVELOPMENT%20OF%20MULTIMEDIA%20LEARNING%20RESOURCES.pdf

Lele, S. R., & Richtsmeier, J. T. (2001). *An invariant approach to statistical analysis of shape, interdisciplinary statistics*. Chapmand and Hall/CRC Press.

Lester, J., Choudhury, T., & Borriello, G. (2006). A practical approach to recognizing physical activities. In Fishkin, K. P., Schiele, B., Nixon, P., & Quigley, A. J. (Eds.), *Pervasive* (pp. 1–16). Springer. doi:10.1007/11748625_1

Lester, J. C., Converse, S. A., Stone, B. A., Kahler, S. E., & Barlow, S. T. (1997). *Animated pedagogical agents and problem-solving effectiveness: A large-scale empirical evaluation.*

Levenson, R. W., Ekman, P., Heider, K., & Friensen, W. V. (1992). Emotion and autonomic nervous system activity in the Minangkabau of West Sumatra. *Journal of Personality and Social Psychology, 62,* 972–988. doi:10.1037/0022-3514.62.6.972

Li, Y.-Z., Wang, L., Wu, X.-M., & Zhang, Y.-T. (2008). Experimental analysis on radio transmission and localization of a Zigbee-based wireless healthcare monitoring platform. In the *Proceedings of 5th International Conference on Information Technology and Application in Biomedicine, in conjunction with The 2nd International Symposium & Summer School on Biomedical and Health Engineering* (pp. 488-490). Shenzhen. *China, ISBN-7,* 9781424422555.

Liberman, R. P. (2007). Dissemination and adoption of social skills training: Social validation of an evidence-based treatment for the mentally disabled. *Journal of Mental Health (Abingdon, England), 16*(5), 595–623. doi:10.1080/09638230701494902

Lin, D. T. (2006). Facial expression classification using PCA and hierarchical radial basis function network.

Littlewort, G. C., Bartlett, M. S., & Lee, K. (2007). *Faces of pain: Automated measurement of spontaneous facial expressions of genuine and posed pain.* International Conference on Multimodal Interfaces. Oral session 1: Spontaneous behaviour (pp. 15-21).

Lombardi, J., & McCahill, M. P. (2004). Enabling social dimensions of learning through a persistent, unified, massively multi-user, and self-organizing virtual environment. *Proceedings of the Second International Conference on Creating, Connecting and Collaborating through Computing,* (pp. 166-172). Washington DC: IEEE.

Long, S., Aust, D., Abowd, G. D., & Atkeson, C. (1996). Cyberguide: Prototyping context-aware mobile applications. In *CHI '96 Conference Companion,* (pp. 293-294).

Loomis, J. W. (2008). *Staying in the game: Providing social opportunities for children and adolescents with autism spectrum disorder and other developmental disabilities.* Shawnee Mission, KS: Autism Asperger Publishing Company.

Loomis, J. M., Golledge, R. G., & Klatzky, R. L. (2001). GPS-based navigation system for the visually impaired. In Barfield, W., & Caudell, T. (Eds.), *Fundamentals of wearable computers and augmented reality* (pp. 429–446). Mahwah, NJ: Lawrence Erbaum Associates.

Lorincz, K., Malan, D. J., Fulford-Jones, T. R. F., Nawoj, A., Clavel, A., & Shnayder, V. … Moulton, S. (2004). *Sensor networks for emergency response: Challenges and opportunities.* Pervasive Computing Conference (pp. 16-23). ISBN: 15361268

Lupton, D., & Seymour, W. (2000). Technology, selfhood and physical disability. *Social Science & Medicine, 50*(12), 1851–1862. doi:10.1016/S0277-9536(99)00422-0

Lynch, K. (1960). *The image of the city.* Cambridge, MA: MIT Press.

Lyons, M., Budynek, J., Plante, A., & Akamatsu, S. (2000). Classifying facial attributes using a 2-D gabor wavelet representation and discriminant analysis. In *Proceedings of the 4th international conference on automatic face and gesture recognition,* (pp. 202–207).

Ma, L., & Khorasani, K. (2004). Facial expression recognition using constructive feed forward neural networks. *IEEE Transactions on Systems, Man, and Cybernetics, Part B, 34*(3). Macsolvers' Blog. (2009). *Testing the text to speech function.* Retrieved October 12, 2009 from http://macsolvers.wordpress.com/2009/03/24/text2speech/

MacKenzie, C. M., Laskey, K., McCabe, F., Brown, P. F., & Metz, R. (2006). *Reference model for service oriented architecture 1.0.* Tech. rep., 2006. Retrieved March 25, 2010, from http://docs.oasis-open.org/soa-rm/v1.0/soa-rm.pdf

Majumdar, R., Laisram, N., & Chowdhary, S. (2006). Associated handicaps in cerebral palsy. *IJPMR, 17*(1), 11–13.

Mancil, G. R., Haydon, T., & Whitby, P. (2009). Differentiated effects of paper and computer-assisted social stories™ on inappropriate behavior in children with autism. *Focus on Autism and Other Developmental Disabilities, 20*(10), 1–11.

Manohar, U. (2008). Why is communication important? *Buzzle.com.* Retrieved November 3, 2009, from http://www.buzzle.com/articles/why-is-communication-important.html

Mäntyjärvi, J. (2003). *Sensor-based context recognition for mobile applications.* Unpublished doctoral dissertation, University of Oulu.

Mantyjarvi, J., Himberg, J., & Seppanen, T. (2001). Recognizing human motion with multiple acceleration sensors. In *Proceedings of 2001 IEEE International Conference on Systems, Man, and Cybernetics* (Vol. 2, pp. 747–752).

Margaryan, A., & Littlejohn, A. (2008). *Are digital natives a myth or reality? Students' use of technologies for learning.* Retrieved December 16, 2009 from http://www.academy.gcal.ac.uk/anoush/documents/Digital Natives Myth Or Reality Margaryan And Little john- draft- 11208.pdf

Martino, A. D., & Tuchman, R. F. (2001). Antiepileptic drugs: Affective use in autism spectrum disorders. *Pediatric Neurology, 25*(3), 199–207. doi:10.1016/S0887-8994(01)00276-4

Mason, H. (2007). *Experiential education in Second Life.* Second Life Education Workshop 2007, Part of Second Life Community Convention, (pp.14-19). Chicago, IL: WordPress.

Massaro, D. W. (2004). Symbiotic value of an embodied agent in language learning. In R.H. Sprague Jr. (Ed.), *IEEE Proceedings of the 37th Annual Hawaii International Conference on System Sciences* (10 pages). Washington, DC: IEEE Computer Society.

Matic, A., Mehta, P., Rehg, J. M., Osmani, V., & Mayora, O. (2010). *aid-me: Automatic identification of dressing failures through monitoring of patients and activity evaluation.* In 4th International Conference on pervasive computing technologies for healthcare 2010 (pervasive health 2010).

Matson, J. L., & Neal, D. (2009). History and overview. In Matson, J. L. (Ed.), *Applied behavior analysis for children with autism spectrum disorders* (pp. 1–13). New York, NY/ Dordrecht, The Netherlands/ Heidelberg, Germany/ London, UK: Springer. doi:10.1007/978-1-4419-0088-3_1

Matsugu, M., Mori, K., Mitari, Y., & Kaneda, Y. (2003). Subject independent facial expression recognition with robust face detection using a convolutional neural network. *Neural Networks, 16*, 555–559. doi:10.1016/S0893-6080(03)00115-1

Mayer-Johnson. (2009). *Boardmaker plus! Adapt your curriculum to the needs of your students*. DynaVox Mayer-Johnson. Retrieved October 29, 2009, from http://www.mayer-johnson.com/products/boardmaker-plus/default.aspx

McArdle, G., Monahan, T., Bertolotto, M., & Mangina, E. (2004). *A Web-based multimedia virtual reality environment for e-learning*. Proceedings Eurographics 2004. Grenoble, France.

McCullough, C., & Beauchamp, M. (2009). *Proposal for the creation of a disability liasion*. Retrieved February 15, 2010, from http://jira.second life.com/ browse/ MISC-2867.

Mcintosh, E. (2006). Podcasting and wikis. In Freedman, T. (Ed.), *Coming of age: An introduction to the new World Wide Web*. Ilford, UK: Terry Freedman Ltd.

Meadows, S. (2009). How was school today? Software helps Scottish children overcome communication difficulties. *Optimist News*. Retrieved October 19, 2009, from http://optimistworld.com/Articles.aspx?id=9668562c-f119-4c92-8080-c39101198362&style=news

Mehrabian, A. (1968). Communication without words. *Psychology Today, 2*(4), 53–56.

Michels, P. (2008). *Universities use Second Life to teach complex concepts*. Retrieved January 21, 2010, from http://www.govtech.com/ gt/252550? topic=118264

Microsoft. (2009). *Threads and threading*. Retrieved May 15, 2009, from http://msdn.microsoft.com/en-us/library/6kac2kdh(VS.71).aspx

Milgram, P., & Kishino, F. (1994). A taxonomy of mixed reality visual displays. *IEICE Transactions on Information and Systems, 77*(12), 1321–1329.

Miller, F. (2005). *Cerebral palsy*. New York, NY: Springer.

Miyake, Y., Yohei, O., & Ernst, P. (2004). Two types of anticipation in synchronization tapping. *Acta Neurologica, 64*, 415–426.

Mladenov, M., & Mock, M. (2009). A step counter service for Java-enabled devices using a built-in accelerometer. In *Cams '09: Proceedings of the 1st International Workshop on Context-Aware Middleware and Services* (pp. 1–5). New York, NY: ACM.

Mobitek System. (2008). *SMS gateway development kit*. Mobitek System. Retrieved February 24, 2010, from http://www.mobitek.com.my/SMS_Gateway/SMS%20Gateway.html

Mollman, S. (2007). *Online a virtual business option for disabled*. Retrieved January 25, 2010, from http://edition.cnn.com/ 2007/ BUSINESS/ 07/10/ virtual. disabled/ index.html

Montello, D. R. (1993). Scale and multiple phychologies of space. In Frank, A., & Campari, I. (Eds.), *Spatial information theory: A theoretical basis for GIS* (pp. 312–321). Berlin/ Heidelberg, Germany & New York, NY: Springer.

Moore, D., Cheng, Y. F., McGrath, P., & Powell, N. J. (2005). Collaborative virtual environment technology for people with autism. *Focus on Autism and Other Developmental Disabilities, 20*(4), 231–243. doi:10.1177/10883576050200040501

Nardi, D. (2001). *Multiple intelligences & personality type: Tools and strategies for developing human potential.* Telos Publications.

National Autistic Society. (2008). *Picture symbols: For professional and students.* Retrieved October 30, 2009, from http://www.nas. org.uk/ nas/ jsp/ polopoly. jsp?d= 297&a= 3642

Nehmer, J., Becker, M., Karshmer, A., & Lamm, R. (2006). Living assistance systems: An ambient intelligence approach. In *Icse '06: Proceedings of the 28th International Conference on Software Engineering* (pp. 43–50). New York, NY: ACM.

Nesson, R. (2007). *Virtual worlds.* Harvard Extension School. Retrieved March 15, 2010, from http://www.eecs.harvard.edu/ ~nesson/e4/

Niagara, F. (2005). ZigBee networks open the door to more wireless medical devices. *Medical Design, 92*(4), 57–64.

Nielsen, J. (1993). *Usability engineering.* San Francisco, CA: Morgan Kaufman.

Noma, H., & Miyasato, T. (1998). Design for locomotion interface in a large scale virtual environment, ATLAS. *ATR Locomotion Interface for Active Self Motion, ASME-DSC, 64*, 111–118.

Novita Children's Services. (2006). *Alternative and augmentative communication* (AAC). Retrieved October 23, 2009 from http://www. novita.org.au/Content.aspx?p=64

Oblinger, D., & Oblinger, J. (2005). Is it age or IT: First steps towards understanding the net generation? In Oblinger, D., & Oblinger, J. (Eds.), *Educating the Net generation* (pp. 2.1–2.20). Boulder, CO: EDUCAUSE.

Ofstad, A., Nicholas, E., Szcodronski, R., & Choudhury, R. R. (2008). Aampl: Accelerometer augmented mobile phone localization. *Proceedings of the First ACM International Workshop on Mobile Entity Localization and Tracking in GPS-Less Environments,* (pp. 13-18).

Oliveira, J. C., Shen, X., & Georganas, N. D. (2000). *Collaborative virtual environment for industrial training and e-commerce.* Workshop on Application of Virtual Reality Technologies for Future Telecommunication Systems, IEEE Globecom 2000 Conference, Nov-Dec. 2000, San Fransisco, CA.

Oliver, M. (1993). *Social work: Disabled people and disabling environments.* Jessica Kingsley Pub.

Online Nursing. (2008). *First paramedic course to use Second Life.* Retrieved January 25, 2009, from http://www.yournursing.com/ 2008/10/16/ first-paramedic- course-to-use-second-life/

Open Mobile Alliance. (2010). *Released enablers.* Retrieved March 25, 2010, from http://www.openmobilealliance.org/technical/released enablers.aspx

Origins of Cerebral Palsy. (2009). Forms of cerebral palsy. *Origins of Cerebral Palsy.* Retrieved August 27, 2009, from http://www. originsofcerebralpalsy.com/index.php

Paganelli, F., & Giuli, D. (2007). A context-aware service platform to support continuous care networks for home-based assistance. In *Uahci '07: Proceedings of the 4th International Conference on Universal access in Human-Computer Interaction* (pp. 168–177). Berlin/Heidelberg, Germany: Springer-Verlag.

Pantic, M., & Rothkrantz, J. M. L. (2000). Expert system for automatic analysis of facial expression. *Image and Vision Computing Journal, 18*(11), 881–905. doi:10.1016/S0262-8856(00)00034-2

Pantic, M., & Patras, I. (2006). Dynamics of facial expression: Recognition of facial actions and their temporal segments from face profile image sequences. *IEEE Transactions on Systems, Man and Cybernetics—Part B, 36*(2).

Papatheodorou, T., & Rueckert, D. (2005). *Evaluation of 3D face recognition using registration and PCA*. International Conference on Audio and Video-based Biometric Person Authentication, (pp. 35-46).

Parker, Q. (2008). *Second Life: Disability charity sets up virtual advice service*. Society Guardian.

Parsons, S., & Mitchell, P. (2002). The potential of virtual reality in social skills training for people with autistic spectrum disorders. *Journal of Intellectual Disability Research, 46*(5), 430–443. doi:10.1046/j.1365-2788.2002.00425.x

Parsons, S., Beardon, L., Neale, H. R., Reynard, G., Eastgate, R., Wilson, J. R., et al. Hopkins, E. (2000). Development of social skills amongst adults with Asperger's syndrome using virtual environments: The AS interactive project. In P. Sharkey, A. Cesarani, L. Pugnetti & A. Rizzo (Eds.), *3rd International Conference of Disability, Virtual Reality and Associated Technology. 2000 ICDVRAT* (pp. 163-170). Alghero, Italy: University of Reading.

Paulos, E., Joki, A., Vora, P., & Burke, A. (2007). AnyPhone: Mobile applications for everyone. *Proceedings of the 2007 Conference on Designing for User eXperiences, 1.*

Pausch, R., Crea, T., & Conway, M. (1992). A literature survey for virtual environments: Military flight simulator visual systems and simulator sickness. *Presence (Cambridge, Mass.), 1*(3), 344–363.

Pease, B., & Pease, A. (1998). *Why men won't listen and women can't read maps*. Mona Vale, NSW: Pease Training International.

Peeters, M., Verhoeven, L., Moor, J., & Balkom, H. V. (2009). Importance of speech production for phonological awareness and word decoding: The case of children with cerebral palsy. *Research in Developmental Disabilities, 30*(4), 712–726. doi:10.1016/j.ridd.2008.10.002

Petrie, H. (1995). User requirements for a GPS-based travel aid for blind people. In Gill, J. M., & Petrie, H. (Eds.), *Orientation and navigation systems for blind persons* (pp. 1–2). UK: February. RNIB.

Phillips, P. J., Moon, H., Rizvi, S. A., & Rauss, P. J. (2000). The feret evaluation methodology for face recognition algorithms. *IEEE Transactions on Pattern Analysis and Machine Intelligence, 22*(10), 1090–1104. doi:10.1109/34.879790

Pighin, F., Hecker, J., Lischinski, D., & Szeliski, R. (1998). *Synthesizing realistic facial expressions from photographs. SIGGRAPH Computer graphics* (pp. 75–84). Orlando, FL: ACM Press.

Pighin, F., Szeliski, R., & Salesin, D. (1999). Resynthesizing facial animation through 3D model-based tracking. *IEEE International Conference on Computer Vision, 1*, 143–150.

Plutchik, R. (1980). *Emotion: A psychoevolutionary synthesis.* New York, NY: Harper and Row.

Polvinen, E. (2007). *Teaching fashion in a virtual environment.* Retrieved January 2, 2010, from http://fitsl.wordpress.com/2007/12/05/elaine-polvinen- teaching-fashion- in-a-virtual- environment/

Prenksy, M. (2001). Digital natives, digital immigrants. *Horizon, 9*(5), 1–6. doi:10.1108/10748120110424816

Prensky, M. (2007). *How to teach with technology: Keeping both teachers and students comfortable in an era of exponential change. Emerging Technology for Learning, 2(1).* BEC.

Price, J. R., & Gee, T. F. (2005). Face recognition using direct, weighted linear discriminant analysis and modular subspaces. *Pattern Recognition, 38*, 209–219. doi:10.1016/S0031-3203(04)00273-0

Pun, T., Roth, P., Bologna, G., Moustakas, K., & Tzovaras, D. (2007). Image and video processing for visually handicapped people. *EURASIP Journal on Image and Video Processing*, 1–12. doi:10.1155/2007/25214

Pyle, D. (1999). *Data preparation for data mining.* San Francisco, CA: Morgan Kaufmann Publishers Inc.

Radegast Metaverse Client. (2010). Retrieved April 10, 2010, from http://radegastclient.org/wp/

Ragozzino, M. E. (2007). The contribution of the medial prefrontal cortex, orbitofrontal cortex, and dorsomedial striatum to behavioral flexibility. *Annals of the New York Academy of Sciences, 1121*, 355–375. .doi:10.1196/annals.1401.013

Rajab, A., Yoo, S. Y., Abdulgalil, A., Kathiri, S., Ahmed, R., & Mochida, G. H. (2006). An autosomal recessive form of spastic cerebral palsy (CP) with microcephaly and mental retardation. *American Journal of Medical Genetics. Part A, 140*(14), 1504–1510. doi:10.1002/ajmg.a.31288

Ran, L., Helal, S., & Moore, S. (2004). *Drishti: An integrated indoor/outdoor blind navigation system and service.* Paper presented at the Second IEEE Annual Conference on Pervasive Computing and Communications.

Raubal, M., & Worboys, M. (1999). A formal model for the process of wayfinding in built environments. In C. Freksa & D. M. Mark (Eds.), *Spatial information theory (Proceedings of COSIT 99).* (pp. 381–399). Berlin/Heidelberg, Germany & New York, NY: Springer.

Ravi, N., Dandekar, N., Mysore, P., & Littman, M. L. (2005). *Activity recognition from accelerometer data*. American Association for Artificial Intelligence.

Reid, D. T. (2002). Benefits of a virtual play rehabilitation environment for children with cerebral palsy on perceptions of self-efficacy: A pilot study. *Pediatric Rehabilitation, 5*(3), 141–148.

Resource4 Cerebral Palsy. (2007). Cerebral palsy types. *Resource4 Cerebral Palsy.* Retrieved October 01, 2009, from http://www.resource4cerebralpalsy.com/topics/typesof-cerebralpalsy.html

Results, V., Sysko, H. B., & Sysko, H. B. (2010). Antecedent assessment and intervention: Supporting children and adults with developmental disabilities in community settings. *Education & Treatment of Children, 33*(1).

Riaz, Z., Mayer, C., Wimmer, M., Beetz, M., & Radig, B. (2009). A model based approach for expression invariant face recognition. In Tistarelli, M., & Nixon, M. S. (Eds.), *Advances in biometrics: Third International Conferences* (pp. 289–298). Alghero, Italy: Springer Berlin. doi:10.1007/978-3-642-01793-3_30

Richardson, W. (2006). *Blogs, wikis, podcasts, and other powerful web tools for classrooms*. Corwin Press.

Rickenbacker, D. (2009). *Some hints on taking pictures in Second Life*. Retrieved January 2, 2010, from http://drickenbacker. wordpress.com/ 2007/08/27/ some-hints- on-taking-pictures-in- second-life/

Rieser, J. J. (1989). Access to knowledge of spatial structure at novel points of observation. *Journal of Experimental Psychology. Learning, Memory, and Cognition, 15*(6), 1157–1165. doi:10.1037/0278-7393.15.6.1157

Riopka, T., & Boult, T. (2003). *The eyes have it*. ACM SINGMM Multimedia Biometrics Methods and Applications Workshop, (pp. 9–16).

Rizzo, A., & Kim, G. (2005). A SWOT analysis of the field of virtual reality rehabilitation and therapy. *Presence (Cambridge, Mass.), 14*(2), 119–146. doi:10.1162/1054746053967094

Robbins, S. (2007). *A futurist's view of Second Life education: A developing taxonomy of digital spaces*. Second Life Education Workshop 2007, Part of the Second Life Community Convention, (pp. 27-34). Chicago, IL: WordPress.

Roger, M. F., & Myles, B. S. (2001). Using social stories and comic strip conversations to interpret social situations for an adolescent with Asperger syndrome. *Intervention in School and Clinic, 36*(5), 310–313. doi:10.1177/105345120103600510

Roy, N., Roy, A., & Das, S. K. (2006). Context-aware resource management in multi-inhabitant smart homes: A Nash h-learning based approach. In *Percom '06: Proceedings of the Fourth Annual IEEE International Conference on pervasive computing and communications* (pp. 148–158). Washington, DC: IEEE Computer Society.

Russell, S., & Novig, P. (2002). *Artificial intelligence: A modern approach* (2nd ed.). Prentice Hall.

Russell, J. (1980). A circumplex model of effect. *Journal of Personality and Social Psychology, 39*, 1161–1178. doi:10.1037/h0077714

Rutten, A., Cobb, S., Neale, H., Kerr, S., Leonard, A., Parsons, S., & Mitchell, P. (2003). The AS interactive project: Single-user and collaborative virtual environment for people with high-functioning autistic spectrum disorders. *The Journal of Visualization and Computer Animation, 14*(5), 233–241. doi:10.1002/vis.320

Ryan, N. S., Pascoe, J., & Morse, D. R. (1998). Enhanced reality fieldwork: The context-aware archaeological assistant. In Gaffney, V., van Leusen, M., & Exxon, S. (Eds.), *Computer applications in archaeology 1997*. Oxford, UK: Tempus Reparatum.

Ryokia, K., Vaucelle, C., & Cassell, J. (2003). Virtual peers as partners in storytelling and literacy learning. *Journal of Computer Assisted Learning, 19*, 195–208. doi:10.1046/j.0266-4909.2003.00020.x

Sabelman, E. E., Burgar, C. G., Curtis, G. E., Goodrich, G., Jaffe, D. L., Mckinley, J. L., et al. Apple, L. G. (1994). *Personal navigation and wayfinding for individuals with a range of disabilities*. Project report: Device development and evaluation. Retrieved from http://guide.stanford.edu/Publications/dev3.html

Samal, A., & Iyergar, P. A. (1992). Automatic recognition and analysis of human faces and facial expressions: A survey. *Pattern Recognition, 25*(1), 102–141. doi:10.1016/0031-3203(92)90007-6

Sansosti, F. J., & Powell-Smith, K. A. (2008). Using computer-presented social stories and video models to increase the social communication skills of children with high-functioning autism spectrum disorders. *Journal of Positive Behavior Interventions, 10*(3), 162–178. doi:10.1177/1098300708316259

Sansosti, F. J., Powell-Smith, K. A., & Kincaid, D. (2004). A research synthesis of social story intervention for children with autism spectrum disorders. *Focus on Autism and Other Developmental Disabilities, 19*(4), 194–204. doi:10.1177/10883576040190040101

Scherer, R., & Ekman, P. (1984). *Approaches to emotion*. Hillsdale, NJ: Lawrence Erlbaum Associates.

Schilit, B. N., & Theimer, M. (1994). Disseminating active map information to mobile hosts. *Network, IEEE, 8*(5), 22–32. doi:10.1109/65.313011

Schilit, B. N., Adams, N. I., & Want, R. (1994). Context-aware computing applications. In *Proceedings of the Workshop on Mobile computing systems and applications, 1994*. (p. 85-90).

Schmidt, A., Beigl, M., & Gellersen, H. W. (1999). There is more to context than location. *Computers & Graphics, 23*(6), 893–901. doi:10.1016/S0097-8493(99)00120-X

Schmidt, A., & Laerhoven, K. V. (2001). How to build smart appliances. *IEEE Personal Communications, 8*, 66–71. doi:10.1109/98.944006

Schneider, N., & Goldstein, H. (2009). Using social stories and visual schedules to improve socially appropriate behaviors in children with autism. *Journal of Positive Behavior Interventions, 20*(10), 1–12.

Schultheis, M., & Rizzo, A. (2001). The application of virtual reality technology for rehabilitation. *Rehabilitation Psychology, 46*(3), 296–311. doi:10.1037/0090-5550.46.3.296

ScienceDaily. (2008). *Facial expression recognition software developed.*

Scopes, A., & Lesley, J. M. (2009). *Learning archetypes as tools of cybergogy for a 3D educational landscape: A structure for e-teaching in Second Life.* Unpublished Master's thesis, University of Southampton, School of Education.

Scurlock, M. (2008). *Using social stories with children with Asperger syndrome.* Unpublished Master's thesis, Ohio University, Athens, Ohio, United States.

Sebe, N., Lew, M. S., Sun, Y., Cohen, I., Gevers, T., & Huang, T. S. (2007). Authentic facial expression analysis. *Image and Vision Computing, 25*(12), 1856–1863. doi:10.1016/j.imavis.2005.12.021

Semwal, S. K., & Evans-Kamp, D. L. (2000). *Virtual environments for visually impaired.* Paper presented at the 2nd International Conference on Virtual worlds, Paris, France.

Shan, C., Gong, S., & McOwan, P. W. (2005). *Robust facial expression recognition using local binary patterns.* IEEE International Conference, Image Processing, 2005. ICIP 2005.

Shen, X., Wang, Z., & Sun, Y. (2005). *Connectivity and RSSI based localization scheme for wireless sensor networks.* Paper presented at the meeting of Computer Science ICIC 2005, Hefei, China.

Shepherd, J. (2007). It's a world of possibilities. *The Guardian.*

Shi, J., Samal, A., & Marx, D. (2006). How effective are landmarks and their geometry for face recognition? *Computer Vision and Image Understanding, 102*, 117–133. doi:10.1016/j.cviu.2005.10.002

Shih, Y.-C., & Yang, M.-T. (2008). A collaborative virtual environment for situated language using VEC3D. *Journal of Educational Technology & Society, 11*(1), 56–68.

Sibert, L., Templeman, J., Page, R., Barron, J., McCune, J., & Denbrook, P. (2004). *Initial assessment of human performance using the gaiter interaction technique to control locomotion in fully immersive virtual environments. (Technical Report).* Washington, DC: Naval Research Laboratory.

Siegel, B. (2003). *Helping children with autism learn: Treatment approaches for parents and professionals.* USA: Oxford University Press.

Siegel, A. W., & White, S. H. (1975). The development of spatial representations of large-scale environments. In Rees, H. W. (Ed.), *Advances in child development and behavior* (*Vol. 10*, pp. 9–55). New York, NY: Academic Press.

Sigafoos, J., Schlosser, R. W., O'Reilly, M. F., & Lancioni, G. E. (2009). Communication. In Matson, J. L. (Ed.), *Applied behavior analysis for children with autism spectrum disorders* (pp. 109–127). New York, NY: Springer. doi:10.1007/978-1-4419-0088-3_6

Sigg, S. (2008). *Development of a novel context prediction algorithm and analysis of context prediction schemes.* Unpublished doctoral dissertation, University of Kassel.

SimTeach. (2009). *Institutions and organizations in SL*. Retrieved October 15, 2009, from http://simteach.com/ wiki/index. php?title= Institutions_and_ organizations_ in_sl#universities.2c_colleges_.26_schools

Singh, S. K., Chauhan, D. S., Vatsa, M., & Singh, R. (2003). A robust skin color based face detection algorithm. *Tamkang Journal of Science and Engineering, 6*(4), 227–234.

Skiba, D. (2007). Nursing education 2.0: Second Life. *Nursing Education Perspectives, 28*, 156–158.

Slater, M., Usoh, M., & Steed, A. (1995). Taking steps: The influence of a walking metaphor on presence in virtual reality. *ACM Transactions on Computer-Human Interaction, 2*(3), 201–219. doi:10.1145/210079.210084

Smith, B. L., & MacGregor, J. T. (1992). What is collaborative learning? In Goodsell, A., Mahler, M., Tinto, V., Smith, B. L., & MacGregor, J. (Eds.), *Collaborative learning: A sourcebook for higher education* (pp. 9–22). University Park, PA: National Center on Postsecondary Teaching, Learning, and Assessment.

Smith, K. (2009). *Disability and virtual worlds: Universal life*. Retrieved February 15, 2010, from http://www.headstar.com/ eablive/?p=366

Softpedia. (2009). *Y speak*. Retrieved October 20, 2009, from http://mac.softpedia. com/progScreenshots/Y-Speak-Screenshot-10550.html

Solomon, G., & Schrum, L. (2007). *Web 2.0: New tools, new schools*. Intl Society for Technology.

Sorrows, M. E., & Hirtle, S. C. (1999). The nature of landmarks in real and electronic spaces. In C. Freksa & D. M. Mark (Eds.), *Spatial information theory (Proceedings of COSIT 99)*, (pp. 37–50). Berlin/Heidelberg, Germany & New York, NY: Springer.

Sparks, B. F., Friedman, S. D., Shaw, D. W., Aylward, E. H., Echelard, D., & Artru, A. A. (2002). Brain structural abnormalities in young children with autism spectrum disorder. *Neurology, 59*, 184–192.

Standen, P. J., & Brown, D. J. (2006). Virtual reality and its role in removing the barriers that turn cognitive impairments into intellectual disability. *Virtual Reality (Waltham Cross), 10*, 241–252. doi:10.1007/s10055-006-0042-6

Standen, P. J., Brown, D. J., & Cromby, J. J. (2001). The effective use of virtual environments in the education and rehabilitation of students with intellectual disabilities. *British Journal of Educational Technology, 32*(3), 289–299. doi:10.1111/1467-8535.00199

Standen, P. J., Cromby, J. J., & Brown, D. J. (1998). Playing for real. *Mental Health Care, 1*, 412–415.

Standup. (2006). *The STANDUP system*. Retrieved October 12, 2009 from http:// www.csd.abdn.ac.uk/research/standup/ software.php

Stein, M. A., & Waterstone, M. (2006). Disability, disparate impact and class actions. *Duke Law Journal, 56*, 861–922.

Sternberg, S. (1969). The discovery of processing stages: Extensions of Bonders' method. *Acta Psychologica, 30*, 216–315. doi:10.1016/0001-6918(69)90055-9

Strang, T., & Linnhoff-Popien, C. (2004). *A context modeling survey*. In First International Workshop on advanced context modelling, reasoning and management, Nottingham, England.

Strothotte, T., Fritz, S., Michel, R., Raab, A., Petrie, H., Johnson, V., et al. Schalt, A. (1996). Development of dialogue systems for the mobility aid for blind people: Initial design and usability testing. *ASSETS '96*, Vancouver, British Columbia, Canada, (pp. 139-144).

Su, M. C., Hsieh, Y. J., & Huang, D. Y. (2007). Facial expression recognition using optical flow without complex feature extraction. *WSEAS Transactions on Computers, 6*(5), 763–770.

Susani, M. (2009). Mobile interaction design in the age of experience ecosystems. *Human-Computer Interaction: Design Issues, Solutions, and Applications, 131.*

Sutterer, M., Droegehorn, O., & David, K. (2008). Upos: User profile ontology with situation-dependent preferences support. In *Achi '08: Proceedings of the First International Conference on advances in computer-human interaction* (pp. 230–235). Washington, DC: IEEE Computer Society.

Suwa, M., Sugie, N., & Fujimura, K. (1978). *A preliminary note on pattern recognition of human emotional expression*. International Joint Conference on Pattern Recognition, (pp. 408–410).

Talamasca, A. (2009). *Proposal for the creation of a disability liaison*. Retrieved April 5, 2010, from http://jira.second life.com/browse/ MISC-2867

Tang, F., & Deng, B. (2007). *Facial expression recognition using AAM and local facial features*. Third International Conference Natural Computation, 2007. ICNC 2007. (p. 632).

Tao, Q., & Veldhuis, R. N. J. (2006). *Verifying a user in a personal face space*. Conference on Control, Automation, Robotics and Vision.

Tapia, E. M., Intille, S. S., Haskell, W., Larson, K., Wright, J., & King, A. (2007). *Real-time recognition of physical activities and their intensities using wireless accelerometers and a heart rate monitor*. In Wearable computers, 2007 11th IEEE international symposium (pp. 37–40).

Tartaro, A. (2007). Authorable virtual peers for children with autism. In *CHI '07 extended abstracts on Human factors in computing system, Conference on Human Factors in Computing Systems* (pp. 1677-1680). New York, NY: ACM.

Tartaro, A., & Cassell, J. (2008). Playing with virtual peers: Bootstrapping contingent discourse in children with autism. In *Proceedings of the Eighth International Conference for the Learning Sciences: Vol. 2. International Conference on Learning Sciences* (pp. 382-389). Utrecht, The Netherlands: International Society of the Learning Sciences.

Teehan, K. (2006). *Digital storytelling: In and out of the classroom*. London, UK: LuLu Inc.

Terzopoulos, D., & Waters, K. (1993). Analysis and synthesis of facial image sequences using physical and anatomical models. *IEEE Transactions on Pattern Analysis and Machine Intelligence, 15*(6), 569–579. doi:10.1109/34.216726

Theng, Y., & Paye, A. (2009). Effects of avatars on children's emotion and motivation in learning. In G. Siemens & C. Fulford (Eds.), *Proceedings of World Conference on Educational Multimedia, Hypermedia and Telecommunications 2009* (pp. 927-936). Chesapeake, VA: AACE.

Thiemann, K. S., & Goldstein, H. (2001). Social stories, written text cues, and video feedback: Effects on social communication of children with autism. *Journal of Applied Behavior Analysis, 34*(4), 425–446. doi:10.1901/jaba.2001.34-425

Thomas, D., & Brown, J. S. (2009). Why virtual worlds can matter. *International Journal of Media and Learning, 1*(1).

Thorup, A., Petersen, L., Jeppesen, P., Øhlenschlæger, J., Christensen, T., & Krarup, G. (2006). Social network among young adults with first-episode schizophrenia spectrum disorders. *Social Psychiatry and Psychiatric Epidemiology, 41*(10), 761–770. doi:10.1007/s00127-006-0098-3

Tian, Y. L., Kanade, T., & Cohn, J. (2001). Recognising action units for facial expression analysis. *IEEE Transactions on Pattern Analysis and Machine Intelligence, 23*(2), 1–19. doi:10.1109/34.908962

Tian, Y. L., Kanade, T., & Cohn, J. (2002). *Evaluation of Gabor-wavelet-based facial action unit recognition in image sequences of increasing complexity*. IEEE International Conference on Automatic Face and Gesture Recognition.

Tian, Y. L., Kanade, T., & Cohn, J. (2005). Facial expression analysis. In *Springer handbook of face recognition*.

Tobler, W. (1976). The geometry of mental maps. In Golledge, R. G., & Rushton, G. (Eds.), *Spatial choice and spatial behavior* (pp. 69–82). Columbus, OH: Ohio State University Press.

Tolman, E. (1948). Cognitive maps in rats and men. *Psychological Review, 55*, 189–208. doi:10.1037/h0061626

Trinder, J. (2005). Mobile technologies and systems. In *Mobile learning: A handbook for educators and trainers*. London, UK: Routledge.

Turk, M., & Pentland, A. (1991). Eigenfaces for recognition. *Journal of Cognitive Neuroscience, 1*(3), 71–86. doi:10.1162/jocn.1991.3.1.71

Tversky, B. (1993). Cognitive maps, cognitive collages, and spatial mental models. In *Spatial Information Theory: A Theroretical Basis for GIS, COSIT'93*, (pp. 14–24).

Ungar, S., Blades, M., & Spencer, S. (1996). The construction of cognitive maps by children with visual impairments. In Portugali, J. (Ed.), *The construction of cognitive maps* (pp. 247–273). Dordrecht, The Netherlands: Kluwer Academic Publishers. doi:10.1007/978-0-585-33485-1_11

United Cerebral Palsy. (2009). Cerebral palsy fact sheet. *United Cerebral Palsy*. Retrieved September 04, 2009, from http://www.ucp.org/uploads/cp_fact_sheet.pdf

Universiteit van Amsterdam. (2008). *eMotion: Emotion recognition software*. Retrieved October 12, 2009, from http://www.visual-recognition.nl/eMotion.html

Valente, J. A. (1983). *Creating a computer-based learning environment for physically handicapped children.* Unpublished doctoral dissertation, Massachusetts Institute of Technology, United States.

Vales-Alonso, J., Egea-Lopez, E., Muoz-Gea, J. P., García-Haro, J., Belzunce-Arcos, F., Esparza-García, M. A., et al. (2008). Ucare: Context-aware services for disabled users in urban environments. In *Ubicomm '08: Proceedings of the 2008 the Second International Conference on mobile ubiquitous computing, systems, services and technologies* (pp. 197–205). Washington, DC: IEEE Computer Society.

Valstar, M. F. (2008). *Timing is everything, a spatio-temporal approach to the analysis of facial action.* Unpublished doctoral dissertation, Imperial College London.

Valstar, M., Pantic, M., & Patras, I. (2004). *Motion history for facial action detection in video.* International Conference on Systems, Man and Cybernetics.

Varshney, U. (2007). Pervasive healthcare and wireless health monitoring. *Mobile Networks and Applications, 12*(2), 113–127. doi:10.1007/s11036-007-0017-1

Verry, D. (2001). *Economics and finance of lifelong learning.* London, UK: Organization for Economic Co-operation and Development.

Vince, J. (2004). *Introduction to virtual reality.* London, UK: Springer-Verlag.

Viola, P., & Jones, M. J. (2004). Robust real-time face detection. *International Journal of Computer Vision, January 10, 52*(2), 137-154.

Vivian, K. (2007). *Disability aid: Brain-computer interface for Second Life.* Retrieved March 30, 2010, from http://dove-lane.com/blog/?p=186

Vygotsky, L. (1978). Interaction between learning and development. In *Mind in Society.* (Trans. M. Cole, pp. 79-91). Cambridge, MA: Harvard University Press.

Waller, A., Black, R., O'Mara, D. A., Pain, H., Ritchie, G., & Manurung, R. (2009). Evaluating the STANDUP Pun generating software with children with cerebral palsy. *ACM Transactions on Accessible Computing, 1*(3), 1–27. doi:10.1145/1497302.1497306

Wallin, J. M. (n.d.). Social stories: An introduction to social stories. *polyxo.com, teaching children with autism,* 2001-2004. Retrieved December 17, 2009, from http://www.polyxo.com/ socialstories/ introduction.html

Wang, J., Plataniotis, K. N., & Venetsanopoulos, A. N. (2005). Selecting discriminate eigenfaces for face recognition. *Pattern Recognition Letters, 26,* 1470–1482. doi:10.1016/j.patrec.2004.11.029

Wang, Y., Pan, G., & Wu, Z. (2007). *3D face recognition in the presence of expression: A guidance-based constraint deformation approach.* IEEE Conference on Computer Vision and Pattern Recognition.

Want, R., Hopper, A., Falc, V., & Gibbons, J. (1992). The active badge location system. *ACM Transactions on Information Systems, 10*(1), 91–102. doi:10.1145/128756.128759

Warren, D., & Strelow, E. (1985). *Electronic spatial sensing for the blind.* Boston, MA: Martinus Nijhoff.

Waterman, J., Curtis, D., Goraczko, M., Shih, E., Sarin, P., & Pino, E. …Stair, T. (2005). Demonstration of SMART (Scalable Medical Alert Response Technology). In the *Proceedings of AMI 2005 Annual Symposium*, (pp. 1182–1183). Washington, DC. ISBN: 1942-597X

Weinstein, I. M. (2005). The arrival of the virtual office: Immediate access to colleagues and customers through an always-on virtual work environment. *Wainhouse Research*. Retrieved January 12, 2010, from http://www.wrplatinum.com/downloads/4256.aspx?relo=1

Weiser, M. (1991). The computer for the 21st century. *Scientific American, 265*(3), 66–75. doi:10.1038/scientificamerican0991-94

Weiss, M. J., LaRue, R. H., & Newcomer, A. (2009). Social skills and autism: Understanding and addressing the deficits. In Matson, J. L. (Ed.), *Applied behavior analysis for children with autism spectrum disorders* (pp. 129–144). New York, NY/ Dordrecht, The Netherlands/ Heidelberg, Germany/ London, UK: Springer. doi:10.1007/978-1-4419-0088-3_7

Werner, D. (1987). *Disabled village children: A guide for health workers, rehabilitation workers and families: Cerebral Palsy* (pp. 87–108). The Hesperian Foundation.

Werner, S., Krieg-Bruckner, B., Mallot, H. A., Schweizer, K., & Freksa, C. (1997). Spatial cognition: The role of landmark, route, and survey knowledge in human and robot navigation. In Jarke, M. (Ed.), *Informatik '97 GI Jahrestagung* (pp. 41–50). Berlin/Heidelberg, Germany & New York, NY: Springer.

Westervelt, H. J., Ruffolo, J. S., & Tremont, G. (2005). Assessing olfaction in the neuropsychological exam: The relationship between odor identification and cognition in older adults. *Archives of Clinical Neuropsychology: The Official Journal of the National Academy of Neuropsychologists, 20*(6), 761–769. doi:. doi:10.1016/j.acn.2005.04.010

Wheelwright, S., Baron-Cohen, S., Goldenfeld, N., Delaney, J., Fine, D., & Smith, R. (2006). Predicting autism spectrum quotient (AQ) from the systemizing quotient-revised (SQ-R) and empathy quotient (EQ). *Brain Research, 1079*(1), 47–56. .doi:10.1016/j.brainres.2006.01.012

White, G. R., Fitzpatrick, G., & McAllister, G. (2008). Toward accessible 3D virtual environments for the blind and visually impaired. In *Proceedings of the 3rd international Conference on Digital interactive Media in Entertainment and Arts*, (pp.134-141). Athens, Greece.

Whitehill, J. R. (2006). *Automatic real-time facial expression recognition for signed language translation*.

Wikipedia. (2009). *Project-SE-integrated development toolset for sensory RSC 4x microcontrollers*. Retrieved March 13, 2009, from http://www.phyton.com/htdocs/tools_se/PICE-SE.pdf

Williams, K. (1995). Understanding the student with Asperger syndrome: Guidelines for teachers. *Focus on Autism and Other Developmental Disabilities, 10*(2), 9. doi:10.1177/108835769501000202

Williams, C., & Wood, R. L. (2009). Impairment in the recognition of emotion across different media following traumatic brain injury. *Journal of Clinical and Experimental Neuropsychology*, 1-11. doi:10.1080/13803390902806543

Wood, D. (2009). Experiential learning through real world placements undertaken in 3D virtual world spaces, same places, different spaces. *Proceedings of ascilite*. Auckland.

World Health Organization[WHO]. (2009). *Visual impairment and blindness*. Retrieved June 7, 2008, from http://www.who.int/mediacentre/factsheets/fs282/en/

Xie, X., & Lam, K. M. (2009). Facial expression recognition based on shape and texture. *Pattern Recognition*, *42*(5), 1003–1011. doi:10.1016/j.patcog.2008.08.034

Yang, G. Z. (2006). *Body sensor network*. Berlin, Germany: Springer. doi:10.1007/1-84628-484-8

Yifenghu, Z. (2010). Second Life & disability. *New Media Square*. Retrieved April 10, 2010, from http://yifenghu. wordpress.com/2010/02/01/ secondlife disability/

Yoo, H., & Min-Yong, K., & Kwon, Ohbyung. (2011). Emotional index measurement method for context-aware service. *Expert Systems with Applications*, *38*, 785–793. doi:10.1016/j.eswa.2010.07.034

Zhan, Y., & Zhou, G. (2007). Facial expression recognition based on hybrid features and fusing discrete HMM. In Shumaker, R. (Ed.), *Virtual reality, HCII 2007, (LNCS 4563)* (pp. 408–417). Berlin/ Heidelberg, Germany: Springer-Verlag.

Zhan, C., Li, W., Ogunbona, P., & Safaei, F. (2006). A real-time facial expression recognition system for online games. *ACM International Conference Proceeding Series, 207*.

Zhang, Y., & Ji, Q. (2005). Active and dynamic information fusion for facial expression understanding from image sequence. *Pattern Analysis and Machine Intelligence, 27*.

Zhang, Z., Lyons, M., Schuster, M., & Akamatsu, S. (1998). *Comparison between geometry-based and Gabor-wavelets-based facial expression recognition using multilayer perceptron*. Third IEEE International Conference, (pp. 454–459).

Zhao, W., Chellappa, R., & Rosenfeld, A. (2003). Face recognition: A literature survey. *IEEE Transactions on Pattern Analysis and Machine Intelligence, 24*(1).

Zielke, M., Roome, T., & Krueger, A. (2009). A composite adult learning model for virtual world residents with disabilities: A case study of the virtual ability Second Life island. Pedagogy, education and innovation in 3-D virtual worlds. *Journal of Virtual Worlds Research, 2*(1).

ZigBee Alliance. (2006). *ZigBee specification 2006. (ZigBee Alliance Document 053474r13)*. CA: San Ramon.

ZigBee Alliance. (2007). *ZigBee-2007 layer PICS and stack profiles*. Retrieved from http://www.zigbee.org/zigbee/en/spec_download/spec_download. asp?AccessCode=1249307135

About the Contributors

Lau Bee Theng is a senior lecturer at Swinburne University of Technology Sarawak Campus. She obtained her PhD from Universiti Malaysia Sarawak in 2005. Her research interests are in the areas of assistive and alternative tools for communication and learning mainly focus on disabled children. She has authored several papers in refereed journals and international conferences.

* * *

Chin Ann Ong received his Bachelor degree of Multimedia majoring in Multimedia Software Development from Swinburne University of Technology in 2009 and pursuing his Master degree of Science by research at the same university currently. His research interests are in the field of Artificial Intelligence, Biometrics Information and Image Processing especially in Facial Expression Recognition.

Duncan F. Gillies is a Professor of Biomedical Data Analysis in the Department of Computing at Imperial College London, United Kingdom. He graduated from Cambridge University with a degree in Engineering Science in 1971. He worked for three years as a control engineer in industry, before returning to full time study and obtaining an MSc Degree in Computing from Birkbeck College London and a PhD in the area of artificial intelligence from Queen Mary College. His research work has mostly concerned the application of computers in medicine and biology. In particular he has worked on interactive graphics for simulation of endoscopic procedures, geometric and physical modelling of the upper human airway, the use of Bayesian inference in visual diagnosis, and statistical analysis of microarray data. To date he has published over 120 papers, been granted five patents, and awarded 24 research grants.

Georgios Dafoulas is a Principal Lecturer in Business Information Systems at School of Engineering & Information Sciences, Middlesex University. He is the Program Leader for BSc. Business Information Systems, BSc. Business Information Systems with Management and all undergraduate BIS transitional programs, the

Curriculum Leader in Pedagogy for Global Campus and a member of the University's e-Learning Strategy Group. He holds a BSc., MPhil and PhD in Computation, a PG Certificate in Academic Practice and near completion of an executive MBA. He was recently awarded a Teaching Fellowship and Associate Membership for the Institute of Work Based Learning. Georgios Dafoulas has authored several research papers for refereed journals and peer-reviewed international conferences, mainly in the fields of software engineering and computer-supported cooperative work. He is the co-author of six books and learning guides.

Jacey-Lynn Minoi is a Senior Lecturer, Faculty of Computer Science and Information Technology, Universiti Malaysia Sarawak, Malaysia. PhD in Computer Engineering, Imperial College London, UK 2009. MSc in Multimedia Technology, Computer Science Department, University of Manchester Institute of Science and Technology, UK 2001. BIT (Hons) in Computational Science, Faculty of Computer Science and Information Technology, Universiti Malaysia Sarawak, Malaysia 1999. She is current at the Royal College of Surgeons in Ireland undergoing a research under the Wellcome Trust working on 3D face analysis on schizophrenia patients. Her research interests include: 3D face and facial expression recognition, statistical discriminant analysis, pattern recognition.

Jonathan Bishop is a Chartered IT Professional and Chair of the Centre for Research into Online Communities and E-Learning Systems. In 1999 he developed the Circle of Friends social networking technology, which has formed part of most online communities he has built since. In 2004 he was recognized as a Top 10 UK Innovator by the New Statesman for developing PARLE, an e-learning system for people with autism, which was part of the Digital Classroom of Tomorrow Project and the forerunner to Vois, proposed in his chapter. Jonathan aims though his work to inspire others to think differently about how technology is used to help minority groups overcome their difficulties and realize their strengths. In his spare time he enjoys photography, listening to music and taking part in speaking and debating competitions.

Kah Phooi Seng received her Ph.D and Bachelor degrees from the University of Tasmania, Australia in 2001 and 1997 respectively. She is currently an Associate Professor at the University of Nottingham Malaysia Campus. Her research interests are in the fields of intelligent visual processing, biometrics and multi-biometrics, artificial intelligence, and signal processing.

Kanubhai K. Patel is an Assistant Professor at the Schools of ICT of Ahmedabad University, Ahmedabad, India. He was previously a faculty member at GLS

ICA, Gujarat University, Ahmedabad. He is pursuing PhD degree from the Faculty of Technology at Dharmsinh Desai University, Nadiad. He received his MCA from Gujarat Vidyapith, Ahmedabad in June 1997. His research interests include assistive technology, spatial cognition, human-computer interaction and virtual learning environments. He has authored over nine publications, including a refereed journal paper and two book chapters. He has also authored a book – "Data Structures: Theory and Problems".

Klaus David has 12 years of industrial experience in with HP, Bell Northern Research, IMEC, T-Mobile (as Head of Group) and IHP (as Head of Department). Since 1998 he is Professor at the Technical Universtity of Brandenburg and since 2000 he is the head of the Chair for Communication Technology (ComTec) at the University of Kassel. His research interests include mobile applications and context awareness. He has published to-date over 140 publications and registered over 10 patents. He is also active in leading international organizations such as IEEE and WWRF (Wireless World Research Forum) and as a technology consultant in companies.

Li-minn Ang received his Ph.D and Bachelor degrees from Edith Cowan University, Australia in 2001 and 1996 respectively. He is currently an Associate Professor at the University of Nottingham Malaysia Campus. His research interests are in the fields of signal, image, vision processing, intelligent processing techniques, hardware architectures, and reconfigurable computing.

Nia Valeria received her Degree of Multimedia (Multimedia Software Development), in September 2009, from Swinburne University of Technology. She has been awarded scholarship by Swinburne University to pursue her Master by Research (Master of Science). Her research interests are more into assistive technology, virtual reality, web, and multimedia. Currently, she is working as teaching assistant in Swinburne University.

Noha Saleeb is a Researcher in Business Information Systems at School of Engineering and Information Sciences, Middlesex University; and Lecturer at Computer Science department, American University in Cairo. She teaches under graduates and post graduates, delivering education and guidance in a variety of topics in programming, architecture and graphics design. Noha holds a BSc., MSc. in engineering and is near completion of her PhD. Also works as a practicing architect and graphic designer both in the physical world and 3D virtual world of Second Life. Being at the intersection of several disciplines namely education, architecture/graphics design and computer science, has been an incentive to research the effect of these areas on student learning, for example a previously completed research focused on evaluating e-learning sites qualitatively creating a framework and prototype to do so. Furthermore, Noha has several publications connected to education and usability in Virtual worlds in several peer reviewed international conferences, journals and book chapters.

Sanjay K. Vij received his PhD degree from IIT, Bombay, in 1974. He is currently a Director in the Department of CE-IT-MCA, Sardar Vallabhbhai Patel Institute of Technology (SVIT), Vasad. His research interests include Text Mining, Knowledge Management, and NLP. He has authored over twenty publications, including over seven refereed journal papers and two book chapters. He is a registered PhD guide with Dharmsinh Desai University, Nadiad. He is Member Board of Studies at MS University, Baroda and Dharmsinh Desai University, Nadiad. He had been a panel of experts/advisor in GSLET and GPSC. He is reviewer in couple of peer reviewed journals. He has been Chairman of Computer Society of India, Vadodara Chapter.

Sian Lun Lau received his bachelor degree in Electronics and Telecommunications at the Universiti Malaysia Sarawak (UNIMAS) in 2000 and his masters' degree in Electrical Communication Engineering at the University of Kassel in 2004. After his graduation, he works as a scientific researcher at the Chair for Communication Technology (ComTec) at the University of Kassel. Throughout the years he was active in various national and international research projects such as Zellular, IST-MobiLife and ITEA-S4ALL. He currently participates in the project MATRIX, a German Federal Ministry of Education and Research (BMBF) funded research project with the focus of context aware telemedicine middleware. His research interests focus in the area of context awareness and end user programming.

Vivi Mandasari is currently doing her Master of Science in Swinburne University of Technology. Prior to her Master degree, she has completed a Bachelor degree in Multimedia Software Development from the same University in 2009. Her research interest includes application in helping the children with Autism Spectrum Disorder.

Zhi Heng Tee received his Bachelor degree from the University of Nottingham Malaysia Campus in 2007. He is currently pursuing his MPhil at the same university. His research interests are in the fields of wireless sensor network, reconfigurable computing and intelligent processing techniques.

Index

Copyright © 2011, IGI Global. Copying or distributing in print or electronic forms without written permission of IGI Global is prohibited.

Copyright © 2011, IGI Global. Copying or distributing in print or electronic forms without written permission of IGI Global is prohibited.

Copyright © 2011, IGI Global. Copying or distributing in print or electronic forms without written permission of IGI Global is prohibited.

P

packets error rate (PER) 276
partially overlapping (PO) 198
peer-to-peer (P2P) 173
personal area networks 275
Personal Digital Assistants (PDA) 106, 107, 112, 255
Pervasive Developmental Disorders – Not Otherwise Specified (PDD-NOS) 4
physical defects 71
Portable Affect Recognition Learning Environment (PARLE) 248, 249, 255, 259, 260, 261, 262, 263, 265, 271, 272
positional variance 235
Principal Component Analysis (PCA) 75, 76, 83, 99, 102
Principle Component Analysis (PCA) 229, 230, 238, 243, 244

Q

Quantum Opportunity Programme (QOP) 259

R

radio-frequency identification (RFID) 105, 106, 107, 109, 111, 112, 114, 115, 120, 124
Radio Frequency (RF) 201, 219
reciprocal social interaction 3, 5
region connection calculus (RCC) 198
remote healthcare monitoring 274
remote monitoring devices 277

S

Scalable Medical Alert and Response Technology (SMART) 274, 286
Second Life (SL) 25, 26, 27, 29, 30, 31, 32, 33, 35, 36, 37, 39, 40, 41, 42, 43, 44, 46, 47, 49, 50, 54, 55, 56, 58, 60, 62, 63, 64, 65, 66, 67, 69
Secure and Safety Mobility Network (SES-AMONET) 105, 106, 107, 108
service execution environment (SEE) 174
service oriented architecture (SOA) 173

Service-Oriented Context aware Middle-ware (SOCAM) 167, 173
short messaging system (SMS) 70, 72, 77, 78, 86, 94, 95, 99, 174, 182, 184
Simulator Sickness Questionnaire (SSQ) 213
smart home 273
smartphone 159, 161, 162, 174, 175, 176, 177, 178, 180, 182, 186
social cognition 5
social communication 2, 3, 9, 19, 22, 23
social detachment 5
social reasoning 4
social skills 253, 258, 259, 267, 268, 269
social stimuli 5
spatial cognition 193, 195, 196
spatial environment 195
spatial knowledge 194, 195, 196, 197, 216, 222
spatial learning 193, 194, 195, 200, 203, 204, 211, 216
Special Educational Needs and Disability Act 2001 (SENDA) 254
special educational needs (SEN) 129
speech modules 112
speech recognition 105, 109, 117
speech recognition technology 105
Support Vector Machine (SVM) 75, 76, 83
Surface Mount Devices (SMD) 123
Systemising Quotient (SQ) 270, 271
system-on-chip (SOC) 117

T

tangential proper part inverse (TPPi) 198
tangential proper part (TPP) 198
Thin Slim Small Outline Package (TSSOP) 123
three-dimensional (3D) 224, 225, 226, 229, 230, 231, 233, 234, 240, 243, 244, 245, 247

U

Ultra Mobile PCs (UMPCs) 256
unified communication (UC) 249, 250
universal design principles 30
Universal Design (UD) 31

Copyright © 2011, IGI Global. Copying or distributing in print or electronic forms without written permission of IGI Global is prohibited.

Copyright © 2011, IGI Global. Copying or distributing in print or electronic forms without written permission of IGI Global is prohibited.